T0248882

Recovery and Management of Brain Injury

Recovery and Management of Brain Injury

Edited by **Craig Smith**

FOSTER
ACADEMICS

New Jersey

Published by Foster Academics,
61 Van Reypen Street,
Jersey City, NJ 07306, USA
www.fosteracademics.com

Recovery and Management of Brain Injury
Edited by Craig Smith

International Standard Book Number: 978-1-63242-354-2 (Hardback)

Contents

Preface

This book includes a unique overview of latest and essential information regarding various aspects of brain injury. The book is aimed at rehabilitation and preventive measures of traumatic brain injuries, and it also describes management approaches. It is a compilation of contributions by experts in this field to provide readers with a rich and valuable account of information to upgrade their knowledge about brain injury.

This book is the end result of constructive efforts and intensive research done by experts in this field. The aim of this book is to enlighten the readers with recent information in this area of research. The information provided in this profound book would serve as a valuable reference to students and researchers in this field.

At the end, I would like to thank all the authors for devoting their precious time and providing their valuable contribution to this book. I would also like to express my gratitude to my fellow colleagues who encouraged me throughout the process.

Editor

Part 1

Protective Mechanisms and Recovery

Mechanisms of Neuroprotection Underlying Physical Exercise in Ischemia – Reperfusion Injury

David Dornbos III and Yuchuan Ding
Wayne State University Department of Neurological Surgery
USA

1. Introduction

Cerebrovascular accidents carry significant morbidity and mortality and are vastly present in current society. One of the most prevalent causes of death and long-term disability within the United States, stroke was found to directly cause 6 million deaths in 2006 and was found to be indirectly attributed to $73.7 billion in health care costs in 2010 (Lloyd-Jones et al., 2010). Current standard of care requires that patients present to a health care facility very early in disease onset so thrombolytic therapy can be initiated; however, this therapy, focusing on the establishment of reperfusion is not ideal as reperfusion often worsens ischemic injury (Yang and Betz, 1994). Clearly, new therapeutic and pharmacologic interventions are needed.

Exercise has long been known to provide protection for ischemic stroke through the amelioration of stroke risk factors. Through its beneficial effects on hypertension, lipid profiles, obesity, and diabetes, exercise training has been associated with decreased stroke incidence and better outcomes after stroke (Evenson et al., 1999; Gillum et al., 1996; Hu et al., 2004). Despite risk factor management, exercise has also been shown to provide endogenous neuroprotection, preserving neuronal viability in the setting of ischemia/ reperfusion injury, resulting in decreased infarct volume and improved neurologic recovery (Chaudhry et al., 2010; Curry et al., 2009; Davis et al., 2007; Ding et al., 2004a, 2004b, 2005, 2006a, 2006b; Guo et al., 2008a; Liebelt et al., 2010; Zwagerman et al., 2010a, 2010b). These beneficial endogenous effects of exercise preconditioning have been seen even after multivariate analysis has controlled for risk factor alterations (Hu et al., 2005).

Multiple studies have shown the endogenous protection of rat myocardium following exercise preconditioning (Powers et al., 2002; Siu et al., 2004) through attenuation of apoptosis and better outcomes following reperfusion. Similarly, endogenous neuroprotection has been shown to take place through multiple mechanisms, including upregulation of neurotrophin expression, strengthening of the blood brain barrier (BBB), enhancing the cerebral capillary and arterial networks, decreasing inflammation and apoptosis, and improving cerebral metabolism. Through these mechanisms, exercise preconditioning provides valuable insight into the science of endogenous neuroprotection and its potential therapeutic and clinical implications.

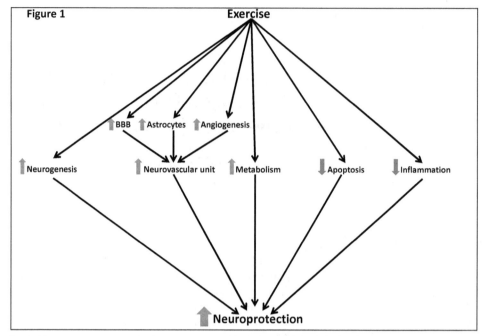

Fig. 1. Exercise generates endogenous neuroprotection through the development of neurogenesis, improved integrity of the neurovascular unit, enhanced metabolism, decreased apoptosis, and amelioration of inflammation.

2. Methods of preconditioning

To date, no specific guidelines have been established through human studies to convey adequate or optimal neuroprotection. Although exercise has been shown to convey endogenous neuroprotection and innate cardioprotection (Hu et al., 2004; Kloner, 2001), the extent, duration, and type of exercise has not been conclusively studied. Despite this, a previous study revealed that moderate intensity and duration of exercise, as opposed to mild or strenuous, correlates with better outcomes and life improvements (Larson et al., 2006). There are specific exercise modalities which convey more potent neuroprotection, and exercise of any duration appears to be neuroprotective. Certainly more studies, especially with human subjects, need to be performed in order to determine exercise regimens resulting in maximal neuroprotection.

2.1 Duration of preconditioning

Despite its known neuroprotective effects, no specific duration of exercise has been shown to provide maximal neuronal survival or lead to better neurologic outcomes. Through multiple studies in rats, it can be seen that exercise preconditioning prior to ischemia/reperfusion injury for a duration of as little as 2 weeks and up to 12 weeks provides similar levels of neuroprotection (Ang et al., 2003; Curry et al., 2009; Davis et al., 2007; Ding et al., 2004a; Stummer et al., 1994; Wang et al., 2001). In addition to the duration of exercise needed, another important factor revolves around the extent of neuroprotection after exercise has stopped. Another study revealed that the neuroprotective effects of exercise preconditioning appear to be long-lasting, showing that 3 weeks after cessation of exercise, rats still maintained lower levels of neurologic deficit and decreased stroke volume when compared to non-exercise rats (Ding et al., 2004b). Future human studies ought to determine the exact duration needed for maximal endogenous neuroprotection.

2.2 Preconditioning modalities

While various modalities, such as treadmill running, voluntary running, simple and complex exercise, have been shown to provide variable amounts of neuroprotection. When comparing forced exercise on a treadmill to voluntary running on a running wheel, rats forced to exercise on a treadmill tend to have better neurologic outcomes after stroke (Hayes et al., 2008). Previous studies have shown that forced exercise on a treadmill is slower but more constant than voluntary exercise occurs in shorter spurts with faster speed, although the total distance is equal in the two groups (Noble et al., 1999). This neuroprotection in forced exercise subjects led to decreased stroke volume, lessened neurologic deficit, upregulation of heat shock proteins, increased neurogenesis and cerebral metabolism (Hayes et al., 2008; Kinni et al., 2011; Leasure and Jones, 2008). These findings show that moderate exercise over a longer time period conveys more efficient and greater neuroprotection than more vigorous exercise over shorter time periods.

In addition to the studies assessing forced and voluntary exercise, differences have also been established when comparing simple and complex exercise. This study analyzed simple exercise as the repetitive movements of treadmill running, whereas complex exercise constituted enriched activities which required both balance and coordination (Ding et al., 2003). Following ischemia/reperfusion injury, rats preconditioned with complex exercise demonstrated increased synaptogenesis and improved neurologic outcomes when compared to simple treadmill exercise (Ding et al., 2003; Jones et al., 1999). Simple exercise training also alleviates much of the injury following ischemia/reperfusion, but its benefit is less pronounced than what is observed with complex exercise training. Although no human studies have definitively shown the most effective means of exercise for enhanced neuroprotection, these animal studies provide a solid framework for the development of appropriate exercise regimens. Moderate exercise intensity, including components of balance, coordination and stress, taking place over a sustained duration seem to be the most neuroprotective when compared to other exercise modalities and intensities.

3. Mechanisms of neuroprotection

Exercise clearly provides substantial endogenous neuroprotection in addition to its role in risk factor reduction for ischemia/reperfusion injury. These effects have been shown through a wide variety of neuroprotective mechanisms all which increase neuronal survival in the setting of ischemic stroke. These protective effects revolve around the neurovascular unit, composed of neuronal, glial, and vascular cells. This unit is significantly enhanced through exercise training and is injured through ischemia/reperfusion. As such, its integrity is paramount for proper cerebral functioning and is the focal point of the neuroprotective effects of exercise in ameliorating ischemic injury. This neuroprotection is, in part, conveyed through the upregulation of neurotrophin expression, including brain derived neurotrophic factor (BDNF) and nerve growth factor (NGF). These important regulatory proteins increase neurogenesis, providing a richer neuronal network prior to injury and a more potent neuronal regenerative ability.

In addition to enhanced neurogenesis, exercise neuroprotection also serves to enhance neurovascular unit integrity through strengthening of the blood brain barrier (BBB). Exercise has been shown to enhance the expression of basal lamina proteins and to increase astrocytosis, effectively providing greater stability to the BBB and the neurovascular unit. Matrix metalloproteinases have also been shown to be downregulated following exercise, enzymes which normally degrade the BBB. Furthermore, angiogenic factors, such as vascular endothelial growth factor (VEGF) and angiopoietins (Ang1 and Ang 2), are upregulated following exercise and correlated with increased blood vessel density and increased cerebral blood flow (CBF). These changes provide further stability to the neurovascular unit and have been shown to provide better outcomes following ischemia/reperfusion injury.

Exercise also regulates apoptotic pathways in such a way as to tip the balance in favor of anti-apoptotic to pro-apoptotic gene expression. Carried out through mediators, such as tumor necrosis factor (TNF)-α, extracellular regulated kinase (ERK)-1/2, and heat shock protein (HSP)-70, increasing the anti:pro-apoptotic ratio effectively decrease apoptosis and prolongs neuronal survival, providing obvious benefit following ischemia/reperfusion injury. Furthermore, exercise preconditioning decreases the expression of vascular adhesion molecules (ICAM-1), which decreases leukocyte infiltration and secondary damage following ischemic stroke. These changes ameliorate much of the neuronal damage and death after hypoxic conditions. Finally, neuronal metabolism is upregulated following chronic exercise, correlating with increased ATP production in the acute phase following ischemia/reperfusion injury. This is done through upregulation of glucose transport enzymes, glycolytic enzymes, and the upstream regulator protein hypoxia-inducible factor (HIF)-1α. The pathways underlying these mechanistic changes in response to exercise preconditioning will be defined in detail as each provides valuable clues to understanding the protective ability of exercise following ischemia/reperfusion injury.

3.1 Neurotrophin expression

Neurotrophins are well known to enhance neurogenesis and synaptogenesis while working to promote cerebral integrity at its most basic unit. Multiple human and animal studies have revealed that brain derived neurotrophic factor (BDNF) and nerve growth factor (NGF) facilitate this process (Cohen-Cory et al., 2010; Kim et al., 2004; Kuipers and Bramham, 2006). These trophic factors generate more abundant neuronal and synaptic networks, and they have also been shown to be protective of the neural and cerebrovascular systems. BDNF and NGF mRNA levels have been shown to be upregulated following several weeks of continuous exercise (Ding et al., 2004b), which has been specifically seen in astrocytes and neuronal cells. In addition, providing exercise in an enriched environment, including running wheels, toy balls, ladders, and wooden planks, increased synaptogenesis and neurologic functioning even more than previously seen with basic exercise preconditioning, which was also associated with an increase in BDNF and NGF mRNA levels (Neeper et al., 1996; Ickes et al., 2000). This further implies that complex exercise, requiring balance and coordination, transmits greater neuroprotection that basic repetitive exercise.

Upregulation of these proteins following chronic exercise generates increased neurogenesis, which is protective in advance of ischemia/reperfusion injury. Several studies have shown that exercise preconditioned rats have elevated levels of BDNF and NGF following ischemia/reperfusion injury, which correlates with decreased neurologic deficit and decreased stroke volume when compared to non-exercised rats (Ang et al., 2003; Ding et al., 2004a). Another study has shown these factors to be upregulated within the reperfusion stage as well (Schabitz et al., 2007), suggesting a possible reparative role post-ischemic insult. The ability to upregulate these neurogenic factors in the reperfusion stage provides the potential for cell survival and regeneration, especially within the ischemic penumbra zone. These results suggest a temporally duel role of BDNF and NGF in exercise preconditioning in which their upregulation via chronic exercise training strengthens the neurovascular unit before and after injury. Altogether, the upregulation of BDNF and NGF seen following exercise preconditioning promotes neuronal survival following ischemia/reperfusion injury.

3.2 Integrity of the neurovascular unit

In addition to neuronal health and viability, integrity of the neurovascular unit as a whole requires maintenance of the blood brain barrier (BBB), structural support provided by astrocytic glial cells, and an intact cerebrovascular network. Composed of capillary endothelial cells, the basal lamina, and astrocytic end-feet, the BBB provides a robust filtration mechanism which serves as the functional barrier for neurovascular unit integrity in the setting of ischemic stroke. Also the first structure injured after ischemia/reperfusion injury, the strength of the BBB is of utmost importance and is a key component to the neuroprotection afforded by exercise training.

While viewing the neurovascular unit as the most basic structure for neuroprotection and stability, astrocytes also play a key role in maintaining the cerebral architecture. Seen following chronic exercise, astrocytosis strengthens the BBB and neurovascular unit, providing a rigid framework to withstand ischemia/reperfusion insults against the neurovascular unit.

Not only does exercise promote neuronal health, BBB integrity, and astrocytic structure, but it also generates an increased blood vessel density. Increased collateral circulation coupled with richer capillary beds allows a more efficient and effective response to ischemia. The angiogenesis and arteriogenesis seen after exercise allow the brain to be rapidly reperfused. In exercised subjects with enhanced BBB integrity, this elevated reperfusion potential occurs much more proficiently and with less damage than is seen in non-exercised subjects. These neuroprotective changes in exercised animals in the setting of ischemia/reperfusion injury underlie the importance of pre-ischemic exercise conditioning and provide potential novel therapeutic interventions.

3.2.1 Blood Brain Barrier integrity

The integrity of the blood brain barrier (BBB) is paramount to maintaining proper filtration of nutrients from the vascular system and in providing the necessary structure to the neurovascular unit. Composed of endothelial cell walls, the basal lamina, and astrocytic end-feet, this filtration barrier is the first structure injured during ischemia/reperfusion injury (del Zoppo and Hallenbeck, 2000; del Zoppo and Mabuchi, 2003), making its integrity a key focal point in the neuroprotective nature of exercise. While an intact endothelial cell wall and astrocytic end-feet are necessary for proper BBB functionality, the basal lamina provides the central structural support and selective permeability necessary to maintain a healthy cerebral environment. The basal lamina is composed of various proteins of the extracellular matrix, including collagen type IV, laminin, heparan sulphate, proteoglycan, and fibronectin, which are produced by surrounding endothelial cells and astrocytes. The importance for proper integrity and functionality of this structure has been repeatedly established (Lo et al., 2003, Lo et al., 2005). When this barrier is damaged, as is the case following ischemia/reperfusion injury, its ability to selectively discriminate products of the cerebrovascular system is compromised, which is clinically evident as vasogenic edema.

In a hypoxic setting, this loss of BBB integrity and introduction of cerebral edema further disturbs cerebral homeostasis in a step-wise manner. Soon after arterial occlusion, the endothelial permeability barrier is lost and matrix proteins, primarily fibronectin, collagen, and laminin, also begin to lose their integrity (del Zoppo and Mabuchi, 2003). As ischemia continues, a lack of selective permeability and continued vasogenic edema lead to cellular swelling. Swelling of astrocytes and endothelial cells separates them further from the basal lamina, further promoting leakage of vascular contents into the cerebral interstitial spaces (del Zoppo and Mabuchi, 2003). Reperfusion tends to worsen this damage, despite its role as the current mainstay of therapy for ischemic stroke. These alterations in the ischemic phase severely damage the integrity of the BBB, and the sudden increase in cerebrovascular flow in the reperfusion stage leads to excessive leakage of water and generation of oxygen free radicals, further promoting cerebral damage (Ayata and Ropper, 2002; Yang and Betz, 1994). Studies have shown that exercise training increases basal lamina thickness, adding both strength and stability to the BBB (Davis et al., 2007). These changes were associated with decreases cerebral edema, decreased stroke volume, and improved neuronal recovery following ischemia/reperfusion injury. Collage type IV, a major component of the basal lamina, was found to be upregulated in exercise preconditioned rats, and these subjects maintained a decreased net loss of collagen type IV levels after stroke as well (Davis et al., 2007). Also confirmed by immunocytochemistry, elevated levels of collagen type IV-positive cells were observed in previously exercise rats, and these rats had significantly lower levels of neurologic deficit following stroke (Davis et al., 2007).

In a similar manner to collagen expression, integrin proteins also provide stability to the basal lamina and BBB, providing additional support to the neurovascular unit. Composed of α and β heterodimers, these proteins serve as cell adhesion molecules within the basal lamina and extracellular matrix, anchoring astrocytes and endothelial cells together, ultimately maintaining the integrity of these structures and the neurovascular unit as a whole (Dans and Giancotti, 1999; Hynes, 1992). Integrins, which are anchored to astrocytic and endothelial cytoskeletons, serve as receptors for numerous ligands and proteins within the basal lamina matrix, primarily collagen and laminin (del Zoppo and Mabuchi, 2003; Tawil et al., 1994). These structural proteins also serve as signalling receptors for astrocytes and endothelial cells, allowing for dynamic alterations of the BBB in response to exercise, ischemia, and other noxious stimuli (Hynes, 1992). Following ischemic/reperfusion injury, these proteins rapidly lose affinity for their associated ligands within the basal lamina, decreasing the connective integrity between endothelial and astrocytic cells and the extracellular matrix (Tagaya et al., 2001; Wagner et al., 1997). However, in exercised-trained rats, integrin expression was found to be significantly higher in astroglia and endothelium following ischemic stroke (Ding et al., 2005; Tawil et al., 1994), which correlated with a decrease in neurologic deficit (Ding et al., 2006b). These changes suggest that integrin expression is uniquely important to BBB integrity as it serves to bind all three components together, and this increased expression following exercise serves as another mechanism of its neuroprotective nature. Through both increased collagen and integrin expression following exercise preconditioning, the enhanced integrity of the BBB decreases vasogenic edema, secondary damage, and neuronal death following ischemia/reperfusion.

While it can clearly be seen that exercise increases the thickness and integrity of the basal lamina and BBB as a whole, pre-ischemic exercise also improves integrity of the neurovascular unit by decreasing BBB breakdown. Matrix metalloproteinase (MMP) is an enzyme produced by endothelial cells, microglia, and astrocytes with a primary function to degrade extracellular matrix and basal lamina proteins (Lo et al., 2003). Expression of MMPs increases exponentially following cerebral damage and, as a result, has been heavily implicated following ischemia/reperfusion injury (Lo et al., 2003). Upregulation of MMP following stroke has been implicated in multiple animal and human studies (Clark et al., 1997; Gasche et al., 1999), leading to increased BBB permeability and vasogenic edema. In addition to these damaging changes, MMP expression has also been correlated with increased inflammation and leukocyte infiltration (Romanic et al., 1998). Pharmacologic inhibition (Romanic et al., 1998) and genetic knockout (Asahi et al., 2001) of MMPs leads to a dramatic decrease in associated edema and neurologic damage. MMP-induced damage following ischemia/reperfusion is mechanistically linked to extracellular matrix breakdown, including degradation of collagen, leading to loss of integrity of the BBB and the neurovascular unit.

Following exercise preconditioning, rats were found to have reduced MMP-9 expression, which correlated with elevated collagen IV levels (Davis et al., 2007), and similar results were seen following pharmacologic inhibition. This neuroprotective effect of exercise is mediated by improved microvascular integrity and basal lamina reinforcement, ultimately decreasing neurologic deficit, infarct volume, and leukocyte infiltration following ischemia/reperfusiom injury (Curry et al., 2009). Interestingly, when these same rats were treated with tumor necrosis factor (TNF)-α antibody or inhibition of extracellular regulated kinase (ERK), MMP-9 levels were not decreased, and the positive effects on neurologic outcome and infarct volume were no longer seen (Curry et al., 2009; Hosomi et al., 2005), suggesting that TNF-α and ERK serve as regulators of MMP expression. Further studies have shown that ERK1/2 mediates a TNF-α induced an increase in MMP-9 expression in the acute setting (Arai et al., 2003), while the gradual increases in TNF-α and ERK1/2 have been shown to decrease MMP-9 expression and lead to decreased neuronal cell death (Chaudhry et al., 2010). These gradual changes are seen following exercise training, in which gradual upregulation of TNF-α and ERK1/2 lead to decreased levels of MMP-9 expression, which also correlates with better outcomes following ischemia/reperfusion injury (Chaudhry et al., 2010). In this study, following ischemic injury, neuronal apoptosis was seen to be reduced in association with decreased levels of MMP-9 expression in exercise preconditioned rats (Chaudhry et al., 2010). Following pharmacologic inhibition of both ERK1/2 and MMP-9, similar effects were also seen, resulting in less neuronal apoptosis and better neurologic outcomes; however, when only ERK1/2 was inhibited, MMP expression returned to the level of non-exercised control rats, suggesting a pathway involving regulation by ERK1/2 and TNF-α of MMP-9 expression (Chaudhry et al., 2010). ERK1/2 has previously been shown to also work through upregulation of tissue inhibitors of metalloproteinases (TIMPs) (Tong et al., 2004), and TIMPs have been previously shown to be upregulated following chronic exercise in association with decreased MMP-9 levels (Guo et al., 2008a). The upregulation of ERK1/2 and TNF-α following exercise preconditioning, leads to decreased MMP-9 expression, decreased BBB dysfunction, improved neurovascular unit integrity, and better neurologic outcomes. In addition to these important findings regarding the role of ERK1/2 and TNF-α, heat shock proteins (HSP-70) are also thought to play a synergistic role in the downregulation of MMP-9 expression (Liebelt et al., 2010). HSP-70 works in concert with TNF-α to decreased MMP-9 expression and has been shown to be increased following chronic exercise training.   Taken together, these various pathways reveal multiple synergistic pathways which function to reduce the breakdown of the BBB, reinforcing the integrity of the neurovascular unit and the cerebral environment.

3.2.2 Astrocytosis
Another vital player in the neurovascular unit is the astrocyte, which also forms the cerebral side of the blood brain barrier (BBB). Astrocytic glial cells are well known to induce strengthening of the BBB (Park et al., 2003; Petty and Lo, 2002). Specifically, these cells have been shown to cover 90% of the cerebrovascular surface and primary function to restrict the permeability across the BBB, providing crucial integrity to the neurovascular unit (Igarashi et al., 1999; Janzer and Raff, 1987; Kondo et al., 1996; Willis et al., 2004). The density and integrity of astrocytes within the brain have also been shown to maintain neurovascular integrity in the setting of acute ischemic stroke (del Zoppo and Mabuchi, 2003; Lo et al., 2005).   The damaging effects of ischemia/reperfusion are primarily seen at the BBB, classically affecting endothelial cells and astrocytes and their corresponding adherence to the extracellular matrix. This interaction between endothelial cells, the extracellular matrix, and astrocytes provides the central trigger for neuronal injury and death in the setting acute stroke (Petty and Wettstein, 2001).   In addition to its other effects, pre-ischemic exercise conditioning has been shown to upregulate the degree of astrocytosis, and this upregulation has been shown to be correlated with better outcomes following ischemic/reperfusion injury (Li et al., 2005). An increased number of astrocytes within the neurovascular unit, provided by exercise training, cover a greater percentage of the BBB. This increased coverage allows the neurovasculature to be more restricted in the blood products that are allowed to permeate the BBB, providing important integrity in the setting of ischemia/reperfusion injury.

3.2.3 Angiogenesis and arteriogenesis
Exercise training transforms the neurovascular system of the neurovascular unit, developing a vital metabolic response network in response to ischemia/reperfusion injury. Under normal conditions, angiogenesis and endothelial cell proliferation is scant in the adult brain (Ogunshola et al., 2000). Nonetheless, as a major element of the neurovascular unit, it plays a crucial role in maintaining an appropriate and healthy cerebral environment. Previous studies have shown that physical activity on a treadmill increases blood vessel density in the brain (Black et al., 1990; Isaacs et al., 1992; Kleim et al., 2002; Swain et al., 2003), and forced exercise on a treadmill induces cortical and striatal angiogenesis (Ding et al., 2004a, 2004b). In addition to these increases in angiogenesis, exercise preconditioning also increases arteriogenesis, which promotes cerebral blood flow (CBF), increases collateral circulation, and ameliorates neuronal injury and death following ischemia/reperfusion injury (Lloyd et al., 2003, 2005). Closely linked to the metabolic requirements needed by the brain during levels of high activity, the amount of blood supply provides the necessary avenue to

produce the needed glucose and oxygen. Through increasing this metabolic demand, exercise leads to permanent structural alterations, such as angiogenesis and arteriogenesis, and these changes allow the increased delivery of vital nutrients to active neurons (Isaacs et al., 1992; Vissing et al., 1996). These structural changes not only facilitate increased glucose and oxygen delivery, but they have also been shown to reduce brain damage as well (Ding et al., 2004a).

The structural alterations seen with angiogenesis are driven by several regulator proteins, namely vascular endothelial growth factor (VEGF) and angiopoietins (Ang) 1 and 2. VEGF and Ang1/2 are known to be expressed in greater abundance following exercise training, and these changes lead to increased blood vessel density (Ding et al., 2004b). Expression of Ang 1 and 2 mRNA has been shown to be increased as early as 1 week after the onset of exercise training (Ding et al., 2006b), and VEGF mRNA expression has been shown to be mildly increased at 1 week but exponentially higher after 3 weeks of exercise training (Matsumori et al., 2005; Nawashiro et al., 1997; Sawatzky et al., 2006; Yong et al., 2001). Exercise-induced angiogenesis was also seen in aging rats with associated increases in VEGF and Ang1/2 mRNA levels (Ding et al., 2006b), suggesting that angiogenesis can be expected in the adult brain. Although most proliferation of the neurovascular system occurs during cerebral development, these findings reveal that VEGF and Ang1/2 drive this process in aging brains as well, further promoting the endogenous neuroprotection afforded by exercise preconditioning.

These changes occurring after chronic exercise also lead to better outcomes following ischemia/reperfusion injury. In addition to correlating with increased cerebral blood flow and glucose utilization, the angiogenesis and arteriogenesis observed following exercise preconditioning is associated with decreased neuronal cell death following ischemia/reperfusion injury (Li et al., 2005). The process of angiogenesis provides considerably denser cerebrovascular networks, which bathes the brain in a network of vessels more apt to deliver the vital nutrients necessary for proper brain health and functioning. The additional benefit seen from arteriogenesis, following exercise preconditioning underscores the importance of increased collateral circulation, particularly vital in saving vital brain volume in the ischemic penumbra. Especially when coupled with astrocytosis, the angiogenesis seen following exercise preconditioning substantially contributes to the development and integrity of the BBB, further promoting the neurovascular unit and protecting against ischemic/reperfusion injury.

3.2.4 Cerebral blood flow and glucose uptake

As previously discussed, exercise training increases angiogenesis and arteriogenesis, providing more avenues for potential blood delivery to the cerebral system. Previous studies with Laser Doppler flowmtery (LDF) and ^{15}O-H_2O positron emission tomography (PET) have shown that preischemic exercise preserves the cerebral blood flow (CBF) during the reperfusion stage in ischemia/reperfusion injury (Zwagerman et al., 2010b). Although CBF was similar in exercised and non-exercised groups during ischemia, CBF was significantly higher in the exercise preconditioned animals during reperfusion and was associated with a decreased volume of the infarct. This increase in perfusion during the reperfusion stage in preconditioned animals suggests that this training may partial ameliorate the "no reflow" phenomenon often seen following ischemia/reperfusion injury.

In the same study, intracerebral glucose uptake was also assessed using an ^{18}F-fluorodeoxy-D-glucose (FDG) radiotracer (Zwagerman et al., 2010b). Following ischemia/reperfusion injury, cerebral metabolism was significantly reduced as evidenced by a decrease in glucose uptake. However, in rats preconditioned with physical exercise, brain glucose uptake and metabolism was substantially preserved following reperfusion and was associated with a decrease in infarct volume and functional neurologic deficit. CBF and metabolism also increase during the act of physical exercise, signifying the increased metabolic demand on neuronal cells during training (Hellstrom et al., 1996; Ide and Secher, 2000; Vissing et al., 1996; Williamson et al., 1997) and the likely underlying mechanism through which neuroprotection is obtained. The angiogenic changes that occur following exercise preconditioning provide the brain with an enriched vascular bed with an enhanced ability for proper cerebral blood flow and glucose delivery to neurons, yielding more tolerance to reperfusion injury in the setting of ischemia/reperfusion.

3.3 Inflammatory response
The "no reflow" phenomenon refers to the tendency towards hypoperfusion during the reperfusion stage following ischemia. This hypoperfusion following transient ischemia is thought to stem from multiple mechanisms, including microvascular damage and cerebrovascular occlusion from cellular elements (Aspey et al., 1989; Dietrich et al., 1987; Mori et al., 1992; Nishigaya et al., 1991). In addition to these observed changes, hemoconcentration, red blood cell sludging, hyperviscosity, and platelet plugging tend to occur as well in the reperfusion phase, further exacerbating the damage seen in ischemia/reperfusion injury (Choudhri et al., 1998). While these effects of reperfusion injury causes significant damage, the accumulation of polymorphonuclear leukocytes are the primary contributors to the perfusion abnormalities observed following transient ischemia. The secondary inflammation after ischemia/reperfusion injury plays a major role in secondary brain damage through increased leukocyte infiltration, microvascular damage, and free radical accumulation during reperfusion.

3.3.1 Adhesion molecules and toll-like receptors
In the setting of ischemia/reperfusion injury, cytokines tend to stimulate the expression of cellular adhesion molecules, attracting leukocytes to the cerebrovascular system and promoting their diapedesis into the interstitial space. Two central cytokines in this process, interleukin-1β (IL-1β) and tumor necrosis factor-α (TNF-α), are known to be upregulated following periods of hypoxia and promote the expression of intercellular adhesion molecule 1 (ICAM-1), P-selectin, and E-selectin on leukocytes and endothelial cells. These changes lead to the leukocyte accumulation classically seen in ischemia/reperfusion, leading to adhesion of leukocytes to the damaged vascular endothelium, clogging of the neurovascular vessels, and infiltration into the brain parenchyma. Previous studies have shown that pre-ischemic exercise training reduces the expression of ICAM-1, leading to decreased leukocyte infiltration and accumulation, in the reperfusion stage (Ding et al., 2005). This downregulation leads to decreased inflammation following ischemia/reperfusion injury and serves as another neuroprotective mechanism of exercise preconditioning.
Another mechanism underlying the inflammatory damage in the reperfusion stage pertains to the expression of toll-like receptors. These cell surface receptors are found within the brain and throughout the body and are actively involved in the immune response by

binding endogenous and foreign materials and triggering a cytokine cascade (Gleeson et al., 2006). Previous research studies have also revealed that exercise preconditioning reduces the expression of Toll-like receptor-4 (McFarlin et al., 2006), and reduction of these receptors in Toll-like receptor-4 deficient mice has been shown to decrease tissue damage and neurologic deficits following ischemia/reperfusion injury (Cao et al., 2007). Another study looking at both of these factors has indicated that exercise preconditioning simultaneously reduces expression of Toll-like receptor-4, which leads to a reduction in brain injury following ischemic stroke (Zwagerman et al., 2010a).

3.3.2 Leukocyte invasion

Through the downregulation of adhesion molecules and toll-like receptors, exercise preconditioning is able to significantly reduce the amount of damage seen following ischemia/reperfusion injury. The underlying mechanism through which this process works focuses on the decreased leukocyte migration and diapedesis often seen in the reperfusion stage following stroke. Decreased leukocyte infiltration decreases many of the secondary changes such as free radical formation and subsequent edema formation. Ultimately, the decreased leukocyte invasion seen in exercise preconditioned subjects leads to better neurologic outcome following ischemia/reperfusion injury.

3.4 Neuronal death and survival signalling pathways

Neuronal survival depends on both external and internal stimuli and environments. Many of the changes following exercise preconditioning, involving inflammation, strengthening of the blood brain barrier, and increased integrity of the neurovascular unit, improve the cerebral environment in the setting of acute ischemia/reperfusion injury. In addition, internal cellular stimuli and pathways have a profound effect on neuronal survival. Following exercise preconditioning, apoptosis is attenuated and heat shock proteins are upregulated through a variety of biomolecular mechanisms following ischemia/reperfusion injury. Likewise, external stimuli through tumor necrosis factor (TNF)-α protect the brain during hypoxia. These changes seen in rats preconditioned with physical exercise are neuroprotective in the setting of ischemia/reperfusion injury, decreasing neuronal death and improving neurologic outcomes.

3.4.1 Anti:Pro apoptotic ratio

Neuronal apoptosis following ischemia/reperfusion injury is regulated by cascades of pro- and anti-apoptotic proteins. Notable among these include pro-apoptotic Bax, Bad, and Bak and anti-apoptotic Bcl-2 and Bcl-xL (Lazou et al., 2006; Mayer and Oberbauer, 2003). Upregulation of anti-apoptotic proteins (Bcl-2, Bcl-xL) and corresponding downregulation of pro-apoptotic proteins (Bax, Bad, and Bak) are seen following exercise preconditioning and are protective in the event of cerebral ischemia (Rybnikova et al., 2006; Wu et al., 2003). In addition to these key regulatory proteins, both caspase-dependent and caspase independent pathways appear to be involved in cerebral ischemia and neuronal death (Cao et al., 2003; Joza et al., 2001; Zhu et al., 2003), and apoptosis induced factor (AIF) also plays a key role in pro-apoptosis (Daugas et al., 2000; Susin et al., 1999).

Exercise preconditioning has been shown to not only enhance the expression of anti-apoptotic Bcl-xL, but to also decrease the expression of pro-apoptotic AIF and Bax, ultimately leading to decreased apoptosis and prolonged neuronal survival (Chaudhry et al., 2010). Following ischemia/reperfusion injury, this increased anti:pro apoptotic ratio generates decreased neuronal death and smaller infarct size. While these neuroprotective mechanisms of exercise are newly evolving, they provide a possible point of therapeutic intervention. While neuroprotective agents that target cell death pathways have been tried in the past, the potential for increasing cell survival reveals a potential novel strategy for improving outcomes following ischemia/reperfusion (Chan, 2004). This could provide a neuroprotective therapy that would simultaneously promote cell survival and decrease neuronal death, thus ameliorating much of the functional loss following acute ischemic stroke.

3.4.2 TNF-α and TNF-α receptor

Tumor necrosis factor (TNF)-α is a major deleterious pro-inflammatory cytokine found throughout the systemic circulation and upregulated following stroke and traumatic brain injury (Botchkina et al., 1997; Sairanen et al., 2001). Despite its inflammatory and injurious effects, evidence also points to TNF-α as a beneficial factor in tissue repair and neuroprotection (Bruce et al., 1996; Feuerstein and Wang, 2001; Wang et al., 2000). Furthermore, this cytokine may serve to induce endogenous neuroprotection following chronic exercise preconditioning. It is believed that exercise training produces a chronic low grade increase in TNF-α concentration, ultimately generating neuronal tolerance and protection in the setting of ischemia/reperfusion injury (Ginis et al., 1999; Liu et al., 2000; Wang et al., 2000). In a similar manner, TNF-α concentration was chronically elevated following exercise, which resulted in reduced myocardial infarction (Yamashita et al., 1999); however, acutely elevated levels of TNF-α following ischemia results in harmful myocardial remodelling (Jobe et al., 2009).

In the brain, exercise preconditioning also chronically increases the level of TNF-α that is exposed to neuronal cells, an effect which prevents the downstream inflammatory reaction which is induced by acutely elevated levels of TNF-α following cerebral ischemia/reperfusion injury (Ding et al., 2005). Furthermore, TNF-α has also been shown to reduce blood brain barrier injury and neuronal damage following ischemic stroke (Guo et al., 2008b). This scenario reveals two sides to the effect of TNF-α on neuronal survival and cerebral integrity. With chronic low levels of the cytokine, it is profoundly beneficial and neuroprotective; however, following ischemia/reperfusion, the acute increase of TNF-α into the cerebrovascular circulation destroys the integrity of the neurovascular unit, increases cell death, and enlarges the infarct volume. Exercise preconditioning enhances the former effect, increasing chronic low grade levels of the cytokine, which ameliorates the latter effect and dampens the injury following acute increases of TNF-α.

Mechanisms underlying this complex picture of TNF-α have not been completely uncovered, but are thought to involve the expression of TNF-α receptors. Previous studies have shown that the chronic exercise-induced levels of TNF-α serve to reduce the expression of TNF-α receptor after ischemia/reperfusion (Reyes, Jr. et al., 2006). Following ischemic injury in a rat model, pre-ischemic exercise was indeed found to decrease the expression of TNF-α receptors I and II, leading to reduced brain damage and enhance neurologic recovery (Reyes, Jr. et al., 2006). These results indicate a classic desensitization of the TNF-α receptor following exercise preconditioning, promoting neuronal tolerance to acutely elevated levels of TNF-α following ischemia/reperfusion injury.

3.4.3 Heat shock proteins

Neuronal survival and neuroprotection appears to be further driven by heat shock protein (HSP)-70, a highly inducible protein of 70 kDa. HSP-70 is well known to respond to various types of stress, including heat shock, hypoxia, oxidative stress, and exposure to metals and toxins (Kiang and Tsokos, 1998). Constitutively expressed, this molecular chaperone protein assists in the folding both nascent and denatured proteins during times of neuronal stress (Schlesinger, 1990). Overexpression of HSP-70 has previously been shown to be neuroprotective in the setting of ischemia/reperfusion (Giffard and Yenari, 2004). This neuroprotective protein interferes with apoptosis inducing factor (AIF), a pro-apoptotic protein. HSP-70 also increases the levels of anti-apoptotic proteins, Bcl-2 and Bcl-xL, thus serving as another mechanism to increase the anti:pro apoptotic ratio and push neurons toward cellular survival, especially in the setting of ischemia/reperfusion (Liebelt et al., 2010; Ohtsuka and Suzuki, 2000).

Multiple studies have shown that ischemic preconditioning induces HSP-70 expression and promotes neuroprotection (Chen and Simon, 1997; Kirino et al., 1991; Masada et al., 2001). Despite these benefits, the effects of HSP-70 are limited. If the insult is very severe or if expression of HSP-70 is too low, the beneficial effects may not be seen (Giffard and Yenari, 2004; Lee et al., 2001; Matsumori et al., 2005). Nonetheless, HSP-70 mice convey more potent neuroprotection than wild type mice, underlying its importance as a key factor in exercise-induced neuroprotection for ischemia/reperfusion injury (Matsumori et al., 2005). In addition to its neuroprotective effects, HSP-70 has also been seen to be cardioprotective following upregulation after exercise preconditioning (Hamilton et al., 2003; Lennon et al., 2004).

Also, HSP-70 alone does not appear to be neuroprotective, but it requires other proteins for optimal neuroprotection (Lee et al., 2001). Upregulation of TNF-α appears to be critical for HSP-70 to effectively reduce apoptosis and prolong neuronal survival (Liebelt et al., 2010). Furthermore, TNF-α and HSP-70 appear to work in concert through an ERK1/2 signal transduction pathway to increase the expression of anti-apoptotic genes and decrease the expression of pro-apoptotic genes (Goel et al., 2010). These results reveal the neuroprotective nature of HSP-70, but they also reveal its limitations. For HSP-70 to truly be effective in the setting of ischemia/reperfusion injury, it requires a large insult, significant HSP-70 expression, and the upregulation of other proteins as well, including TNF-α. Despite these constraints, HSP-70 does appear to induce neuroprotection in ischemia/reperfusion injury following exercise preconditioning.

3.5 Extracellular signal-regulated kinase

Extracellular signal-regulated kinases (ERK1/2) are involved in mitogen-activated protein kinase pathways and are constitutively expressed in the adult brain (Fiore et al., 1993; Sharony et al., 2005). These ERK1/2-regulated pathways are pivotal in signal transduction and neuroprotection in the setting of ischemia/reperfusion injury. Numerous studies have shown a pro-apoptotic role for ERK1/2 in neurons and other cells as well (Chu et al., 2004; Shackelford and Yeh, 2006; Zhuang and Schnellmann, 2006). Although ERK1/2 has been shown to push cells towards death, a protective and beneficial role has also been established (Rybnikova et al., 2006). Activation of this regulatory kinase has been shown to enable tissue repair in the setting of ischemia/reperfusion injury, thus decreasing cell death (Cavanaugh, 2004; Hetman and Gozdz, 2004; Ostrakhovitch and Cherian, 2005; Sawatzky et al., 2006). Furthermore, exercise preconditioning appears to upregulate ERK1/2, leading to an ischemic neuronal tolerance under hypoxic condition (Gu et al., 2001; Jones and Bergeron, 2004; Shamloo and Wieloch, 1999). While ERK1/2 is upregulated following ischemic preconditioning (Lecour et al., 2005), ERK1/2 activation also is detrimental following stroke, trauma and degenerative disease (Chu et al., 2004). This dual role of ERK1/2, being both beneficial and detrimental, may be similar in mechanism to the effects of TNF-α in which chronic upregulation following exercise preconditioning generates neuronal tolerance and improved outcome following ischemia/reperfusion injury.

Following inhibition of ERK1/2 in exercise preconditioned animals, neuroprotection was substantially reduced in ischemia/reperfusion, suggesting the pertinent role of ERK1/2 in exercise-induced neuroprotection (Guo et al., 2008b). However, exercise preconditioned animals did have elevated levels of ERK1/2 and TNF-α following exercise training, which correlated with decreased neurologic deficit, smaller brain infarcts, and less inflammation (Curry et al., 2009). A recent study has shown that ERK1/2 activation also helps to regulate apoptosis (Liebelt et al., 2010). Again, pre-ischemic exercise led to minor increases in ERK1/2, which was neuroprotective against the large acute elevations seen following ischemia/reperfusion injury. In the setting of hypoxic injury, ERK1/2 regulates the anti- and pro-apoptotic pathways involving such regulators as Bcl-xL, Bax, and AIF. Following exercise preconditioning, the upregulation of ERK1/2 served to promote anti-apoptosis, leading to decreased neuronal apoptosis and infarct volume.

ERK1/2, while shown to ameliorate ischemia/reperfusion through its apoptotic regulatory effects and inflammatory changes, has also been linked with HSP-70 and TNF-α. Several studies have shown these three important proteins to be fundamentally linked in a relationship where TNF-α and HSP-70 activate the MEK/ERK signalling pathway, leading to neuroprotection (Gortz et al., 2005; Lee et al., 2001,2005). While ischemic preconditioning has been shown to induce ERK1/2-mediated neuroprotection, pharmacologic pre-treatment with TNF-α has not shown similar results (Lecour et al., 2005), suggesting that multiple interacting pathways and proteins are likely necessary to observe the full neuroprotective effect. It seems likely that a cross talk between TNF-α, HSP-70, and ERK1/2 occurs in exercise training, allowing for a greater neuroprotective response following ischemia/reperfusion injury. Nonetheless, these studies have clarified a dual role of ERK1/2 in neuroprotection, in which chronic low levels protect against acute elevations of the protein and ameliorate the damage and neuronal loss following ischemia/reperfusion injury.

3.6 Metabolic enhancement
The association between exercise preconditioning and neuroprotection in ischemia/reperfusion has been well established. In addition to the aforementioned mechanisms, chronic exercise training also affects cerebral metabolism and energy production, allowing neurons to re-establish homeostasis more rapidly following acute ischemic stroke. A recent study revealed that forced exercise resulted in enhanced cerebral glycolysis and cerebral metabolism (Kinni et al., 2011). In addition to increasing glycolysis, exercise preconditioning is also well known to increase cerebral blood flow (CBF) and adenosine triphosphate (ATP) production (Ide and Secher, 2000; McCloskey et al., 2001; Ogoh and Ainslie, 2009). Exercise can be best viewed as a chronic state of metabolic stress, which requires increased glucose delivery, glycolysis, and ATP production in order to match the energy demand. Chronic exercise preconditioning enables the neuronal cells to accumulate the necessary machinery for mass ATP production, which elevates the metabolic and ATP production potential in these cells. In the setting of ischemia/reperfusion injury,

these preconditioned neurons have an increased metabolic capacity and are better able to avoid hypoxic damage.

3.6.1 ATP production

The process of ATP production requires several key steps, involving detection of low ATP stores, glucose transport and glycolysis. 5'-AMP-activated protein kinase (AMPK) serves as an energy sensor and is capable of detecting low ATP stores in cells (Minchenko et al., 2003). The protein is a heterotrimeric serine/threonine kinase, which becomes activated in times of metabolic stress and decreased ATP stores (Emerling et al., 2007; Hardie et al., 2003; Zorzano et al., 2005). When ATP concentrations drop, AMPK activates glycolysis in order to restore the cell's energy balance, allowing it to serve as an excellent marker of metabolic demand (Kahn et al., 2005). Following exercise training, levels of the active phosphorylated form of AMPK are increased in response to the elevated metabolic demand (Aschenbach et al., 2004; Kinni et al., 2011). Following ischemia/reperfusion injury, the active phosphorylated form of AMPK has been shown to be upregulated in preconditioned rats, suggesting an increased metabolic response to hypoxia in these exercised animals (unpublished data). This increased capacity for metabolism upregulation is mirrored in elevated levels of glucose transporters and glycolytic enzymes, which are also seen following exercise training and correlate with better outcomes following ischemia/reperfusion injury.

While increases in cerebral blood flow associated with exercise facilitate greater transport of glucose to the neurovascular system, transport across the BBB and neuronal membrane are controlled by glucose transporters (GLUT). GLUT1 is primarily found in the endothelial cells of the BBB and generates a basal glucose level, while GLUT3 is found exclusively in neurons, and both of these glucose transporters have previously been shown to increase in response to hypoxia and elevated metabolic demand (Maurer et al., 2006). The increased need for energy production following hypoxia requires more glucose to be available within neurons, and these two glucose transporters work together to shuttle glucose from the circulation into neurons. GLUT1 and GLUT3 are known to have increased expression following exercise preconditioning (Kinni et al., 2011). Following ischemia/reperfusion injury, GLUT1 and GLUT3 levels are elevated in the first 4 hours after reperfusion is established in exercise preconditioned rats, but expression is equal to control at 24 hours after injury (unpublished data). This elevation in GLUT expression in the acute phase of reperfusion indicates that these preconditioned animals have the cellular machinery in place immediately when it is needed. Non-exercised rats take longer to transcribe and translate the needed metabolic proteins, leading to increased metabolic dysfunction. Thus, exercise preconditioning provides neuroprotection by increasing the levels of available glucose within neurons, providing the necessary substrate for ATP production.

Once inside neurons, glucose must be metabolized to produce ATP for the cell. The initial steps of glycolysis are primarily regulated by the key rate limiting step of phosphofructokinase (PFK), which catalyzes the phosphorylation of fructose-6-phosphate to fructose-1,6-bisphosphonate. PFK expression is known to be upregulated following increased metabolism and glycolysis and is has been shown to be neuroprotective in hypoglycemic conditions (Minchenko et al., 2003). Another study has revealed PFK is increased following exercise preconditioning (Kinni et al., 2011), and this enzyme is increased following ischemia/reperfusion injury, leading to increased neuronal metabolism and decreased neurologic deficits (unpublished data). The elevated ability of neurons to process glucose through glycolysis in exercise preconditioned animals underlies another key component of exercise-induced neuroprotection. Not only does exercise training increase glucose delivery to cells through angiogenesis and glucose transport, it also upregulates the machinery needed for glucose breakdown and ATP production.

Ultimately, these processes work to increase ATP production to meet the energy demand of neurons. One test used to assess the ATP production capacity of a neuron is an ADP:ATP ratio, which has been found to be decreased following ischemia/reperfusion injury in exercise preconditioned rats (unpublished data). A lower ADP:ATP ratio indicates a lower level of metabolic dysfunction and increased capacity for ATP production in exercise trained rats. Through the increased expression of various metabolic proteins, including AMPK, GLUT1, GLUT3, and PFK, exercise preconditioning upregulates multiple stages of ATP production, providing cells with the important energy substrate. The increased capacity for ATP production allows neurons in exercise trained rats to decrease their energy deficit following ischemia/reperfusion injury. In turn, this promotes neuronal survival and decreases infarct size, leading to better outcomes following ischemia/reperfusion.

3.6.2 HIF-1α and metabolism

Hypoxic-induced factor-1α (HIF-1α) is a transcription factor, which is normally inhibited by oxygen-dependent hydroxylase enzymes, but in hypoxic conditions, these hydroxylase enzymes lose their ability to function and allow HIF-1α to initiate gene transcription (Bracken et al., 2006). HIF-1α is known to be neuroprotective in rats following ischemia/reperfusion injury (Bernaudin et al., 2002; Schubert, 2005). Not only is HIF-1α increased following hypoxia, but it also is increased in rats that are chronically exposed to hypoxic events (Bernaudin et al., 2002; Bracken et al., 2006). The expression of HIF-1α is also known to be increased following exercise preconditioning (Kinni et al., 2011). In addition to these findings, the transcription factor has also been shown to increase the expression of genes and proteins involved in angiogenesis and glycolysis, revealing its metabolism promoting activity (Bergeron et al., 1999; Bernaudin et al., 2002; Iyer et al., 1998; Jones and Bergeron, 2001; Schubert, 2005; Semenza, 2009). HIF-1α is known to increase the expression of VEGF, glucose transporters and enzymes involved in glycolysis, such as PFK (Bergeron et al., 1999; Jones and Bergeron, 2001; Kim et al., 2006). HIF-1α is not only involved in enhanced expression of metabolic enzymes and pathways, but the expression of HIF-1α is also increased by AMPK, a master regulator of neuronal metabolism (Emerling et al., 2007; Lee et al., 2003; Neurath et al., 2006). In fact, studies in chronically exercised rats have demonstrated that increased levels of AMPK induce HIF-1α to increase the expression of glucose transporters and PFK (Emerling et al., 2007; Hardie et al., 2003; Kahn et al., 2005; McGee and Hargreaves, 2006).

HIF-1α, through its multiple mechanistic pathways, can increase metabolism and angiogenesis in an oxygen-deficient state, allowing it to simultaneously increase the mode of glucose delivery and the mechanism of ATP production. In addition to being increased following exercise preconditioning (Kinni et al., 2011), HIF-1α is also increased in exercise trained animals following ischemia/reperfusion injury, which correlated with better neurologic outcomes and decreased infarct size (unpublished data). These results indicate that exercise equips neurons with a greater ability to upregulated glucose transport and metabolism, resulting in greater ATP production and decreased metabolic dysfunction, following acute ischemic stroke. This rapid response to an elevated energy demand promotes neuronal recovery and survival and serves as another mechanism of exercise-induced neuroprotection in the setting of ischemia/reperfusion injury.

4. Clinical implications

Exercise-induced preconditioning is useful in prevention and amelioration of neuronal loss and neurologic dysfunction following ischemia/reperfusion injury, but it also has many therapeutic implications as well. The potential for future drug targets at various levels of the neuroprotective mechanisms are abundant as the effects of neurotrophic factors, neurovascular unit integrity, inflammatory markers, and metabolic changes provide potential avenues for future pharmacologic intervention. Particularly evident in patients with a history of ischemic stroke, traumatic brain injury, or transient ischemic attacks, pharmacologic interventions that could increase metabolism, strengthen the neurovascular unit, or decrease inflammation could have profound effects on morbidity and mortality associated with cerebrovascular accidents. Finally, the implications for exercise preconditioning prior to neurosurgical intervention can clearly be seen. Through its ability to strengthen the neurovascular unit and decrease brain inflammation, exercise training should be strongly encouraged in any individuals prior to neurosurgical intervention.

5. Conclusion

Exercise preconditioning clearly is neuroprotective in the setting of ischemia/reperfusion injury, and these protective effects are conveyed through multiple mechanisms. The neuroprotection derived as a result of exercise training is an endogenous effect that occurs independently of the risk factor modification that is also seen following exercise. Innate neuroprotection from exercise is derived from elevated levels of neurotrophin proteins, which increase neuronal abundance and strength. Furthermore, enhanced integrity of the neurovascular unit occurs through strengthening of the blood brain barrier, astrocytosis, angiogenesis, and arteriogenesis. Exercise preconditioning also decreases the inflammatory response and leukocyte invasion following ischemia/reperfusion injury, thus decreasing much of the secondary damage seen following the reperfusion stage. Neuronal apoptosis is reduced as exercise training increases anti-apoptotic factors and simultaneously decreases pro-apoptotic factors, pushing neurons towards a state of survival rather than programmed cell death. Finally, exercise increases the metabolic capacity of neurons through upregulation of cerebral blood flow, glucose transport, glycolysis, and ATP production. Altogether, these changes seen following exercise preconditioning decreased neuronal loss, reduce infarct volume, and improve neurologic outcomes after ischemia/reperfusion injury.

6. References

Ang, E. T., P. T. Wong, S. Moochhala, and Y. K. Ng, 2003, Neuroprotection associated with running: is it a result of increased endogenous neurotrophic factors?: Neuroscience, v. 118, no. 2, p. 335-345.

Arai, K., S. R. Lee, and E. H. Lo, 2003, Essential role for ERK mitogen-activated protein kinase in matrix metalloproteinase-9 regulation in rat cortical astrocytes: Glia, v. 43, no. 3, p. 254-264.

Asahi, M., X. Wang, T. Mori, T. Sumii, J. C. Jung, M. A. Moskowitz, M. E. Fini, and E. H. Lo, 2001, Effects of matrix metalloproteinase-9 gene knock-out on the proteolysis of blood-brain barrier and white matter components after cerebral ischemia: J Neurosci, v. 21, no. 19, p. 7724-7732.

Aschenbach, W. G., K. Sakamoto, and L. J. Goodyear, 2004, 5' adenosine monophosphate-activated protein kinase, metabolism and exercise: Sports Med., v. 34, no. 2, p. 91-103.

Aspey, B. S., C. Jessimer, S. Pereira, and M. J. Harrison, 1989, Do leukocytes have a role in the cerebral no-reflow phenomenon?: J Neurol Neurosurg Psychiatry, v. 52, no. 4, p. 526-528.

Ayata, C., and A. H. Ropper, 2002, Ischaemic brain oedema: J Clin Neurosci, v. 9, no. 2, p. 113-124.

Bergeron, M., A. Y. Yu, K. E. Solway, G. L. Semenza, and F. R. Sharp, 1999, Induction of hypoxia-inducible factor-1 (HIF-1) and its target genes following focal ischaemia in rat brain: Eur.J.Neurosci., v. 11, no. 12, p. 4159-4170.

Bernaudin, M., A. S. Nedelec, D. Divoux, E. T. MacKenzie, E. Petit, and P. Schumann-Bard, 2002, Normobaric hypoxia induces tolerance to focal permanent cerebral ischemia in association with an increased expression of hypoxia-inducible factor-1 and its target genes, erythropoietin and VEGF, in the adult mouse brain: J.Cereb.Blood Flow Metab, v. 22, no. 4, p. 393-403.

Black, J. E., K. R. Isaacs, B. J. Anderson, A. A. Alcantara, and W. T. Greenough, 1990, Learning causes synaptogenesis, whereas motor activity causes angiogenesis, in cerebellar cortex of adult rats: Proceedings of the National Academy of Sciences of the United States of America, v. 87, no. 14, p. 5568-5572.

Botchkina, G. I., M. E. Meistrell, I. L. Botchkina, and K. J. Tracey, 1997, Expression of TNF and TNF receptors (p55 and p75) in the rat brain after focal cerebral ischemia: Mol Med, v. 3, no. 11, p. 765-781.

Bracken, C. P., A. O. Fedele, S. Linke, W. Balrak, K. Lisy, M. L. Whitelaw, and D. J. Peet, 2006, Cell-specific regulation of hypoxia-inducible factor (HIF)-1alpha and HIF-2alpha stabilization and transactivation in a graded oxygen environment: J.Biol.Chem., v. 281, no. 32, p. 22575-22585.

Bruce, A. J., W. Boling, M. S. Kindy, J. Peschon, P. J. Kraemer, M. K. Carpenter, F. W. Holtsberg, and M. P. Mattson, 1996, Altered neuronal and microglial responses to excitotoxic and ischemic brain injury in mice lacking TNF receptors: Nat Med, v. 2, no. 7, p. 788-794.

Cao, C. X., Q. W. Yang, F. L. Lv, J. Cui, H. B. Fu, and J. Z. Wang, 2007, Reduced cerebral ischemia-reperfusion injury in Toll-like receptor 4 deficient mice: Biochem.Biophys.Res.Commun., v. 353, no. 2, p. 509-514.

Cao, G., R. S. Clark, W. Pei, W. Yin, F. Zhang, F. Y. Sun, S. H. Graham, and J. Chen, 2003, Translocation of apoptosis-inducing factor in vulnerable neurons after transient cerebral ischemia and in neuronal cultures after oxygen-glucose deprivation: J Cereb.Blood Flow Metab, v. 23, no. 10, p. 1137-1150.

Cavanaugh, J. E., 2004, Role of extracellular signal regulated kinase 5 in neuronal survival: Eur.J.Biochem., v. 271, no. 11, p. 2056-2059.

Chan, P. H., 2004, Future targets and cascades for neuroprotective strategies: Stroke, v. 35, no. 11 Suppl 1, p. 2748-2750.

Chaudhry, K. et al., 2010, Matrix metalloproteinase-9 (MMP-9) expression and extracellular signal-regulated kinase 1 and 2 (ERK1/2) activation in exercise-reduced neuronal apoptosis after stroke: Neuroscience Letters, v. 474, no. 2, p. 109-114.

Chen, J., and R. Simon, 1997, Ischemic tolerance in the brain: Neurology, v. 48, no. 2, p. 306-311.

Choudhri, T. F., B. L. Hoh, H. G. Zerwes, C. J. Prestigiacomo, S. C. Kim, E. S. Connolly, Jr, G. Kottirsch, and D. J. Pinsky, 1998, Reduced microvascular thrombosis and improved outcome in acute murine stroke by inhibiting GP IIb/IIIa receptor-mediated platelet aggregation: Journal of Clinical Investigation, v. 102, no. 7, p. 1301-1310.

Chu, C. T., D. J. Levinthal, S. M. Kulich, E. M. Chalovich, and D. B. DeFranco, 2004, Oxidative neuronal injury. The dark side of ERK1/21: Eur.J Biochem., v. 271, no. 11, p. 2060-2066.

Clark, A. W., C. A. Krekoski, S. S. Bou, K. R. Chapman, and D. R. Edwards, 1997, Increased gelatinase A (MMP-2) and gelatinase B (MMP-9) activities in human brain after focal ischemia: Neurosci Lett, v. 238, no. 1-2, p. 53-56.

Cohen-Cory, S., A. H. Kidane, N. J. Shirkey, and S. Marshak, 2010, Brain-derived neurotrophic factor and the development of structural neuronal connectivity: Dev.Neurobiol., v. 70, no. 5, p. 271-288.

Curry, A. et al., 2009, Exercise pre-conditioning reduces brain inflammation in stroke via tumor necrosis factor-alpha, extracellular signal-regulated kinase 1/2 and matrix metalloproteinase-9 activity: Neurological Research.

Dans, M. J., and F. G. Giancotti, 1999,Dans, M. J., and F. G. Giancotti Guidebook to the extracellular matrix, anchor, and adhesion proteins: Oxford, Sambrook & Tooze Publication at Osford University Press.

Daugas, E. et al., 2000, Mitochondrio-nuclear translocation of AIF in apoptosis and necrosis: FASEB J, v. 14, no. 5, p. 729-739.

Davis, W., S. Mahale, A. Carranza, B. Cox, K. Hayes, D. Jimenez, and Y. Ding, 2007, Exercise pre-conditioning ameliorates blood-brain barrier dysfunction in stroke by enhancing basal lamina: Neurological Research, v. 29, no. 4, p. 382-387.

del Zoppo, G. J., and J. M. Hallenbeck, 2000, Advances in the vascular pathophysiology of ischemic stroke: Thromb Res, v. 98, no. 3, p. 73-81.

del Zoppo, G. J., and T. Mabuchi, 2003, Cerebral microvessel responses to focal ischemia: J Cereb Blood Flow Metab, v. 23, no. 8, p. 879-894.

Dietrich, W. D., R. Busto, S. Yoshida, and M. D. Ginsberg, 1987, Histopathological and hemodynamic consequences of complete versus incomplete ischemia in the rat: J Cereb Blood Flow Metab, v. 7, no. 3, p. 300-308.

Ding,Y, Y H Ding, J Li, J A Rafols. Exercise induces integrin overexpression and improves neurovascular integrity in ischemic stroke. Stroke 36[2], 470. 2005. Ref Type: Abstract

Ding, Y., J. Li, J. Clark, F. G. Diaz, and J. A. Rafols, 2003, Synaptic plasticity in thalamic nuclei enhanced by motor skill training in rat with transient middle cerebral artery occlusion: Neurological Research, v. 25, p. 189-194.

Ding, Y., J. Li, X. Luan, Y. H. Ding, Q. Lai, J. A. Rafols, J. W. Phillis, J. Clark, and F. G. Diaz, 2004a, Exercise Pre-conditioning Reduces Brain Damage in Ischemic Rats That May be Associated with Regional Angiogenesis and Cellular Overexpression of Neurotrophin: Neuroscience, v. 124, p. 583-591.

Ding, Y. H., Y. Ding, J. Li, D. A. Bessert, and J. A. Rafols, 2006a, Exercise pre-conditioning strengthens brain microvascular integrity in a rat stroke model: Neurol Res, v. 28, no. 2, p. 184-189.

Ding, Y. H., J. Li, W. X. Yao, J. A. Rafols, J. C. Clark, and Y. Ding, 2006b, Exercise preconditioning upregulates cerebral integrins and enhances cerebrovascular integrity in ischemic rats: Acta Neuropathol.(Berl), v. 112, no. 1, p. 74-84.

Ding, Y. H., X. Luan, J. Li, J. A. Rafols, M. Guthikonda, F. G. Diaz, and Y. Ding, 2004b, Exercise-induced overexpression of angiogenic factors and reduction of ischemia/reperfusion injury in stroke: Current Neurovascular Research, v. 1, no. 5, p. 411-420.

Emerling, B. M., B. Viollet, K. V. Tormos, and N. S. Chandel, 2007, Compound C inhibits hypoxic activation of HIF-1 independent of AMPK: FEBS Lett., v. 581, no. 29, p. 5727-5731.

Evenson, K. R., W. D. Rosamond, J. Cai, J. F. Toole, R. G. Hutchinson, E. Shahar, and A. R. Folsom, 1999, Physical activity and ischemic stroke risk. The atherosclerosis risk in communities study: Stroke, v. 30, no. 7, p. 1333-1339.

Feuerstein, G. Z., and X. Wang, 2001, Inflammation and stroke: benefits without harm?: Arch Neurol, v. 58, no. 4, p. 672-674.

Fiore, R. S., V. E. Bayer, S. L. Pelech, J. Posada, J. A. Cooper, and J. M. Baraban, 1993, p42 mitogen-activated protein kinase in brain: prominent localization in neuronal cell bodies and dendrites: Neuroscience, v. 55, no. 2, p. 463-472.

Gasche, Y., M. Fujimura, F. Morita, J. C. Copin, M. Kawase, J. Massengale, and P. H. Chan, 1999, Early appearance of activated matrix metalloproteinase-9 after focal cerebral ischemia in mice: a possible role in blood-brain barrier dysfunction: J Cereb Blood Flow Metab, v. 19, no. 9, p. 1020-1028.

Giffard, R. G., and M. A. Yenari, 2004, Many mechanisms for hsp70 protection from cerebral ischemia: J Neurosurg Anesthesiol., v. 16, no. 1, p. 53-61.

Gillum, R. F., M. E. Mussolino, and D. D. Ingram, 1996, Physical activity and stroke incidence in women and men. The NHANES I Epidemiologic Follow-up Study: Am J Epidemiol, v. 143, no. 9, p. 860-869.

Ginis, I., U. Schweizer, M. Brenner, J. Liu, N. Azzam, M. Spatz, and J. M. Hallenbeck, 1999, TNF-alpha pretreatment prevents subsequent activation of cultured brain cells with TNF-alpha and hypoxia via ceramide: Am J Physiol, v. 276, no. 5 Pt 1, p. C1171-C1183.

Gleeson, M., B. McFarlin, and M. Flynn, 2006, Exercise and Toll-like receptors: Exerc.Immunol.Rev., v. 12, p. 34-53.

Goel, G., M. Guo, J. Ding, D. Dornbos, III, A. Ali, M. Shenaq, M. Guthikonda, and Y. Ding, 2010, Combined effect of tumor necrosis factor (TNF)-alpha and heat shock protein

(HSP)-70 in reducing apoptotic injury in hypoxia: a cell culture study: Neuroscience Letters, v. 483, no. 3, p. 162-166.

Gortz, B., S. Hayer, B. Tuerck, J. Zwerina, J. S. Smolen, and G. Schett, 2005, Tumour necrosis factor activates the mitogen-activated protein kinases p38alpha and ERK in the synovial membrane in vivo: Arthritis Res Ther., v. 7, no. 5, p. R1140-R1147.

Gu, Z., Q. Jiang, and G. Zhang, 2001, Extracellular signal-regulated kinase 1/2 activation in hippocampus after cerebral ischemia may not interfere with postischemic cell death: Brain Research, v. 901, no. 1-2, p. 79-84.

Guo, M., B. Cox, S. Mahale, W. Davis, A. Carranza, K. Hayes, S. Sprague, D. Jimenez, and Y. Ding, 2008a, Pre-ischemic exercise reduces matrix metalloproteinase-9 expression and ameliorates blood-brain barrier dysfunction in stroke: Neuroscience, v. 151, no. 2, p. 340-351.

Guo, M., V. Lin, W. Davis, T. Huang, A. Carranza, S. Sprague, R. Reyes, D. Jimenez, and Y. Ding, 2008b, Preischemic induction of TNF-alpha by physical exercise reduces blood-brain barrier dysfunction in stroke: J.Cereb.Blood Flow Metab, v. 28, no. 8, p. 1422-1430.

Hamilton, K. L., J. L. Staib, T. Phillips, A. Hess, S. L. Lennon, and S. K. Powers, 2003, Exercise, antioxidants, and HSP72: protection against myocardial ischemia/reperfusion: Free Radic.Biol Med, v. 34, no. 7, p. 800-809.

Hardie, D. G., J. W. Scott, D. A. Pan, and E. R. Hudson, 2003, Management of cellular energy by the AMP-activated protein kinase system: FEBS Lett., v. 546, no. 1, p. 113-120.

Hayes, K., S. Sprague, M. Guo, W. Davis, A. Friedman, A. Kumar, D. F. Jimenez, and Y. Ding, 2008, Forced, not voluntary, exercise effectively induces neuroprotection in stroke: Acta Neuropathologica, v. 115, no. 3, p. 289-296.

Hellstrom, G., C. Fischer, N. G. Wahlgren, and T. Jogestrand, 1996, Carotid artery blood flow and middle cerebral artery blood flow velocity during physical exercise: J Appl Physiol, v. 81, no. 1, p. 413-418.

Hetman, M., and A. Gozdz, 2004, Role of extracellular signal regulated kinases 1 and 2 in neuronal survival: Eur.J.Biochem., v. 271, no. 11, p. 2050-2055.

Hosomi, N., C. R. Ban, T. Naya, T. Takahashi, P. Guo, X. Y. Song, and M. Kohno, 2005, Tumor necrosis factor-alpha neutralization reduced cerebral edema through inhibition of matrix metalloproteinase production after transient focal cerebral ischemia
2: J Cereb.Blood Flow Metab, v. 25, no. 8, p. 959-967.

Hu, G., N. C. Barengo, J. Tuomilehto, T. A. Lakka, A. Nissinen, and P. Jousilahti, 2004, Relationship of physical activity and body mass index to the risk of hypertension: a prospective study in Finland: Hypertension, v. 43, no. 1, p. 25-30.

Hu, G., C. Sarti, P. Jousilahti, K. Silventoinen, N. C. Barengo, and J. Tuomilehto, 2005, Leisure time, occupational, and commuting physical activity and the risk of stroke: Stroke, v. 36, no. 9, p. 1994-1999.

Hynes, R. O., 1992, Integrins: versatility, modulation, and signaling in cell adhesion: Cell, v. 69, no. 1, p. 11-25.

Ickes, B. R., T. M. Pham, L. A. Sanders, D. S. Albeck, A. H. Mohammed, and A. C. Granholm, 2000, Long-term environmental enrichment leads to regional increases in neurotrophin levels in rat brain: Exp Neurol, v. 164, no. 1, p. 45-52.

Ide, K., and N. H. Secher, 2000, Cerebral blood flow and metabolism during exercise: Prog Neurobiol, v. 61, no. 4, p. 397-414.

Igarashi, Y. et al., 1999, Glial cell line-derived neurotrophic factor induces barrier function of endothelial cells forming the blood-brain barrier: Biochem Biophys Res Commun, v. 261, no. 1, p. 108-112.

Isaacs, K. R., B. J. Anderson, A. A. Alcantara, J. E. Black, and W. T. Greenough, 1992, Exercise and the brain: angiogenesis in the adult rat cerebellum after vigorous physical activity and motor skill learning: J Cereb Blood Flow Metab, v. 12, no. 1, p. 110-119.

Iyer, N. V. et al., 1998, Cellular and developmental control of O2 homeostasis by hypoxia-inducible factor 1 alpha: Genes Dev., v. 12, no. 2, p. 149-162.

Janzer, R. C., and M. C. Raff, 1987, Astrocytes induce blood-brain barrier properties in endothelial cells: Nature, v. 325, no. 6101, p. 253-257.

Jobe, L. J., G. C. Melendez, S. P. Levick, Y. Du, G. L. Brower, and J. S. Janicki, 2009, TNF-alpha inhibition attenuates adverse myocardial remodeling in a rat model of volume overload: Am.J.Physiol Heart Circ.Physiol, v. 297, no. 4, p. H1462-H1468.

Jones, N. M., and M. Bergeron, 2004, Hypoxia-induced ischemic tolerance in neonatal rat brain involves enhanced ERK1/2 signaling: Journal of Neurochemistry, v. 89, no. 1, p. 157-167.

Jones, N. M., and M. Bergeron, 2001, Hypoxic preconditioning induces changes in HIF-1 target genes in neonatal rat brain: J.Cereb.Blood Flow Metab, v. 21, no. 9, p. 1105-1114.

Jones, T. A., C. J. Chu, L. A. Grande, and A. D. Gregory, 1999, Motor skills training enhances lesion-induced structural plasticity in the motor cortex of adult rats: J Neurosci, v. 19, no. 22, p. 10153-10163.

Joza, N. et al., 2001, Essential role of the mitochondrial apoptosis-inducing factor in programmed cell death: Nature, v. 410, no. 6828, p. 549-554.

Kahn, B. B., T. Alquier, D. Carling, and D. G. Hardie, 2005, AMP-activated protein kinase: ancient energy gauge provides clues to modern understanding of metabolism: Cell Metab, v. 1, no. 1, p. 15-25.

Kiang, J. G., and G. C. Tsokos, 1998, Heat shock protein 70 kDa: molecular biology, biochemistry, and physiology: Pharmacol.Ther., v. 80, no. 2, p. 183-201.

Kim, H., Q. Li, B. L. Hempstead, and J. A. Madri, 2004, Paracrine and autocrine functions of brain-derived neurotrophic factor (BDNF) and nerve growth factor (NGF) in brain-derived endothelial cells: J.Biol.Chem., v. 279, no. 32, p. 33538-33546.

Kim, H. L., E. J. Yeo, Y. S. Chun, and J. W. Park, 2006, A domain responsible for HIF-1alpha degradation by YC-1, a novel anticancer agent: Int.J.Oncol., v. 29, no. 1, p. 255-260.

Kinni, H., M. Guo, J. Y. Ding, S. Konakondla, D. Dornbos, III, R. Tran, M. Guthikonda, and Y. Ding, 2011, Cerebral metabolism after forced or voluntary physical exercise: Brain Research, v. 1388, p. 48-55.

Kirino, T., Y. Tsujita, and A. Tamura, 1991, Induced tolerance to ischemia in gerbil hippocampal neurons: J Cereb.Blood Flow Metab, v. 11, no. 2, p. 299-307.

Kleim, J. A., N. R. Cooper, and P. M. VandenBerg, 2002, Exercise induces angiogenesis but does not alter movement representations within rat motor cortex: Brain Res, v. 934, no. 1, p. 1-6.

Kloner, R. A., 2001, Preinfarct angina and exercise: yet another reason to stay physically active: J.Am.Coll.Cardiol., v. 38, no. 5, p. 1366-1368.

Kondo, T., H. Kinouchi, M. Kawase, and T. Yoshimoto, 1996, Astroglial cells inhibit the increasing permeability of brain endothelial cell monolayer following hypoxia/reoxygenation: Neurosci Lett, v. 208, no. 2, p. 101-104.

Kuipers, S. D., and C. R. Bramham, 2006, Brain-derived neurotrophic factor mechanisms and function in adult synaptic plasticity: new insights and implications for therapy: Curr.Opin.Drug Discov.Devel., v. 9, no. 5, p. 580-586.

Larson, E. B., L. Wang, J. D. Bowen, W. C. McCormick, L. Teri, P. Crane, and W. Kukull, 2006, Exercise is associated with reduced risk for incident dementia among persons 65 years of age and older: Ann.Intern.Med., v. 144, no. 2, p. 73-81.

Lazou, A., E. K. Iliodromitis, D. Cieslak, K. Voskarides, S. Mousikos, E. Bofilis, and D. T. Kremastinos, 2006, Ischemic but not mechanical preconditioning attenuates ischemia/reperfusion induced myocardial apoptosis in anaesthetized rabbits: the role of Bcl-2 family proteins and ERK1/2: Apoptosis., v. 11, no. 12, p. 2195-2204.

Leasure, J. L., and M. Jones, 2008, Forced and voluntary exercise differentially affect brain and behavior: Neuroscience, v. 156, no. 3, p. 456-465.

Lecour, S., N. Suleman, G. A. Deuchar, S. Somers, L. Lacerda, B. Huisamen, and L. H. Opie, 2005, Pharmacological preconditioning with tumor necrosis factor-alpha activates signal transducer and activator of transcription-3 at reperfusion without involving classic prosurvival kinases (Akt and extracellular signal-regulated kinase): Circulation, v. 112, no. 25, p. 3911-3918.

Lee, J. E., M. A. Yenari, G. H. Sun, L. Xu, M. R. Emond, D. Cheng, G. K. Steinberg, and R. G. Giffard, 2001, Differential neuroprotection from human heat shock protein 70 overexpression in in vitro and in vivo models of ischemia and ischemia-like conditions: Exp.Neurol, v. 170, no. 1, p. 129-139.

Lee, J. S., J. J. Lee, and J. S. Seo, 2005, HSP70 deficiency results in activation of c-Jun N-terminal Kinase, extracellular signal-regulated kinase, and caspase-3 in hyperosmolarity-induced apoptosis: J Biol Chem., v. 280, no. 8, p. 6634-6641.

Lee, M., J. T. Hwang, H. J. Lee, S. N. Jung, I. Kang, S. G. Chi, S. S. Kim, and J. Ha, 2003, AMP-activated protein kinase activity is critical for hypoxia-inducible factor-1 transcriptional activity and its target gene expression under hypoxic conditions in DU145 cells: J.Biol.Chem., v. 278, no. 41, p. 39653-39661.

Lennon, S. L., J. Quindry, K. L. Hamilton, J. French, J. Staib, J. L. Mehta, and S. K. Powers, 2004, Loss of exercise-induced cardioprotection after cessation of exercise: J Appl.Physiol, v. 96, no. 4, p. 1299-1305.

Li, J., Y. H. Ding, J. A. Rafols, Q. Lai, J. P. McAllister, II, and Y. Ding, 2005, Increased astrocyte proliferation in rats after running exercise: Neuroscience Letters, v. 386, p. 160-164.

Liebelt, B. et al., 2010, Exercise preconditioning reduces neuronal apoptosis in stroke by up-regulating heat shock protein-70 (heat shock protein-72) and extracellular-signal-regulated-kinase 1/2: Neuroscience, v. 166, no. 4, p. 1091-1100.

Liu, J., I. Ginis, M. Spatz, and J. M. Hallenbeck, 2000, Hypoxic preconditioning protects cultured neurons against hypoxic stress via TNF-alpha and ceramide: Am J Physiol Cell Physiol, v. 278, no. 1, p. C144-C153.

Lloyd, P. G., B. M. Prior, H. Li, H. T. Yang, and R. L. Terjung, 2005, VEGF receptor antagonism blocks arteriogenesis, but only partially inhibits angiogenesis, in skeletal muscle of exercise-trained rats: Am.J.Physiol Heart Circ.Physiol, v. 288, no. 2, p. H759-H768.

Lloyd, P. G., B. M. Prior, H. T. Yang, and R. L. Terjung, 2003, Angiogenic growth factor expression in rat skeletal muscle in response to exercise training: Am J Physiol Heart Circ.Physiol, v. 284, no. 5, p. H1668-H1678.

Lloyd-Jones, D. et al., 2010, Heart disease and stroke statistics--2010 update: a report from the American Heart Association: Circulation, v. 121, no. 7, p. e46-e215.

Lo, E. H., T. Dalkara, and M. A. Moskowitz, 2003, Mechanisms, challenges and opportunities in stroke: Nat Rev Neurosci, v. 4, no. 5, p. 399-415.

Lo, E. H., M. A. Moskowitz, and T. P. Jacobs, 2005, Exciting, radical, suicidal: how brain cells die after stroke: Stroke, v. 36, no. 2, p. 189-192.

Masada, T., Y. Hua, G. Xi, S. R. Ennis, and R. F. Keep, 2001, Attenuation of ischemic brain edema and cerebrovascular injury after ischemic preconditioning in the rat: J Cereb Blood Flow Metab, v. 21, no. 1, p. 22-33.

Matsumori, Y. et al., 2005, Hsp70 overexpression sequesters AIF and reduces neonatal hypoxic/ischemic brain injury: J Cereb.Blood Flow Metab, v. 25, no. 7, p. 899-910.

Maurer, M. H., H. K. Geomor, H. F. Burgers, D. W. Schelshorn, and W. Kuschinsky, 2006, Adult neural stem cells express glucose transporters GLUT1 and GLUT3 and regulate GLUT3 expression: FEBS Lett., v. 580, no. 18, p. 4430-4434.

Mayer, B., and R. Oberbauer, 2003, Mitochondrial regulation of apoptosis: News Physiol Sci., v. 18, p. 89-94.

McCloskey, D. P., D. S. Adamo, and B. J. Anderson, 2001, Exercise increases metabolic capacity in the motor cortex and striatum, but not in the hippocampus: Brain Res, v. 891, no. 1-2, p. 168-175.

McFarlin, B. K., M. G. Flynn, W. W. Campbell, B. A. Craig, J. P. Robinson, L. K. Stewart, K. L. Timmerman, and P. M. Coen, 2006, Physical activity status, but not age, influences inflammatory biomarkers and toll-like receptor 4: J.Gerontol.A Biol.Sci.Med.Sci., v. 61, no. 4, p. 388-393.

McGee, S. L., and M. Hargreaves, 2006, Exercise and skeletal muscle glucose transporter 4 expression: molecular mechanisms: Clin.Exp.Pharmacol.Physiol., v. 33, no. 4, p. 395-399.

Minchenko, O., I. Opentanova, and J. Caro, 2003, Hypoxic regulation of the 6-phosphofructo-2-kinase/fructose-2,6-bisphosphatase gene family (PFKFB-1-4) expression in vivo: FEBS Lett., v. 554, no. 3, p. 264-270.

Mori, E., G. J. del Zoppo, J. D. Chambers, B. R. Copeland, and K. E. Arfors, 1992, Inhibition of polymorphonuclear leukocyte adherence suppresses no-reflow after focal cerebral ischemia in baboons: Stroke, v. 23, no. 5, p. 712-718.

Nawashiro, H., D. Martin, and J. M. Hallenbeck, 1997, Inhibition of tumor necrosis factor and amelioration of brain infarction in mice: J Cereb Blood Flow Metab, v. 17, no. 2, p. 229-232.

Neeper, S. A., P. Gomez, J. Choi, and C. W. Cotman, 1996, Physical activity increases mRNA for brain-derived neurotrophic factor and nerve growth factor in rat brain: Brain Res, v. 726, no. 1-2, p. 49-56.

Neurath, K. M., M. P. Keough, T. Mikkelsen, and K. P. Claffey, 2006, AMP-dependent protein kinase alpha 2 isoform promotes hypoxia-induced VEGF expression in human glioblastoma: Glia, v. 53, no. 7, p. 733-743.

Nishigaya, K., Y. Yoshida, M. Sasuga, H. Nukui, and G. Ooneda, 1991, Effect of recirculation on exacerbation of ischemic vascular lesions in rat brain: Stroke, v. 22, no. 5, p. 635-642.

Noble, E. G., A. Moraska, R. S. Mazzeo, D. A. Roth, M. C. Olsson, R. L. Moore, and M. Fleshner, 1999, Differential expression of stress proteins in rat myocardium after free wheel or treadmill run training: J.Appl.Physiol, v. 86, no. 5, p. 1696-1701.

Ogoh, S., and P. N. Ainslie, 2009, Cerebral blood flow during exercise: mechanisms of regulation: J.Appl.Physiol, v. 107, no. 5, p. 1370-1380.

Ogunshola, O. O., W. B. Stewart, V. Mihalcik, T. Solli, J. A. Madri, and L. R. Ment, 2000, Neuronal VEGF expression correlates with angiogenesis in postnatal developing rat brain: Brain Res Dev Brain Res, v. 119, no. 1, p. 139-153.

Ohtsuka, K., and T. Suzuki, 2000, Roles of molecular chaperones in the nervous system: Brain Res Bull., v. 53, no. 2, p. 141-146.

Ostrakhovitch, E. A., and M. G. Cherian, 2005, Inhibition of extracellular signal regulated kinase (ERK) leads to apoptosis inducing factor (AIF) mediated apoptosis in epithelial breast cancer cells: the lack of effect of ERK in p53 mediated copper induced apoptosis: J Cell Biochem., v. 95, no. 6, p. 1120-1134.

Park, J. A., K. S. Choi, S. Y. Kim, and K. W. Kim, 2003, Coordinated interaction of the vascular and nervous systems: from molecule- to cell-based approaches: Biochem Biophys Res Commun, v. 311, no. 2, p. 247-253.

Petty, M. A., and E. H. Lo, 2002, Junctional complexes of the blood-brain barrier: permeability changes in neuroinflammation: Prog Neurobiol, v. 68, no. 5, p. 311-323.

Petty, M. A., and J. G. Wettstein, 2001, Elements of cerebral microvascular ischaemia: Brain Res Brain Res Rev, v. 36, no. 1, p. 23-34.

Powers, S. K., S. L. Lennon, J. Quindry, and J. L. Mehta, 2002, Exercise and cardioprotection: Curr.Opin.Cardiol., v. 17, no. 5, p. 495-502.

Reyes, R., Jr., Y. Wu, Q. Lai, M. Mrizek, J. Berger, D. F. Jimenez, C. M. Barone, and Y. Ding, 2006, Early inflammatory response in rat brain after peripheral thermal injury: Neuroscience Letters, v. 407, no. 1, p. 11-15.

Romanic, A. M., R. F. White, A. J. Arleth, E. H. Ohlstein, and F. C. Barone, 1998, Matrix metalloproteinase expression increases after cerebral focal ischemia in rats: inhibition of matrix metalloproteinase-9 reduces infarct size: Stroke, v. 29, no. 5, p. 1020-1030.

Rybnikova, E., N. Sitnik, T. Gluschenko, E. Tjulkova, and M. O. Samoilov, 2006, The preconditioning modified neuronal expression of apoptosis-related proteins of Bcl-2 superfamily following severe hypobaric hypoxia in rats: Brain Res, v. 1089, no. 1, p. 195-202.

Sairanen, T. R., P. J. Lindsberg, M. Brenner, O. Carpen, and A. Siren, 2001, Differential cellular expression of tumor necrosis factor-alpha and Type I tumor necrosis factor receptor after transient global forebrain ischemia: J Neurol Sci, v. 186, no. 1-2, p. 87-99.

Sawatzky, D. A., D. A. Willoughby, P. R. Colville-Nash, and A. G. Rossi, 2006, The involvement of the apoptosis-modulating proteins ERK 1/2, Bcl-xL and Bax in the resolution of acute inflammation in vivo: Am J Pathol., v. 168, no. 1, p. 33-41.

Schabitz, W. R., T. Steigleder, C. M. Cooper-Kuhn, S. Schwab, C. Sommer, A. Schneider, and H. G. Kuhn, 2007, Intravenous brain-derived neurotrophic factor enhances poststroke sensorimotor recovery and stimulates neurogenesis: Stroke, v. 38, no. 7, p. 2165-2172.

Schlesinger, M. J., 1990, Heat shock proteins: J Biol Chem., v. 265, no. 21, p. 12111-12114.

Schubert, D., 2005, Glucose metabolism and Alzheimer's disease: Ageing Res.Rev., v. 4, no. 2, p. 240-257.

Semenza, G. L., 2009, Regulation of oxygen homeostasis by hypoxia-inducible factor 1: Physiology.(Bethesda.), v. 24, p. 97-106.

Shackelford, D. A., and R. Y. Yeh, 2006, Modulation of ERK and JNK activity by transient forebrain ischemia in rats: J Neurosci.Res, v. 83, no. 3, p. 476-488.

Shamloo, M., and T. Wieloch, 1999, Changes in protein tyrosine phosphorylation in the rat brain after cerebral ischemia in a model of ischemic tolerance: J.Cereb.Blood Flow Metab, v. 19, no. 2, p. 173-183.

Sharony, R., G. Pintucci, P. C. Saunders, E. A. Grossi, F. G. Baumann, A. C. Galloway, and P. Mignatti, 2005, Matrix Metalloproteinase Expression in Vein Grafts: Role of Inflammatory Mediators and Extracellular Signal-Regulated Kinases-1 and -2 2: Am.J Physiol Heart Circ.Physiol.

Siu, P. M., R. W. Bryner, J. K. Martyn, and S. E. Alway, 2004, Apoptotic adaptations from exercise training in skeletal and cardiac muscles: FASEB J., v. 18, no. 10, p. 1150-1152.

Stummer, W., K. Weber, B. Tranmer, A. Baethmann, and O. Kempski, 1994, Reduced mortality and brain damage after locomotor activity in gerbil forebrain ischemia: Stroke, v. 25, no. 9, p. 1862-1869.

Susin, S. A. et al., 1999, Molecular characterization of mitochondrial apoptosis-inducing factor: Nature, v. 397, no. 6718, p. 441-446.

Swain, R. A. et al., 2003, Prolonged exercise induces angiogenesis and increases cerebral blood volume in primary motor cortex of the rat: Neuroscience, v. 117, no. 4, p. 1037-1046.

Tagaya, M. et al., 2001, Rapid loss of microvascular integrin expression during focal brain ischemia reflects neuron injury: J Cereb Blood Flow Metab, v. 21, no. 7, p. 835-846.

Tawil, N. J., P. Wilson, and S. Carbonetto, 1994, Expression and distribution of functional integrins in rat CNS glia: J.Neurosci.Res., v. 39, no. 4, p. 436-447.

Tong, L., D. Smyth, C. Kerr, J. Catterall, and C. D. Richards, 2004, Mitogen-activated protein kinases Erk1/2 and p38 are required for maximal regulation of TIMP-1 by oncostatin M in murine fibroblasts: Cell Signal., v. 16, no. 10, p. 1123-1132.

Vissing, J., M. Andersen, and N. H. Diemer, 1996, Exercise-induced changes in local cerebral glucose utilization in the rat: J Cereb Blood Flow Metab, v. 16, no. 4, p. 729-736.

Wagner, S., M. Tagaya, J. A. Koziol, V. Quaranta, and G. J. del Zoppo, 1997, Rapid disruption of an astrocyte interaction with the extracellular matrix mediated by integrin alpha 6 beta 4 during focal cerebral ischemia/reperfusion: Stroke, v. 28, no. 4, p. 858-865.

Wang, R. Y., Y. R. Yang, and S. M. Yu, 2001, Protective effects of treadmill training on infarction in rats: Brain Res, v. 922, no. 1, p. 140-143.

Wang, X., X. Li, J. A. Erhardt, F. C. Barone, and G. Z. Feuerstein, 2000, Detection of tumor necrosis factor-alpha mRNA induction in ischemic brain tolerance by means of real-time polymerase chain reaction: J Cereb Blood Flow Metab, v. 20, no. 1, p. 15-20.

Williamson, J. W., A. C. Nobrega, R. McColl, D. Mathews, P. Winchester, L. Friberg, and J. H. Mitchell, 1997, Activation of the insular cortex during dynamic exercise in humans: J Physiol, v. 503 (Pt 2), p. 277-283.

Willis, C. L., C. C. Nolan, S. N. Reith, T. Lister, M. J. Prior, C. J. Guerin, G. Mavroudis, and D. E. Ray, 2004, Focal astrocyte loss is followed by microvascular damage, with subsequent repair of the blood-brain barrier in the apparent absence of direct astrocytic contact: Glia, v. 45, no. 4, p. 325-337.

Wu, C., H. Fujihara, J. Yao, S. Qi, H. Li, K. Shimoji, and H. Baba, 2003, Different expression patterns of Bcl-2, Bcl-xl, and Bax proteins after sublethal forebrain ischemia in C57Black/Crj6 mouse striatum: Stroke, v. 34, no. 7, p. 1803-1808.

Yamashita, N., S. Hoshida, K. Otsu, N. Taniguchi, T. Kuzuya, and M. Hori, 1999, Monophosphoryl lipid A provides biphasic cardioprotection against ischaemia-reperfusion injury in rat hearts: Br J Pharmacol, v. 128, no. 2, p. 412-418.

Yang, G. Y., and A. L. Betz, 1994, Reperfusion-induced injury to the blood-brain barrier after middle cerebral artery occlusion in rats: Stroke, v. 25, no. 8, p. 1658-1664.

Yong, V. W., C. Power, P. Forsyth, and D. R. Edwards, 2001, Metalloproteinases in biology and pathology of the nervous system: Nat Rev Neurosci, v. 2, no. 7, p. 502-511.

Zhu, C., L. Qiu, X. Wang, U. Hallin, C. Cande, G. Kroemer, H. Hagberg, and K. Blomgren, 2003, Involvement of apoptosis-inducing factor in neuronal death after hypoxia-ischemia in the neonatal rat brain: J Neurochem., v. 86, no. 2, p. 306-317.

Zhuang, S., and R. G. Schnellmann, 2006, A death-promoting role for extracellular signal-regulated kinase: J Pharmacol.Exp.Ther., v. 319, no. 3, p. 991-997.

Zorzano, A., M. Palacin, and A. Guma, 2005, Mechanisms regulating GLUT4 glucose transporter expression and glucose transport in skeletal muscle: Acta Physiol Scand., v. 183, no. 1, p. 43-58.

Zwagerman, N., C. Plumlee, M. Guthikonda, and Y. Ding, 2010a, Toll-like receptor-4 and cytokine cascade in stroke after exercise: Neurological Research, v. 32, no. 2, p. 123-126.

Zwagerman, N., S. Sprague, M. D. Davis, B. Daniels, G. Goel, and Y. Ding, 2010b, Pre-
     ischemic exercise preserves cerebral blood flow during reperfusion in stroke:
     Neurological Research.

Physiological Neuroprotective Mechanisms in Natural Genetic Systems: Therapeutic Clues for Hypoxia-Induced Brain Injuries

Thomas I Nathaniel[1,2], Francis Umesiri[3], Grace Reifler[4],
Katelin Haley[4], Leah Dziopa[4], Julia Glukhoy[4] and Rahul Dani[4]
[1]Center for Natural and Health Sciences, Marywood University
[2]Department of Biomedical Sciences, University of South Carolina
School of Medicine-Greenville, Greenville
[3]Department of Chemistry, University of Toledo, Toledo
[4]Center for Natural and Health Sciences, Marywood University
USA

1. Introduction

Adaptations, conservation or evolution of physiological systems in human indicates that the physiological system for hypoxia tolerance represents an adaptive character that is present in humans, just like in poikilotherms or endotherms(Hochachka 1993; Hochachka et al. 1996). Precisely, brain metabolic organization capability is thought to represent an adaptive physiological system that is present in humans, but composed of so many neurochemical products and physiological mechanisms that make it difficult to account for its plasticity for manipulation to induce protection(Hochachka 1993; Frappell et al. 2002). Evidence that hypoxia tolerating mammals suppressed metabolic demand in response to hypoxia contributed substantially to the understanding of metabolic regulation as a neuroprotective strategy that can be adapted for the protection of tissue hypoxia in humans. In that case, understanding the physiological mechanisms that are involved in such ability in hypoxia tolerating species may provide a clue for specific mechanisms that could be manipulated in the brain of stroke patients to prevent the death of metabolically vulnerable neurons. In this context, knowledge of the specific role of the central neurotransmitter systems and pathways that control metabolic suppression during hypoxia tolerance is important. This is because the neurochemical-mediators that may defend against hypoxic insults during brain injury act through interconnections within the neural systems that are highly protected in hypoxia tolerating species(Mravec et al. 2006). Exposure of non hypoxia tolerating species to severe hypoxia results in the alteration of the connections within the neural systems because of loss control of local microcirculation of oxygen. This leads to ineffectiveness of membrane potentials to modulate neuronal function (Ackland et al. 2007). If this occurs, there is some hope for effective neuropharmacological intervention through neurotransmitter-mediators. The fact that chemical neurotransmitters are part of normal physiology, whether during development or adulthood, means that specific agonists and antagonists that restore physiological homeostasis can lead to pharmacological repair of hypoxia-induced neuronal damage in humans.

2. Physiological strategies that protect the brain during ischemic stroke

Hypothermia is one strategy that can decrease hypoxic/ischemic injury under regulated conditions (Rincon 2008; Statler 2008). This is possible because a decline in brain temperature can prevent the dead of neurons that are deprived of nutrients. Such a protective strategy has been attributed to the reversible protein phosphorylation that regulates suppression of the rates of multiple ATP-production, ATP-utilization and related cellular processes that allow animals to go through a stable hypometabolic state (Storey and Storey 2007; Storey and Storey 2005). A stable hypometabolic state mechanism is known to protect against pathological effects of cortical neuronal pathology or oxidative stress in stroke patients (Ma et al. 2005). Cumulative evidence from studies of hypometabolism during hibernation in small mammals suggests that hypometabolism is a stable metabolic state that allows timely limited energy regulation during hypoxia (Heldmaier et al. 2004). This is because a stable metabolic state activates defense mechanisms, such as antioxidants, proteins, protease inhibitors that stabilize macromolecules and promote long-term neuronal viability in the stable metabolic state (Zhou et al. 2001; Zhao and Zuo 2005). These adaptations can be manipulated in humans to prevent the death of metabolically vulnerable neurons in stroke patients. Although these adaptations do not fully account for the mechanisms that facilitate the suppression of metabolism during exposure to hypoxia (Nathaniel et al. 2009) or during mammalian hibernation (Drew et al. 2007), it has been proposed that hypoxia itself could facilitate a systematic regulation of metabolism through cooling of core body temperature and stabilization of temperature in the new metabolic rate (Barros et al. 2001). Future studies that explore the mechanisms that switch-off energy demand, when supplies become limited during metabolic suppression could provide clues of how to develop metabolic suppression as novel therapy in the clinical management of stroke.

3. Cellular implications of disruption of brain energy balance when oxygen delivery fails to meet demand

The mammalian brain is a highly oxidative organ that accounts for an inexplicably large percentage of the whole body oxygen consumption that provides the major source of energy during aerobic metabolism (Wang et al. 2002). This implies that structural and functional integrity of brain functions strongly depend on a regular oxygen and glucose supply. Therefore, any disruption of the homeostasis of brain energy demand and supply becomes life threatening. This is because a reduction in oxygen availability due to the abnormality in systemic or local blood circulation cannot be endured for a prolonged period by a non hypoxia tolerant species (Zhou et al. 2001a; Barger et al. 2003). The immediate effect is variation in oxygen partial pressure (PO_2), within the brain that is detected by cellular oxygen sensors. The cellular oxygen sensors, such as hypoxia inducible transcription factors (HIFs), are thought to be available to regulate oxygen homeostasis in the brain. In order for the brain to cope with variations in oxygen partial pressure, these sensors induce adaptive mechanisms to avoid, or at least minimize, brain damage (Nawashiro et al. 1996). Any abnormality in cellular oxygen-sensor response is a reflection of the low partial pressure and

Physiological Neuroprotective Mechanisms in Natural Genetic Systems: Therapeutic Clues
for Hypoxia-Induced Brain Injuries

33

concentrations of oxygen in the brain. The abnormality is primarily because of the inability of a specific oxygen-sensor or target system to tailor adaptive responses according to differences in the cellular oxygen availability in a short or long term. In this context, the arising question is how does low cellular oxygen availability affect neuronal and physiological activities? Major cellular operations in the brain are dependent on the oxygen level in the physiological range (Erecinska et al. 2005). Limitation of oxygen supply to the brain below a critical physiological level blocks oxidative phosphorylation, which drastically decreased cellular ATP leading to a collapse in ion gradients. Consequently, neuronal activity stops. If the process of re-oxygenation is not re-introduced quickly, neurons will die(Nawashiro et al. 1996). In the brain of a stroke patient, early interruption of energy homeostasis when oxygen delivery fails to meet oxygen demand is the first step in a surge of events that leads to cell death of metabolically susceptible neurons. If hypoxia does not set in, availability of glucose will help maintain ATP levels through glycolysis. However, if glucose supply is limited, reduction of high-energy phosphates (e.g. ATP) results in loss of cellular ionic homeostasis (Erecińska and Silver 2001). This is because the disruption of ion homeostasis causes an influx of Na^+ and Cl^- ions, the release of neurotransmitters, opening of voltage-gated Ca^{2+} channels, and anoxic depolarization (Erecinska et al. 2005). This finding suggests that anoxic depolarization is directly associated with hypoxia-induced neuronal loss that leads to irreversible brain damage. An interesting question relevant to this idea is how does anoxic depolarization trigger neuronal death during hypoxia? This question has been investigated in the context of the mechanism of anoxic depolarization. For instance, concurrent changes in $(K^+)_0 t$ that lead to failure of (Na^+ ,K^+) ATPase occur during hypoxia due to ATP depletion(Balestrino et al. 1989). In support of this idea, electrophysiological evidence reveals that failure of ATPase causes anoxic depolarization through some intermediate event, such as Na^+-induced cell swelling(Rufini et al. 2009). To clarify the direct relationship between anoxic depolarization and ATP levels, synaptic transmission analysis in rat hippocampus revealed that first, Na^+ influx plays a relatively larger role in ATP consumption during hypoxia than Ca^{2+} influx; second, anoxic depolarization imposes a large and rapid drop in ATP levels(Fowler et al. 1999). Taken together, it then implies that depolarization and increased sodium concentration during hypoxia seem to account for a significant portion of the neuronal damage induced by hypoxia that eventually leads to both necrotic and apoptotic processes (Reshef et al. 2000; Gonchar and Mankovskaya 2009).

4. Stimulation of glutamate, activation of NMDA and AMPA receptors regulate calcium influx and promote neuronal damage

Although increased sodium concentration during hypoxia seems to account for a major part of neuronal damage during hypoxia, additional structural damages develop hours or days later because Ca^{2+} influx into neurons is stimulated by glutamate (He et al. 2009), and amplified by activation of NMDA and AMPA receptors (Zamalloa et al. 2009). Glutamate is one of the most widespread excitatory neurotransmitters in the brain. In small amounts, it is indispensable for neuronal function, while in excessive amounts it is a neuronal poison (excitotoxin) that stimulates Ca^{2+} influx into neurons (Liljequist et al. 1995; Bonde et al. 2005). If the excessive extracellular release of glutamate is not regulated, it could lead to brain damage(Robinson 2006). This idea is strengthened by the observation that overstimulation of glutamate receptors promotes neuronal death(Sheldon and Robinson

2007a). Since excessive glutamate is harmful to the brain, how exactly can excess amounts of glutamate be regulated in the brain cells? It is possible that such regulation could be achieved by controlling a specific effector system that modulates the activities of glutamate. In support of this idea, studies by Pellegrini-Giampietro et al.(1999), Sheldon and Robinson (2007a) suggest that the mechanism that regulates glutamate transporter activity within minutes is a major redistributor of proteins in the plasma. This idea is further strengthened by the finding that glutamate transporters are regulated by the mechanism that redistributes proteins to or from the plasma membrane(Savolainen et al. 1995; Noda et al. 2000; Sheldon and Robinson 2007b). Findings from these studies indicate that longer-term activation of protein kinase C (PKC) decreased the activity and cell surface expression of the predominant forebrain glutamate Glu-1 transporter that is being redistributed from the plasma membrane to an intracellular compartment. Taken together, the existing studies reveal that the cellular machinery required for redistribution is via lysosomal degradation and not proteosomal degradation. Since longer-term activation of PKC results in degradation of GLT-1 that can be blocked by inhibitors of lysosomal but not proteosomal degradation, we speculate that regulation of total GLT-1 levels during hypoxia could play a significant role in hypoxia neuroprotection. Since the stimulative effect of glutamate (Noda et al. 2000) and activation of NMDA and AMPA receptors (Sobczyk et al. 2005) led to calcium overload (Mulvey and Renshaw 2009), our interest in this review to determine whether the different roles of glutamate, NMDA and AMPA receptors are the sole means of extracellular accumulation of calcium following hypoxic insults. By analyzing the influence of a specific ion channel inhibitor on the rise of cytosolic free calcium (Ca^{2+}) during hypoxia in a rat's cerebrocortical brain slices, Bickler (1998) found that the cytosolic calcium changes during hypoxia are due to multiple mechanisms. The changes are incompletely inhibited by a combined ion channel blockade. They are associated with the disruption of the cell membrane integrity. There is evidence that other factors may be at work as well. One factor is oxidative stress that is associated with the activation of microglia. Activation of microglia in turn, releases inflammatory cytokines, nitric oxide and extracellular accumulation of calcium, resulting in stress and neuronal death. Another factor is an increase in reactive oxygen species production. This alters cellular components including calcium levels and contributes to cytotoxic events that lead to cell death.

5. Cellular responses in brain neural systems can help in understanding hypoxia-induced hypometabolism and neuroprotection

In the previous section, we described how the stimulation of glutamate, activation of NMDA and AMPA receptors can regulate calcium influx and promote neuronal damage. It is now important to discuss how cellular responses in brain neural systems can help in understanding hypoxia-induced hypometabolism to initiate neuroprotection. Obviously, this proposal needs an explanation on how the cellular responses in any brain neural network would be a major factor for understanding hypoxia-induced hypometabolism and functional integrity. Indeed, a correlative neurophysiological observation tells us that understanding hypometabolism during neuroprotection should be in the context of functional integrity, because hypoxic response of each neuron can be unexpectedly heterogeneous, even within the same brain region(Boutilier 2001). The heterogeneity might be due to the fact that hypoxia itself leads to considerable downregulation of ion channels inside the brain neuronal systems, such that hypoxic reaction of individual neurons vary

Physiological Neuroprotective Mechanisms in Natural Genetic Systems: Therapeutic Clues
for Hypoxia-Induced Brain Injuries

35

(Pena and Ramirez 2005). The variation, in turn, may help in maintaining functional integrity. The idea is supported by the observation that ion channel arrest does not lead to the shutdown of entire networks, nor can networks operate by all cellular components entering a general hypometabolic-neuroprotective state(Ramirez et al. 2007). For instance, a general shutdown of NMDA or Ca^{2+} dependent processes would not be beneficiary to a hypoxia tolerating animal in a hypometabolic state. This is because such a shutdown would severely compromise higher-brain functions. Therefore, hypoxia research should focus on understanding mechanisms of hypometabolism during neuroprotection in the context of functional integrity, and as expressed by hypoxia tolerating species. This disconnect may explain why the protection against tissue hypoxia during stroke is still a main medical problem. There is no doubt that activation of NMDA receptors or intracellular Ca^{2+} may lead to necrosis and apoptosis. However, restraining these mechanisms is not very helpful because they also affect neuroprotection. Taken together, understanding how hypoxia-tolerant neurons sense changes in oxygen dynamics and create signals that have instant and long-term effects on neuronal survival will be significant in developing new strategies for neuroprotection. Studies of how metabolism is regulated at cellular levels during which energy-producing and energy-consuming processes are balanced, facilitated by neurotransmitters-mediated mechanism would be of considerable interest. Since many of the existing studies support the idea that adenosine induces neuroprotection during hypoxia, we will now focus on the different physiological and molecular mechanisms used by adenosine in inducing protection in natural systems of hypoxia tolerance.

6. Adenosine induces neuroprotection by mediating ion signaling during response to chronic hypoxia

Several lines of evidence indicate that reduced ion leakage is an important mechanism for energy conservation during extreme hypoxia, and adenosine has been implicated in ion channel activity. Precisely, it has been shown that A1 receptor stimulation inhibits the brain's electrical activity through K^+ channel activation (direct coupling *via* G-proteins to ion channels) and/or by inhibiting the high-voltage-activated Ca^{2+} channels (Fowler et al. 1999; Reshef et al. 2000). Extracellular adenosine plays a role in the reduction of K^+ influx (channel arrest) that occurs in a brain that was subjected to chronic hypoxia(Reshef et al. 2000). Monitoring of the changes in extracellular K^+ concentration $(K+)o$ in the in-situ brain of the turtle (*Trachemys scripta*), following inhibition of $Na^+/K(^+)$-ATPase with ouabain revealed that the time to reach full depolarization $(K^+)o$ plateau) was 3 times more in the chronic hypoxic brain than in normoxic controls (Pék and Lutz 1997). The initial rate of K^+ leakage was reduced by approximately 70%. Following superfusing the brain, before the onset of chronic hypoxia with the non selective adenosine receptor blocker, theophylline, or the specific adenosine A1 receptor blocker, 8-cyclopentyltheophylline, there was a significant reduction in the time to full depolarization in the ouabain-challenged hypoxic-brain and an increase in the rate of K^+ efflux(Pék and Lutz 1997). The results indicate that A1 receptors are involved in the expression of chronic hypoxia-induced ion channel arrest in the brain. This finding is supported by other studies that indicated that in a chronic hypoxic tolerant specie, the basic strategy for hypoxia survival is the maintenance of ion gradients to avoid anoxic depolarization (Lutz et al. 1996; Perez-Pinzon and Born 1999). To this extent, an important question that re-occurred in many of the most recent theoretical papers is how does hypoxia tolerant species respond to anoxia? In our physiological perspective of hypoxia neuroprotection, adaption to anoxia (an extreme form of hypoxia) is mainly controlled by hypoxia/ischemic conditioning mechanism(Liu et al. 1991). In addition, the different physiological adaptations for extreme hypoxia have been well described in turtles, one of the species with a unique ability to tolerate extreme hypoxia. In humans, an extreme hypoxia condition causes major histopathological events to the brain. However, in turtles that have the ability to resist extreme form of hypoxia, tolerance is seen when a sublethal ischemic/anoxia insult is induced sometime before a lethal ischemic/anoxia insult is induced(Liu et al. 1991). The mechanisms involved are not well understood. Therefore, a better understanding of the mechanisms that induce extreme tolerance to hypoxia in turtles may provide novel therapeutic interventions that may aide human brain to resist the ravages of extreme hypoxia.

6.1 Adenosine facilitates hypoxia neuroprotection by mediating intracellular signaling pathways

Several lines of evidence indicate that severe hypoxia can cause an imbalance between oxygen supply and consumption. This is   usually accompanied by transportation of adenosine down its concentration gradient from the cell via nucleoside transporters, such as ENT1 and the ENT2. These transporters are equilibrative nucleoside transporters that are expressed in   the CNS (Chaudary et al. 2004b; Chaudary et al. 2004a), to promote the extracellular accumulation of adenosine. In this context, adenosine seems to act as an autocrine signal that indicates the disproportion between cellular oxygen availability and oxygen usage. Since adenosine is also an essential component of ATP synthesis, adenosine pools need to be vigilantly sustained in metabolically active cells in the brain. This could be done by minimizing extracellular release of adenosine, first by down-regulation of ENT activity. This would   aid the restoration of   ATP pools once the hypoxic stress has been removed. It is also important to point out that an ENT activity could lead to reuptake of extracellular adenosine to terminate receptor activation, as uniquely done by the neurotransmitter transporters to help restore intracellular pools of adenosine. The precise nature of the relationship between adenosine transporters, adenosine receptors and intracellular signaling pathways is not well known. Hypoxia is known to regulate the adenosine transporter mENT1 (inhibitor-sensitive), and protein kinase c q (PKCq) is involved in regulation of mENT1(Chaudary et al. 2004a), suggesting that chronic hypoxia regulates ENT1, both in terms of protein and overall reactivity through PKC-mediated hypoxia preconditioning.

The PKC-mediated hypoxia protection occurs when extracellular adenosine interacts with adenosine receptors (A_1, A_{2A}, A_{2B}, and/or A_3), and activation of adenosine receptors stimulate signaling pathways that "resist" the stress caused by hypoxia (David et al. 2002). It then implies that the onset of hypoxia leads to a decrease in cellular ATP stores and subsequent generation of adenosine, which is then released extracellularly. An increase in adenosine levels, in addition to bradykinin and opioids, initiate a series of intracellular signaling events via G-protein-coupled receptor signaling leading to activation of PKC activation (Di-Capua et al. 2003). Several studies have shown that injections of adenosine could protect neuronal cells against hypoxic-type injury via a PKC-mediated mechanism (Dave et al. 2009). A series of intracellular signaling that leads to the adenosine-mediated PKC-induced mechanism of hypoxia protection include; i) adenosine stimulates G-protein-coupled receptors, such as the A1/A3 adenosine receptors which activate phospholipases (phospholipase C; PLC) via G-proteins (Gi/o). ii) Other preconditioning stimulus, such as extracellular glutamate stimulates NMDARs, leading to increased cytosolic calcium and PLC activation. iii) εPKC is activated by PLC, and it increases di-acylglycerol (DAG) production, which in turn activates PKC isozymes including εPKC. Finally, the εPKC activation of extracellular signal-regulated kinase (ERK) promotes survival. Neuronal survival occurs because PKC may induce the opening of K (ATP) channels in the mitochondria ($KATP$) to regulate ATP production, and reduce generation of ROS. Interestingly, mitochondria are ideally located to serve as the cellular oxygen signal and mediator of protective mechanisms, such as ion channel arrest. Thus, regulation of mitochondria based mechanism of ion channel arrest involving ATP-sensitive mitochondrial K(+) channels, cytosolic calcium and ROS concentrations could contribute to neuronal survival.

It is also very important to point out that adenosine-mediated εPKC signaling is mediated in part through ERK, a mitogen-activated protein kinase (MAPK) family member that has been implicated in antiapoptotic signaling(Lange-Asschenfeldt et al. 2004). ERK maintains mitochondrial function by inhibiting deleterious Bcl-2 associated death domain protein BAD activity(Qiu et al. 2001).Taken together, adenosine-mediated εPKC signaling seems to activate ERK. This activation is involved in antiapoptotic signaling and cell survival during the induction of hypoxia preconditioning state, in order to salvage 'at-risk-tissue' with residual energy levels. The role of adenosine-mediated εPKC signaling in altering the expression or activity of calcium/calmodulin-dependent protein kinase II, MAPK family members, c-Jun N-terminal kinase, ERK, protein kinase B and PKC indicates that multiple kinases participate in the response of the tissue to counteract the effect of hypoxia (Obexer et al. 2006). This is important because PKC activity has been implicated in cell injury in the cerebral brain (Bright et al. 2008)indicating that it could be involved in a conserved hypoxia response pathway. εPKC activation delays the collapse of ion homeostasis during ischemia in arctic ground squirrels(Dave et al. 2009). This finding suggests that εPKC mediates 26 collapse of ion homeostasis in Arctic Ground Squirrels. This is possible because εPKC inhibits both 27 Na(+)/K(+)-ATPase and voltage-gated sodium channels, which are primary mediators of 28 the collapse of ion homeostasis during ischemia in Arctic Ground Squirrel (Perez-Pinzon et 29 al. 2005). For this reason, the specific role of εPKC in mediating hypoxia/ischemia-induced brain injury following the onset of stroke will be an interesting area of attention. Even more interesting is that the controversy over whether PKC mediates or is simply activated during hypoxia/ischemia-induced cell injury has been resolved to an extent by studies in ischemic models that suggest that PKC activity occurs via εPKC that mediates adenosine-induced preconditioning via $K^+{}_{ATP}$ function (Chaudary et al. 2004b; Bright et al. 2008).

Several lines of evidence suggest that εPKC can confer cerebral protection partly by maintaining mitochondrial function via ERK activity and by modulating adenosine-induced $mK^+{}_{ATP}$ channel function. It is also possible that εPKC activity inside the mitochondria may facilitate the regulation of $mK^+{}_{ATP}$ channels, which is important for defending mitochondrial membrane potential and robust maintenance of ionic homeostasis. Recently, the role of εPKC as a key mediator of neuroprotection was investigated (Teshima et al. 2003). Finding from this study indicates that epsilonPKC inhibits both Na(+)/K(+)-ATPase and voltage-gated sodium channels, which are primary mediators of the collapse of ion homeostasis during ischemia in Arctic Ground Squirrel. Their results support the hypothesis that εPKC activation is neuroprotective by delaying the collapse of ion homeostasis during ischemia or hypoxia. This probably involves robust maintenance of ion homeostasis, which leads to the conservation of energy by plummeting calcium influx during metabolic challenges. In summary, studies exploring the specific signaling pathways in which PKC participates, including different downstream effectors in different phases of stroke injury will be significant to develop an adenosine-mediated εPKC signaling therapeutic strategy for the clinical management of stroke patients. It is also important to emphasize that continuous cerebral blood flow, maintenance of cerebral oxygen tension and normal mitochondrial function are vital for the maintenance of brain function and tissue viability in the face of chronic hypoxia. The maintenance of normal brain functions require many parameters to work together and contribute to the homeostasis of brain energy demand and supply. Such a combination of parameters that could, in turn, lead to hypoxia protection include regulation of levels of inducible nitric oxide synthase (Thompson and Dong 2005; Thompson et al. 2009)and expression of HIF-1a(Trollmann and Gassmann 2009). Other parameters include the activation of extracellular-signal-regulated kinase(Osorio-Fuentealba et al. 2009; Wilkerson and Mitchell 2009)and c-Jun N-terminal kinase/stress-activated protein kinases (Comerford et al. 2004). Understanding the central mechanism that regulates the combination of the parameters is necessary when developing new approaches to remedying hypoxia-induced brain injuries. This is because there is the possibility that a single central cellular mechanism could invoke a combination of parameters that could lead to the remarkable tolerance to hypoxia as seen in natural genetic models of hypoxia-tolerance.

7. Conclusion

Physiological mechanisms of hypoxia neuroprotection in natural systems of hypoxia tolerance represent the core of our understanding of how the brain of a stroke patient can be made to resist hypoxic insults. Our understanding of physiological adaptations associated with hypoxia tolerance in natural systems, and the diverse cellular implications of disrupting brain energy balance when oxygen delivery fails to meet demand provide the insights of how the human brain can be made tolerant to hypoxia. In this review, we suggest that the physiological mechanisms used by hypoxia-tolerant species offer clues on strategies to adapt for the clinical management of brain injuries where oxygen demand fails to match the supply.

8. References

Ackland GL, Kasymov V, Gourine AV (2007) Physiological and pathophysiological roles of extracellular ATP in chemosensory control of breathing Biochemical Society Transactions 35:1264-1268

Balestrino M, Aitken PG, Somjen GG (1989) Spreading depression-like hypoxic depolarization in CA1 and fascia dentata of hippocampal slices: Relationship to selective vulnerability. Brain Res 497:102–107

Barger JL, Brand MD, Barnes BM, Boyer BB (2003) Tissue-specific depression of mitochondrial proton leak and substrate oxidation in hibernating arctic ground squirrels. Am. J. Physiol. Reg. Integr. Comp. Physiol. 284:1306 -1313

Barros RC, Zimmer ME, Branco LG, Milsom WK (2001) Hypoxic metabolic response of the golden-mantled ground squirrel. J Appl Physiol, 91:603-612.

Bickler PE (1998) Reduction of NMDA receptor activity in cerebrocortex of turtles (Chrysemys picta) during 6 wk of anoxia. Am. J. Physiol. 275:86-91

Bonde C, Noraberg J, Noer H, Zimmer J (2005) Ionotropic glutamate receptors and glutamate transporters are involved in necrotic neuronal cell death induced by oxygen-glucose deprivation of hippocampal slice cultures. . Neuroscience. 136:779-794.

Boutilier RG (2001) Mechanisms of cell survival in hypoxia and hypothermia. J Exp Biol 204:3171-3181

Bright R, Sun GH, Yenari MA, Steinberg GK, Mochly-Rosen D (2008) epsilonPKC confers acute tolerance to cerebral ischemic reperfusion injury. Neurosci Lett. 441:120-124

Chaudary N, Naydenova Z, Shuralyova I, Coe IR (2004a) Hypoxia regulates the adenosine transporter, mENT1, in the murine cardiomyocyte cell line, HL-1. Cardiovasc Res. 61:780-788

Chaudary N, Naydenova Z, Shuralyova I, Coe IR (2004b) PKC regulates ischemic preconditioning and the adenosine transporter, mENT1, in the mouse cardiac myocyte cell line, HL-1. J Pharmacol Exp Ther 310:1190-1198

Comerford KM, Cummins EP, Taylor CT (2004) c-Jun NH2-terminal kinase activation contributes to hypoxia-inducible factor 1alpha-dependent P-glycoprotein expression in hypoxia. Cancer Res 64:9057-9061.

Dave KR, Anthony R, Defazo R, Rava IAP, Dashkin O, Iceman KE, Perez-Pinzon M (2009) Protein kinase C epsilon activation delays neuronal depolarization during cardiac arrest in the euthermic arctic ground squirrel. J Neurochem. 110(4):1170-9

David B, David G, Marie-Christine G, Pablo A, Kadiombo B, Serge NS (2002) The Adenosine A1 Receptor Agonist Adenosine Amine Congener Exerts a Neuroprotective Effect against the Development of Striatal Lesions and Motor Impairments in the 3-Nitropropionic Acid Model of Neurotoxicity. The Journal of Neuroscience 22:9122-9133

Di-Capua N, Sperling O, Zoref-Shani E (2003) Protein kinase C-epsilon is involved in the adenosine-activated signal transduction pathway conferring protection against ischemia-reperfusion injury in primary rat neuronal cultures. J Neurochem. 84:409-412

Drew KL, Buck CL, Barnes BM, Christian SL, Rasley BT, Harris MB (2007) Central nervous system regulation of mammalian hibernation: implications for metabolic suppression and ischemia tolerance. J Neurochem. 102:1713-1726

Erecinska M, Cherian S, Silver A (2005) Brain Development and Susceptibility to Damage; Ion Levels and Movements Current Topics in Developmental Biology 69:139-186

Erecińska M, Silver IA (2001) Tissue oxygen tension and brain sensitivity to hypoxia. Respir Physiol. 128:263-276.

Fowler JC, Partridge LD, Gervitz L (1999) Hydroxylamine blocks adenosine A1 receptor-mediated inhibition of synaptic transmission in rat hippocampus. Brain Res 815:414-418

Frappell PB, Baudinette RV, MacFarlane PM, Wiggins PR, Shimmin G (2002) Ventilation and metabolism in a large semifossorial marsupial: the effect of graded hypoxia and hypercapnia. Physiol. Biochem. Zool. 75:77-82

Gonchar O, Mankovskaya I (2009) Effect of moderate hypoxia/reoxygenation on mitochondrial adaptation to acute severe hypoxia. Acta Biol Hung 60:185-194.

He Z, Lu Q, Xu X, Huang L, Chen J, Guo L (2009) DDPH ameliorated oxygen and glucose deprivation-induced injury in rat hippocampal neurons via interrupting Ca2+ overload and glutamate release. Eur J Pharmacol 28:50-55

Heldmaier G, Ortmann S, Elver R (2004) Natural hypometabolism during hibernation and daily torpor in mammals. Respiratory Physiology & Neurobiology 141:317-329

Hochachka PW (1993) Hypoxia tolerance in Amazon fishes: status of an underexplored biological "goldmine". CRC Press,, Boca Raton

Hochachka WP, Buck LT, Doll CJ, Land SC (1996) Unifying theory of hypoxia tolerance: molecular/metabolic defense and rescue mechanisms for surviving oxygen lack. Biochemistry 93: 9493-9498

Lange-Asschenfeldt C, Raval AP, Dave KR, Mochly-Rosen D, Sick TJ, Perez-Pinzon MA (2004) Epsilon protein kinase C mediated ischemic tolerance requires activation of the extracellular regulated kinase pathway in the organotypic hippocampal slice. J Cereb Blood Flow Metab. 24:636–645

Liljequist S, Cebers G, Kalda A (1995) Effects of decahydroisoquinoline-3-carboxylic acid monohydrate, a novel AMPA receptor antagonist, on glutamate-induced CA2+ responses and neurotoxicity in rat cortical and cerebellar granule neurons. Biochem Pharmacol. 50:1761-1774.

Liu GS, Thornton J, Van Winkle DM, Stanley AW, Olsson RA, Downey JM (1991) Protection against infarction afforded by preconditioning is mediated by A1 adenosine receptors in rabbit heart. Circulation. 84:350–356.

Lutz PL, Nilsson GE, Peréz-Pinzón MA (1996) Anoxia tolerant animals from a neurobiological perspective. Comp Biochem Physiol B Biochem Mol Biol. 113:3-13

Ma YL, Zhu X, Rivera PM (2005) Absence of cellular stress in brain after hypoxia induced by arousal from hibernation in Arctic ground squirrels. Am J Physiol Regul Integr Comp Physiol 289:297–306

Mravec B, Gidron Y, Kukanova B, Bizik J, Kss I, Hulin I (2006) Neural–endocrine–immune complex in the central modulation of tumorigenesis: Facts, assumptions, and hypotheses. Journal of Neuroimmunology. 180:104-116

Mulvey JM, Renshaw GM (2009) GABA is not elevated during neuroprotective neuronal depression in the hypoxic epaulette shark (Hemiscyllium ocellatum). Comp Biochem Physiol A Mol Integr Physiol. 152:273-277

Nathaniel IT, Saras A, Umesiri F, Olajuyigbe F (2009) Tolerance to Oxygen nutrient deprivation in the hippocampous slices of the naked mole rats. Journal of Integrative Neuroscience. 8:123-136

Nawashiro H, Tasaki K, Ruetzler CA, Hallenbeck JM (1996) TNF-alpha pretreatment induces protective effects against focal cerebral ischemia in mice. J Cereb Blood Flow Metab. 17:483-490

Noda M, Nakanishi H, Nabekura J, Akaike N (2000) AMPA-kainate subtypes of glutamate receptor in rat cerebral microglia. J Neurosci. 20:251-258

Obexer P, Geiger K, Ambros PF, Meister B, Ausserlechner MJ (2006) FKHRL1-mediated expression of Noxa and Bim induces apoptosis via the mitochondria in neuroblastoma cells. Cell Death Differ. 14:534-547

Osorio-Fuentealba C, Valdés JA, Riquelme D, Hidalgo J, Hidalgo C, Carrasco MA (2009) Hypoxia stimulates via separate pathways ERK phosphorylation and NF-kappaB activation in skeletal muscle cells in primary culture. J Appl Physiol. 106:1301-1310

Pék M, Lutz PL (1997) Role for adenosine in channel arrest in the anoxic turtle brain. J Exp Biol. 200:1913-1917.

Pellegrini-Giampietro DE, Peruginelli F, E. M, Cozzi A, Albani-Torregrossa S, Pellicciari R, Moroni F (1999) Protection with metabotropic glutamate 1 receptor antagonists in models of ischemic neuronal death: time-course and mechanisms. Neuropharmacology 38:1607-1619.

Pena F, Ramirez JM (2005) Hypoxia-induced changes in neuronal network properties. Mol. Neurobiol. 32:251–283

Perez-Pinzon MA, Born JG (1999) 1999. Rapid preconditioning neuroprotection following anoxia in hippocampal slices: role of the K+ATP channel and protein kinase C. Neuroscience. 89:453-459.

Perez-Pinzon MA, Dave KR, Raval AP (2005) Role of reactive oxygen species and protein kinase C in ischemic tolerance in the brain. . Antioxid Redox Signal 7:1150-1157

Qiu J, Grafe MR, Schmura SM, Glasgow JN, Kent TA, Rassin DK, Perez-Polo JR (2001) Differential NF-kappa B regulation of bcl-x gene expression in hippocampus and basal forebrain in response to hypoxia. J Neurosci Res. 64:223-234.

Ramirez JM, Folkow LP, Blix AS (2007) Hypoxia Tolerance in Mammals and Birds: From the Wilderness to the Clinic

Annu. Rev. Physiol. 69:113-143

Reshef A, Sperling O, Zoref-Shani E (2000) Role of K(ATP) channels in the induction of ischemic tolerance by the "adenosine mechanism" in neuronal cultures. Adv Exp Med Biol. Adv Exp Med Biol 486:217-221

Rincon F (2008) Therapeutic Hypothermia after Cardiac Arrest. , 2008. 148 ANN INTERN MED.:485-486.

Robinson MB (2006) Acute regulation of sodium-dependent glutamate transporters: a focus on constitutive and regulated trafficking. Handb Exp Pharmacol 175:251-275.

Rufini S, Grossi D, Luly P, Tancredi V, Frank C, D'Arcangelo G (2009) Cholesterol depletion inhibits electrophysiological changes induced by anoxia in CA1 region of rat hippocampal slices. Brain Res 1298:178-185.

Savolainen KM, Loikkanen J, Naarala J (1995) Amplification of glutamate-induced oxidative stress. Toxicol Lett. 82:399-405

Sheldon AL, Robinson MB (2007a) The role of glutamate transporters in neurodegenerative diseases and potential opportunities for intervention. Neurochem Int. 51:333-355.

Sheldon AL, Robinson MB (2007b) The role of glutamate transporters in neurodegenerative diseases and potential opportunities for intervention. Neurochem. Int 51:333-355.

Sobczyk A, Scheuss V, Svoboda K (2005) NMDA receptor subunit-dependent [Ca2+] signaling in individual hippocampal dendritic spines. J Neurosci. 25:6037-6046.

Statler KD (2008) Hypothermia to Treat Neonatal Hypoxic Ischemic Encephalopathy. AAP Grand Rounds 19:3-4

Storey JM, Storey KB (2005) Biochemical Adaptation to Extreme Environments Integrative Physiology in the Proteomics and Post-Genomics Age:169-200

Storey KB, Storey JM (2007) putting life on 'pause'--molecular regulation of hypometabolism. J Exp Biol. 10:1700-1714

Teshima Y, Akao M, Li RA, Chong TH, Baumgartner WA, Johnston MV, Marban E (2003) Mitochondrial ATP-sensitive potassium channel activation protects cerebellar granule neurons from apoptosis induced by oxidative stress. Stroke. 2003 34:1796-1802.

Thompson L, Dong Y, Evans L (2009) Chronic hypoxia increases inducible NOS-derived nitric oxide in fetal guinea pig hearts. Pediatr Res. 65:188-192.

Thompson LP, Dong Y (2005) Chronic hypoxia decreases endothelial nitric oxide synthase protein expression in fetal guinea pig hearts. Soc Gynecol Investig. 12:388-395

Trollmann R, Gassmann M (2009) The role of hypoxia-inducible transcription factors in the hypoxic neonatal brain. Brain Dev.45:503-9.

Wang SQ, Lakatta EG, Cheng H, Zhou ZQ (2002) Adaptive mechanisms of intracellular calcium homeostasis in mammalian hibernators. J. Exp. Biol. 205:2957 -2962

Wilkerson JE, Mitchell GS (2009) Daily intermittent hypoxia augments spinal BDNF levels, ERK phosphorylation and respiratory long-term facilitation. Exp Neurol. 217:116-123

Zamalloa T, Bailey CP, Pineda J (2009) Glutamate-induced post-activation inhibition of locus coeruleus neurons is mediated by AMPA/kainate receptors and sodium-dependent potassium currents. Br J Pharmacol. 156:649-661.

Zhao P, Zuo Z (2005) Prenatal hypoxia-induced adaptation and neuroprotection that is inducible nitric oxide synthase-dependent. Neurobiol Dis. 20:871-880.

Zhou F, Braddock JF, Hu Y, Zhu X, Castellani RJ, Smith MA, Drew KL (2001a) Microbial origin of glutamate, hibernation and tissue trauma: an in vivo microdialysis study. J. Neurosci. Meth. 119:121 -128

Zhou F, Zhu X, Castellani JR, Stimmelmayr R, Perry G, Smith MA, Drew KL (2001) Hibernation, a Model of Neuroprotection. American Journal of Pathology. American Journal of Pathology 158:2146-2150.

Part 2

Management Approaches

3

Clinical Neuroprotection Against Tissue Hypoxia During Brain Injuries; The Challenges and the Targets

Thomas I Nathaniel[1], Effiong Otukonyong[2], Sarah Bwint[3], Katelin Haley[3],
Diane Haleem[3], Adam Brager[3] and Ayotunde Adeagbo[4]
*[1]Department of Biomedical Sciences, University of South Carolina
School of Medicine - Greenville, Greenville
[2]Department of Health Sciences, East Tennessee State University, Johnson City
[3]Center for Natural and Health Sciences, Marywood University
[4]Department of Pharmacology and Physiology
The Commonwealth Medical College, Scranton
USA*

1. Introduction

1.1 Understanding hypoxia tolerance and the challenge of clinical neuroprotection

Most of the existing research on brain hypoxia mainly focused mainly on understanding the mechanisms of neuronal death as the means of identifying targets for therapy. This approach has not been helpful in understanding how the brain of humans can be made to resist tissue hypoxia. This is a major factor that leads to neuronal death during stroke, for example. Hypoxia tolerance is a robust fundamental adaptation to low oxygen supply and represents a novel neuroscience problem with significance to mammalian physiology as well as human health. Physiological and molecular changes during hypoxia are critical to the prevention, management, and treatment of many important health conditions, such as stroke and cardiac arrest. However, the initiation and maintenance of physiological changes during hypoxia tolerance can be very difficult, and even those interventions that succeed in laboratory animals and controlled clinical trials do not always translate into clinical therapy. Transformative advances in the science of mammalian physiology, especially those that can connect mammalian physiological, molecular changes and diseases are urgently needed. In this review, we discussed major molecular and physiological adaptations during hypoxia tolerance that can be developed for the induction of clinical neuroprotection to tissue hypoxia during brain injuries.

2. Convergence between a specific neurotransmitter system and physiological mechanisms maybe critical for tissue hypoxia during brain injuries

Comparative studies of adaptive physiology demonstrated that hypoxia tolerant animal species represent potential sources of new strategies in our search for brain protection. This is because studies on the neurons of these animals repeatedly reminded us that we are closer to understand how cells and tissues develop resistance to hypoxia. Hypoxia tolerant species are very valuable models for understanding oxygen signaling processes simply because the responses to hypoxia are well developed. The possibility of separating adaptive signaling or defense responses from injury is a major benefit of studying hypoxia tolerant cells. They also serve as models for the slow adaptation of tissues to hypoxia, which humans are clearly capable of, and which might be enhanced to improve adaptation to diseases involving oxygen deficits.

Studies on the pathophysiology of shock-induced disturbances in tissue homeostasis reveal that tissue hypoxia is a consequence of distressed microcirculation that worsens the diffusion geometry, such that tissue hypoxia induced significant physiological changes in brain cells. Measuring the targets that detect tissue hypoxia is known to reveal the immediate effect of the distressed microcirculation. Recent studies on hypoxia neurobiology research have advanced a considerable body of evidence supporting the hypothesis that convergence between neurotransmitter systems and physiological mechanisms is protective in hypoxia tolerant species. Establishing this protective phenotype in response to hypoxic stress depends on a convergence response at the genomic, molecular, and cellular and tissue levels (Singer, 2004, Jeffrey, 2006). At the cellular level, studies in mammalian hibernation that explore hypoxia tolerance capability reveal evidence of ion channel arrest, regulation of inhibitory neurotransmission and suppression of substrate oxidation as cellular physiological adaptations (Gentile et al., 1996, Wang et al., 2002). Furthermore, extracellular levels of GABA decline in the striatum during hibernation, while extracellular glutamate remains unchanged during steady-state torpor of hibernation when compared with euthermic animals (Zhou et al., 2001). A decrease in the tissue-specific depression of substrate oxidation is also thought to decrease oxygen consumption, and consequently attenuate cytotoxic events that lead to cell death (Barger et al., 2003). This effect was attributed to a decrease in ATP demand resulting in the maintenance of homeostasis of brain energy demand and supply. The central mechanism that underlies hypoxia preconditioning-induced tolerance, which maintains the homeostasis of brain energy demand and supply, remains unclear. Interestingly, a number of potential neurochemical induction pathways have been proposed to control hypoxia tolerance in natural genetic systems of hypoxia tolerance. Such pathways include neuroactive cytokines (Nawashiro et al., 1996), glutamate receptors (Ravid et al., 2007, Sivakumar et al., 2009), adenosine receptors (Perez-Pinzon et al., 2005), the ATP-sensitive potassium Channel (Reshef et al., 2000), nitric oxide (Gonzalez-Zulueta et al., 2000) and oxidative stress (Dalen et al., 2009).

Taken together, findings from the aforementioned studies indicate that neuroprotective mechanisms against hypoxic insults in natural genetic systems of hypoxia or ischemic tolerance maybe be hinged on the convergence between a specific neurotransmitter system and physiological mechanisms. Although only few of the existing studies have been demonstrated in humans, one of these few studies indicates that elucidation of the central neurochemical mechanism of hypoxia tolerance is in this area of interest because the tolerance has been experimentally induced by clinically approved drugs (Konstantin et al., 2003). In another human study, it was found that adenosine plasma levels strikingly increased, such that the adenosine flow lasted days after transient ischemic or hypoxia attack and weeks after stroke (Moncayo et al., 2000, Pasini et al., 2000). Our view openly acknowledges the existence of hypoxia tolerance capacity in human brains and a possible central endogenous neuroprotective mechanism for hypoxia brain injuries in humans. In this context, considering the roles of adenosine as a molecule, it is possible that adenosine might represent a potential central neurotransmitter system that modulates physiological mechanisms during hypoxia protection. It is also important to emphasize that hypoxia itself could be the driving force for the convergence between a specific neurotransmitter system such as adenosine and physiological mechanisms during protection in hypoxia tolerant species. Since extensive studies have been done on adenosine system in the context of hypoxia protection over the past twenty years, we will now summarize the existing knowledge of specific roles of adenosine (A1) receptor in inducing survival during hypoxia.

3. Specific roles of A1 receptor during hypoxia tolerance

Survival in a severe hypoxic stress during which arterial oxyhemoglobin saturation is equal to 35% or less is connected with the ability of the brain to adapt to low oxygen supply and demand, and is thought to be regulated by a specific neurotransmitter system, such as adenosine (Blood et al., 2002). Studies in young sheep and adult rats indicate that intracerebral A1 concentrations increased during hypoxia. The specific role of A1 was linked to its ability to inhibit neuronal activity (Fowler et al., 1999). In vitro studies on hippocampal slices indicate that elevation of A1 receptors is associated with hypoxia (Jin and Fredholm, 1997), and severe asphyxia *in vivo* (Hunter et al., 2003c), following inhibition of neuronal activity. Studies in the fetal sheep further revealed that breathing movements can be inhibited by hypoxia and that such adaptation could be abolished by adenosine-receptor blockade at the level of the thalamus due to the inhibition of thalamic neurons (Chau and Koos, 1999). In a mouse knocked-out of A1 receptor, there is a significant decrease in tolerance to hypoxia (Johansson et al., 2001). Involvement of adenosine or adenosine triphosphate-sensitive potassium (K_{ATP}) channels in the development of tolerance has been suggested in global ischemia and hypoxia models (Kumral et al., 2010), cross-tolerance models (Xu et al., 2002) and *in vitro* studies (Perez-Pinzon et al., 2005). Activation of A1 receptors directly accelerate neuritogenesis in the primary neuronal precursor cells of rats(Canals et al., 2005). This finding suggests that A1 receptors may play an important role in myelinization and neuronal differentiation with the potential for clinical management of neuronal repair in hypoxic-induced brain injury.

By evaluating the action of hypoxia on synaptic transmission in hippocampal slices Sebastião and Ribeiro (2001) revealed that γ-aminobutyric acid (GABA), acetylcholine, and even glutamate may also have a neuroprotective role; however their action is evident only when activation of adenosine A_1 receptors is impaired. This finding indicates that adenosine A_1 receptors have a pivotal role of neuromodulating during hypoxia, though other substances can enhance adenosine actions when the nucleoside is not operative. A_1 receptors fine tuning neuromodulation is a very restrained change, similar to what *e.g.*, a pianist does, modulating a tune through introduction of another tune to modify the characteristics of the previous tune. A_1 receptors have specificity of interacting with receptors of other neurotransmitters and neuromodulators as well as with adenosine transport systems. A_1 receptors and other cellular elements involved in brain insults act via interconnections between the cellular elements and their secretions, such as the immune system(Ribeiro, 2005). In this manner, the nervous system can be highly regulated in normal physiology to induce neuroprotection against hypoxia. The fact that chemical neuromodulators such as A1 receptors are already part of normal physiology, either during embryonic development or adulthood, implies that their activity can be modified by specific pharmacological agonists and antagonists to restore homeostasis or to promote the safe pathways that can lead to tissue hypoxia protection.

4. Cellular mechanisms that promote neuronal death can be manipulated to promote neuronal survival

It is well known that neuronal death or apoptosis may result from continued activation of damaging molecular processes or pathways set in motion by a series of hypoxic insults, with the ultimate breakdown of the cell as a unit. According to Lipton (1999) such neuronal death is a morphological one, during which the cell cannot recover to perform its anatomical function. The idea is that the study of molecular processes of neuronal death at this point provides an understanding of what leads to these drastic structural changes and what needs to be done to promote neuronal survival. An interesting question in this regard is how can the molecular mechanisms or pathways that promote hypoxia-induced neuronal death be manipulated to promote neuronal survival? By targeting the disruption of the mouse caspase 8 genes, it has been shown that caspase 8 can regulate the activities of death promoting receptor signaling within the TNFR superfamily. For example, the deletion of caspase 8 gene completely abrogated TNFR12 and Fas receptor-induced apoptosis that was enacted via generation of reactive oxygen species during hypoxia (Cobelens et al., 2007). In other studies that explore the mechanisms of hypoxia-induced cell death in primary cortical neurons, it was found that TNFalpha was responsible for inducing cell death in the cortical neurons of cultured rats (Reimann-Philipp et al., 2001). These investigations established that TNF receptors are responsible for neuronal apoptosis because of the formation of an intracellular protein complex induced by hypoxia.

Although TNFalpha is directly implicated in neuronal apoptosis, TNFalpha-induced neuronal death can be inhibited by nerve growth factors (Haviv and Stein, 1999). This finding indicates that that hypoxia-associated apoptotic effects of TNFalpha can be converted by trophic factors (NGFs), and that the survival-promoting effect of NGF is mediated by a specific pathway not shared by all tyrosine kinase receptors. This implies that the manipulation of caspases and NGFs during hypoxia-induced activation of TNFalpha in the cortical neurons can prevent apoptotic effect of TNFalpha during hypoxia. Phosphorylation networks regulating JNK activity have evolved to enable swift and accurate responses, even in the face of hypoxia-induced cellular perturbations (Bakal et al., 2008). The JNK signaling network is thought to maintain cell and tissue integrity during hypoxia-induced cellular stress that involves stress-activated protein kinases (SAPKs), also known as JUN NH$_2$-terminal kinases (JNKs). Hypoxia-induced activation of JNK is an early response to hypoxic stress (Antoniou et al., 2009). When treated with CEP-1347, which inhibits JNK activation, the increase of cellular JNK activity was blocked, such that sympathetic and cortical neurons were saved from hypoxia-induced stress (Qi et al., 2009). Hypoxia-induced cell death can be averted by inhibiting JNK activation(Wardle, 2009). The explanation for this is that C-jun, a transcription factor that controls genes involved in cell death, is a constituent of another transcription factor called AP-1, and when phosphorylated by JNK, c-jun becomes activated and induces apoptosis, by withdrawing survival signals but when inactivated, metabolically vulnerable neurons can be saved from apoptosis.

Apart from JNK, there are other molecular systems that are able to induce apoptosis or neuronal death when in an active form, yet in an inactive form fail to do so. Molecular factors such as CREN, NF-kB (238) and FKHRL1 (Obexer et al., 2006), must be in its inactive form in order to refrain from inducing the expression of death genes in cerebellar granule neurons during hypoxia. These factors (CREN, NF-kB and FKHRL1) can be activated by Akt (Akt is a protein family of the kinases B (PKB) that is involved in cellular signaling to support their continued existence in brain cells to promote apoptosis (Park et al., 2007). Akt can also inhibit the cellular machinery that functions in killing cells. This is possible by phosphorylation at sites both upstream (BAD) and downstream (Caspase 9) of mitochondrial cytochrome c release (Dashniani et al., 2009). Such phosphorylation has been previously suggested to regulate glucose metabolism, thus, helping cells to live rather than die following hypoxic insults (Zhou et al., 2001). In summary, most of the aforementioned studies have been done in rats, exploring similar studies in hypoxia tolerating species will provide an in-depth-understanding of the activities of these molecular mechanisms or pathways during neuronal survival in hypoxia tolerating conditions.

Hormones are chemical substances produced by specialized glands with the primary function of regulating cellular activity. Levels of hormones in the brain demonstrate unique secretory characteristics that are linked to hypoxia. Leptin is a protein hormone with important effects in regulating metabolism functions. Most recent evidence has implicated leptin, the product of the obese gene derived from fat cells and placenta known to regulate body weight and food intake (Otukonyong et al., 2005), and synaptic plasticity during hypoxia neuroprotection (Shanley et al., 2001). More recently, the neuroprotective effects of leptin against tissue hypoxia have been explored (Perez-Pinzon and Born, 1999). This study revealed that leptin receptors are expressed in neurons of the hypothalamus. Another study (Guo et al., 2008),revealed the expression of leptin in the hippocampus and cerebral cortex. Endogenous synthesis and release of leptin by the brain may explain how localized leptin could protect neurons during hypoxia. For instance, cumulative evidence indicate that leptin could exert its neuroprotective effects to enhance neuronal survival both in vitro and in vivo by a mechanism involving stimulation of the Janus kinase (JAK)-signal transducers and activator of transcription (STAT) pathways. It has been shown that leptin protects neurons from neurotoxic 1-methyl-4-pyridinium (MPP+)-induced cell death in a dose dependent manner by activating the phosphatidylinositol 3-kinase (PI3-K)/Akt pathway; Jingnan et al., 2006). In mice model, systemic administration of leptin was shown to decrease infarct volume induced by focal cerebral hypoxia ischemia (Zhang et al., 2007). Apoptosis resulting from hypoxia or global ischemia is involved in the pathology of cerebral infarction and neuronal death. Leptin has been reported to inhibit apoptosis by removing growth factor from neuroblastoma cells utilizing JAK2-STAT3 and P13K/AKT signaling pathways (Guo et al., 2008). In seizures and epilepsy related hypoxia, leptin has been shown to protect hippocampal neurons against excitotoxicity in leptin deficient ob/ob mice, which are more prone to seizures (Erbayat-Atlay et al., 2006). Leptin has been reported as a hypoxic response gene whose transcription is induced by transcription factor HIF-1. Understanding the specific role of leptin in hypoxia conditioning can add leptin to the list of potential molecules for the treatment of hypoxia-associated brain injury.

Ghrelin is another peptide hormone that has been implicated in regulating glucose homeostasis (Andrews, 2011). The discovery of ghrelin was based on its ability to stimulate growth hormone (GH) release by activating the GH secretagogue receptor (GHSR1a) widely distributed in the hypothalamus and the pituitary gland. The neuroprotective effect of ghrelin has been demonstrated in many animal models of hypoxic-induced brain injury and stroke (Donnan et al., 2008). Injection of ghrelin intraperitonealy or intravenously in rats (both in vivo and in vitro) neuroprotects the forebrain by reducing infarct volume and cell death (Liu et al., 2009). Ghrelin has also been shown to attenuate CAI and CA3 hippocampal neuronal loss by inhibiting casp 3 activation in the pilocarpine-model of epilepsy (Xu et al., 2009). It is also important to point out that the crosstalk in leptin and ghrelin secreting sites to contribute to neuroprotection during the period of hibernation. Precisely, during the winter months hibernating mammals, such as the Arctic ground squirrel undergo physiological and behavioral changes to cope with seasonal periods of food scarcity and high energy demand. Before going into hibernation, the Arctic ground squirrel eat a lot and accumulate body fat, such that leptin level increases resulting in the development of leptin resistance without which the process of adipose mass deposition will fail, and hibernation which is also characterized with hypoxia tolerance will be in jeopardy. When hibernating, the Arctic ground squirrels do not eat because food is scarce, body metabolism decreases and hypothermia sets in. Since ghrelin stimulates appetite, and the animals are able to eat after hibernation is over. Leptin resistance is known to allow fat to be stored in anticipation of another season. Therefore, we propose that the understanding of the interconnections between the leptin and ghrelin with the metabolic networks could open new windows on the treatment that identifies the role of leptin and ghrelin in the preservation of metabolically vulnerable neurons during tissue hypoxia following the onset of stroke.

5. Conclusion

Analysis of brain mechanisms that control hypoxia tolerance in natural systems indicate that the physiological and molecular mechanisms of hypoxia neuroprotection represent the core of our understanding of how the brain can be made to resist tissue hypoxic insults. Studies of mammalian hypoxia physiology revealed that hypoxia tolerating models have an intrinsic ability to resist hypoxia. The physiological and intracellular mechanisms underlying such protection are not fully understood. Transformative advances in the science of mammalian physiology, especially those that can connect mammalian physiological and molecular changes and diseases, such as stroke and cardiac arrest, are urgently needed. In this review, we suggest that the protective physiological and molecular mechanisms employed by hypoxia-tolerant species offer clues on strategies to adapt for the clinical management of brain injuries where oxygen demand fails to match the supply.

7. References

Andrews ZB (2011) The extra-hypothalamic actions of ghrelin on neuronal function. . Trends Neurosci 34:31-40.
Antoniou X, Sclip A, Ploia C, Colombo A, Moroy G, Borsello T (2009) JNK Contributes to Hif-1alpha Regulation in Hypoxic Neurons. Molecules 15:114-127.

Bakal C, Linding R, Llense F, Heffern E, Martin-Blanco E, Pawson T, Perrimon N (2008) Phosphorylation networks regulating JNK activity in diverse genetic backgrounds. Science 322:453-456.

Barger JL, Brand MD, Barnes BM, Boyer BB (2003) Tissue-specific depression of mitochondrial proton leak and substrate oxidation in hibernating arctic ground squirrels. . Am J Physiol Reg Integr Comp Physiol 284:1306 -1313.

Blood AB, Hunter CJ, Power GG (2002) The role of adenosine in regulation of cerebral blood flow during hypoxia in the near-term fetal sheep. J Physiol 543:1015–1023.

Canals M, Angulo E, Casadó V, Canela EI, Mallol J, Viñals F, Staines W, Tinner B, Hillion J, Agnati L, Fuxe K, Ferré S, Lluis C, Franco R (2005) Molecular mechanisms involved in the adenosine A and A receptor-induced neuronal differentiation in neuroblastoma cells and striatal primary cultures. . J Neurochem 92:337-348.

Chau A, Koos BJ (1999) Metabolic and cardiorespiratory responses to hypoxia in fetal sheep: adenosine receptor blockade. . Am J Physiol 276:1805–1811.

Cobelens PM, Kavelaars A, Heijnen CJ, Ribas C, Mayor F, Penela P (2007) Hydrogen peroxide impairs GRK2 translation via a calpain-dependent and cdk1-mediated pathway. . Cell Signal 19:269-277.

Dalen ML, Frøyland E, Saugstad OD, Mollnes TE, Rootwelt T (2009) Post-hypoxic hypothermia is protective in human NT2-N neurons regardless of oxygen concentration during reoxygenation. . Brain Res 1259:80-90.

Dashniani MG, Chkhikivishvili NT, Naneïshvili TL, Burdzhanadze MA, Maglakelidze G, A. (2009) Regularities of the egocentric spatial memory development in children aged 24-60 months. Georgian Med News 174:65-72.

Donnan GA, Fisher M, Macleod M, Davis SM (2008) Stroke. Lancet 9624:1612-1623.

Otukonyong EE, Dube MG, Torto R, Kalra PS, Kalra SP (2005). Central leptin differentially modulates ultradian secretory patterns of insulin, leptin and ghrelin independent of effects on food intake and body weight. Peptides 26:2559-2566.

Erbayat-Atlay E, Yamada KA, Wong M (2006) Increased severity of pentylentetrazol-induced seizures in leptin deficient ob/ob mice. . Epilepsia 47:303-304.

Fowler JC, Partridge LD, Gervitz L (1999) Hydroxylamine blocks adenosine A1 receptor-mediated inhibition of synaptic transmission in rat hippocampus. . Brain Res 815:414–418.

Gentile NT, Spatz M, Brenner M, McCarron RM, Hallenbeck JM (1996) Decreased calcium accumulation in isolated nerve endings during hibernation in ground squirrels. Neurochem. . Neurochem Res 21:947 -954.

Gonzalez-Zulueta M, Feldman AB, Klesse LJ, Kalb RG, Dillman JF, Parada LF, Dawson TM, Dawson VL (2000) Requirement for nitric oxide activation of p21(ras)/extracellular regulated kinase in neuronal ischemic preconditioning. . Proc Natl Acad Sci USA 9:7436-7441.

Guo Z, Jiang H, Xu X (2008) leptin-mediated cell survival signaling in hippocampal neurons mediated by JAK STAT3 and mitochondrial stabilization. J Biol Chem 1754-1763.

Haviv R, Stein R (1999) Nerve growth factor inhibits apoptosis induced by tumor necrosis factor in PC12 cells. J Neurosci Res 55:269-277.

Hunter CJ, Blood AB, Power GG (2003c) Cerebral metabolism during cord occlusion and hypoxia in the fetal sheep: a novel method of continuous measurement based on heat production. . J Physiol 552:241-251.

Jeffrey MG (2006) Cerebral preconditioning and ischaemic tolerance Nature Reviews Neuroscience 7:437-448.

Jin S, Fredholm BB (1997) Adenosine A1 receptors mediate hypoxia-induced inhibition of electrically evoked transmitter release from rat striatal slices. Eur J Pharmacol 329:107-113.

Jingnan L, Chang-Shin P, Sung-Keun L (2006) leptin inhibits 1-methyl-4- phenylpyridinium-induced cell death in SH-SY5Y cells. . Neurosci Lett 3:240- 243.

Johansson B, Halldner L, Dunwiddie TV, Masino SA, Poelchen W, Giménez-Llort L, Escorihuela RM, Fernández-Teruel A, Wiesenfeld-Hallin Z, Xu XJ, Hårdemark A, Betsholtz C, Herlenius E, Fredholm BB (2001) Hyperalgesia, anxiety, and decreased hypoxic neuroprotection in mice lacking the adenosine A1 receptor. Proc Natl Acad Sci U S A 98:9407-9412.

Konstantin P, A. S, K. R, Löwl D, Muselmann D, Victorov I, Kapinya K, Dirnagl U, Meisel A (2003) Hypoxia-Induced Stroke Tolerance in the Mouse Is Mediated by Erythropoietin. Stroke 34:1981-1986.

Kumral A, Yesilirmak DC, Aykan S, Genc S, Tugyan K, Cilaker S, Akhisaroglu M, Aksu I, Sutcuoglu S, Yilmaz O, Duman N, Ozkan H (2010) Protective Effects of Methylxanthines on Hypoxia-Induced Apoptotic Neurodegeneration and Long-Term Cognitive Functions in the Developing Rat Brain. Neonatology 98: 128-136.

Lipton P (1999) Ischemic cell death in brain neurons. Physiol Rev 79:1431-1568.

Liu Y, Chen L, Xu X, Vicaut E, Sercombe R (2009) Both ischemic preconditioning and ghrelin administration protect hippocampus from ischemia/reperfusion and upregulate uncoupling protein-2. BMC Physiol 9:17-20.

Moncayo J, de Freitas GR, Bogousslavsky J, Altieri M, van Melle G (2000) Do transient ischemic attacks have a neuroprotective effect? Neurology 54:2089-2094.

Nawashiro H, Tasaki K, Ruetzler CA, Hallenbeck JM (1996) TNF-alpha pretreatment induces protective effects against focal cerebral ischemia in mice. . J Cereb Blood Flow Metab 17:483-490.

Obexer P, Geiger K, Ambros PF, Meister B, Ausserlechner MJ (2006) FKHRL1-mediated expression of Noxa and Bim induces apoptosis via the mitochondria in neuroblastoma cells. Cell Death Differ 14:534-547.

Park MK, Kim CH, Kim YM, Kang YJ, Kim HJ, Kim HJ, Seo HG, Lee JH, Chang KC (2007) Akt-dependent heme oxygenase-1 induction by NS-398 in C6 glial cells: a potential role for CO in prevention of oxidative damage from hypoxia. Neuropharmacology 53:542-551.

Pasini FL, Guideri F, Picano E, Parenti G, Petersen C, Varga A, Perri TD (2000) Increase in plasma adenosine during brain ischemia in man: a study during transient ischemic attacks, and stroke. . Brain Res Bull 51:327−330.

Perez-Pinzon MA, Born JG (1999) 1999. Rapid preconditioning neuroprotection following anoxia in hippocampal slices: role of the K+ATP channel and protein kinase C. . Neuroscience 89:453-459.

Perez-Pinzon MA, Dave KR, Raval AP (2005) Role of reactive oxygen species and protein kinase C in ischemic tolerance in the brain. . Antioxid Redox Signal 7:1150-1157.

Qi D, Hu X, Wu X, Merk M, Leng L, Bucala R, Young LH (2009) Cardiac macrophage migration inhibitory factor inhibits JNK pathway activation and injury during ischemia/reperfusion. J Clin Invest 119:3807-3816.

Ravid O, Shams I, Ben Califa N, Nevo E, Avivi A, Neumann D (2007) An extracellular region of the erythropoietin receptor of the subterranean blind mole rat Spalax enhances receptor maturation. Proceedings of the National Academy of Sciences of the United States of America 104:14360-14365.

Reimann-Philipp U, Ovase R, Weigel PH, Grammas P (2001) Mechanisms of cell death in primary cortical neurons and PC12 cells. J Neurosci Res 64:654-660.

Reshef A, Sperling O, Zoref-Shani E (2000) Role of K(ATP) channels in the induction of ischemic tolerance by the "adenosine mechanism" in neuronal cultures. Adv Exp Med Biol. . Adv Exp Med Biol 486:217-221.

Ribeiro JA (2005) What can adenosine neuromodulation do for neuroprotection? Ribeiro JA. Curr Drug Targets CNS Neurol Disord 4:325-329.

Sebastião AM, Ribeiro AJ (2001) Neuroprotection during hypoxic insults: Role of adenosine. Drug Development Research 52:291–295.

Shanley LJ, Irving A, Harvey J (2001) Leptin enhances NMDA receptor receptor function and modulates hippocampal synaptic plasticity. J Neurosci 21:186-190.

Singer D (2004) Metabolic adaptation to hypoxia: cost and benefit of being small. Respiratory Physiology & Neurobiology 141:215-228.

Sivakumar V, Ling EA, Lu J, Kaur C (2009) Role of glutamate and its receptors and insulin-like growth factors in hypoxia induced periventricular white matter injury. Glial 34:45-67.

Wang SQ, Lakatta EG, Cheng H, Zhou ZQ (2002) Adaptive mechanisms of intracellular calcium homeostasis in mammalian hibernators. . J Exp Biol 205:2957 -2962.

Wardle EN (2009) Programmed Cell Death: Apoptosis In: Guide to Signal Pathways in Immune Cells, pp 111-128: Humana Press.

Xu H, Aibiki M, Nagoya J (2002) Neuroprotective effects of hyperthermic preconditioning on infarcted volume after middle cerebral artery occlusion in rats: Role of adenosine receptors. . Crit Care Med 30:1126–1130.

Xu J, Wang S, Lin Y, Cao L, Wang R, Chi Z (2009) Ghrelin protects against cell death of hippocampal neurons in pilocarpine-induced seizures in rats. Neurosci Lett 453:58-61.

Zhang F, Wang SP, Signore AP (2007) Neuroprotective effects of leptin against ischemic injury induced by oxygen-glucose deprivation and transient cerebral ischemia. . Stroke 38:2329-2336.

Zhou F, Zhu X, Castellani JR, Stimmelmayr R, Perry G, Smith MA, Drew KL (2001) Hibernation, a Model of Neuroprotection. American Journal of Pathology. American Journal of Pathology 158:2146-2150.

4

Competing Priorities in the Brain Injured Patient: Dealing with the Unexpected

Jonathan R. Wisler, Paul R. Beery II,
Steven M. Steinberg and Stanislaw P. A. Stawicki
Department of Surgery, Division of Critical Care
Trauma, and Burn, The Ohio State University
Medical Center, Columbus, Ohio
USA

1. Introduction

Management of the multiply injured trauma patient can be defined by its complex nature and the necessity to reconcile multiple competing clinical priorities. Approach to single anatomic region/organ system traumatic injury tends to be relatively straight forward, although increasing severity of any isolated injury can by itself pose a formidable therapeutic challenge. In fact, any such "isolated" injury can be life threatening if severe enough and/or not managed optimally.

When the effects of simultaneous injuries to different anatomic regions and organ systems are combined, the cumulative complexity of trauma management can increase dramatically.[1] This chapter discusses clinical approaches to patients with traumatic brain injury in the context of multiple simultaneous associated injuries, focusing on addressing competing priorities and triage strategies needed to successfully manage these patients.

2. Team management and leadership

Effective diagnostic and therapeutic approaches to the multiply injured patient require the presence of well-functioning trauma systems and integrated specialty teams.[2] The optimal approach to the multiply injured patient involves the involvement of trauma-trained surgeons, intensivists, orthopedic specialists, urologists, neurosurgeons, and interventional radiologists.[3, 4] Highly skilled team management, leadership, and communication skills are of critical importance.[4] Excellent communication between physicians and teams, including awareness of important clinical pitfalls and constant vigilance on the part of all participating teams (i.e., presence of multiple cross-checks), as well as the need for centralized care planning (including multi-disciplinary patient care conferences) are crucial.[5]

3. Physiologic and outcome considerations

Restoration and maintenance of homeostasis is critical in management of the multiply injured patient. This often formidable task requires the achievement of a delicate balance between satisfying individual organ-system physiologic needs while reconciling the frequent necessity for micro-management of often competing specific organ- or body system-oriented considerations (i.e., maintenance of relatively lower blood pressure levels in a patient with concomitant aortic and brain injury *versus* maintenance of higher blood pressures to ensure adequate brain perfusion). The critical nature of clinical decision making is exemplified by the finding that morbidity and mortality in head injured patients can as much as triple in the presence of hypotension.[6] Additionally, when matched for injury severity and age, multiply injured patients with brain trauma have a significantly worse long term outcomes compared to multiply injured patients without brain trauma.[1,2]

Early predictors of outcome from traumatic brain injury (TBI) include age, Glasgow Coma Scale, pupillary exam, computed tomographic (CT) characteristics, and the presence of hypotension (systolic blood pressure <90 mmHg).[7] The key consideration is to maintain homeostasis and to triage clinical management in a manner that optimizes recovery of all affected organ systems. This involves the need for intimate knowledge of individual organ system tolerance limits, the knowledge of common clinical management pitfalls, as well as familiarity with temporal evolution of injuries and injury patterns in the context of overlapping priorities and biomedical parameter ranges.

The overarching goal is to prevent the so-called "secondary hits" that have been shown to adversely affect outcomes.[2] These secondary insults, in contrast to the primary trauma, are amenable to prevention and may be reversible if detected and managed promptly.[8] As many as 40% of patients with TBI exhibit some form of significant neurologic deterioration during their hospital stay, most often from secondary insults.[3] Significant proportion of patients with traumatic brain injury are initially lucid after injury but deteriorate quickly. Therefore, practitioners should always have a high index of suspicion and should avoid potentially dangerous clinical assumptions (i.e., assuming acute intoxication) when approaching patients with possible TBI. One must remember that nearly one-third of all head injured patients who die may belong in this category[9], and up to 75% of these have an identifiable and avoidable secondary insult.[10] Hypotension accompanies severe head trauma in approximately 35% of cases and entails a near doubling of mortality (from 27% to 50%).[10] Hypotension in the setting of hemorrhagic shock is also associated with increased mortality. A hematocrit of less than 30% may be associated with a reduction in blood oxygen carrying capacity and potential worsening of cerebral ischemia. Acute anemia associated with head injuries has been cited to carry an associated mortality of 52%.[10] Despite that, universal blood transfusion triggers continue to be controversial, and there is evidence to suggest that "dosing" blood by unit(s) as opposed to absolute hematocrit targets may be more prudent in the context of brain tissue oxygenation.[11-13] The age of the transfused blood may also be an important consideration, with more favorable cerebral oxygenation responses seen following transfusions of blood stored for fewer than 19 days.[11]

Therapy directed at correcting hypovolemic shock includes prompt volume expansion with crystalloid solutions, followed by administration of blood products as per established trauma guidelines. It is hypothesized that, following traumatic brain injury, cerebrovascular dysfunction results in loss of brain compliance, resulting in increased sensitivity to elevated venous pressures. Increased central venous pressure (CVP) occurring with vigorous crystalloid resuscitation may therefore contribute to the loss of brain compliance and the development of intracranial hypertension.[14] Cerebral perfusion pressure (CPP), defined as the difference between mean arterial pressure (MAP) and intracranial pressure (ICP) is an important factor in determining the adequacy of cerebral blood flow. Cerebrovascular autoregulation, present in the uninjured brain, is lost when the CPP falls below 50 mmHg.[15]

Xenon 133 scanning to measure cerebral blood flow in brain injured patients found that cerebrovascular dysfunction and global cerebral ischemia was seen in 13% of patients with a GCS of 8 or less, and of these patients 63% were in a persistent vegetative state or died.[16] In some cases, patients with spinal cord injury may exhibit hypotension secondary to dysfunction of the sympathetic nervous system and loss of peripheral vascular tone, an important consideration due to the association between the relatively frequent co-occurrence of TBI and spinal injury.[17, 18]

4. Overview of injury mechanisms and related considerations

Blunt trauma is associated with some form of brain injury in as many as 40-50% of patients.[19, 20] Among those with TBI, the incidence of associated injuries can exceed 60%.[19] Moreover, the very presence of TBI and an associated injury approximately doubles the mortality (from ~10% to ~20%) when compared to TBI alone.[19] In patients with a GCS of less than 8, mortality is as high as 45%. In terms of the components of the GCS scale, a motor score of 2 or less was associated with the lowest survival.[5] Certain associated injuries, when combined with TBI carry an especially high mortality, including great vessel (50% mortality), liver (39%), bowel (37%), spleen (34%), lung (34%), spine (26-32%), and various skeletal injuries (18-29%).[21] Of note, many of these "high mortality" concurrent injuries tend to be associated with either blood loss and hemorrhage (i.e., femur fracture, splenic/hepatic laceration) or hypoxia (i.e., pulmonary injury).

5. Concurrent spinal injury

Spinal injuries and TBI frequently occur together. Combination of TBI and spinal injury without neurologic deficit carries an approximate mortality of 25%, which increases to about 33% when neurologic deficit is present.[21] In addition to a defined set of priorities associated with the management of TBI, the trauma practitioner must be aware of important considerations unique to the setting of spinal injury. The overarching consideration is the avoidance of secondary injury by preventing both hypotension and hypoxia.[8] This spans an entire spectrum of preventive measures, including adequate spinal immobilization with spinal precautions, avoidance of excessive manipulation during patient transfers and procedures (i.e., endotracheal intubation), and provision of adequate cardio-respiratory support. Patients with spinal cord injuries (SCI) may be at increased risk of respiratory failure due to diaphragmatic and/or intercostal muscle dysfunction, depending on the level of SCI.[22] The most common causes of spinal cord injuries are motor vehicle crashes (48%), falls (21%), assaults (15%) and sports-related accidents (14%).[4] It is imperative that the practitioner be aware of the possibility of spinal cord injury in the multiply injured patient. Of all trauma patients that die within the first 30 minutes after injury, 20-25% have a cervical SCI.[6]

A distinct set of complicating factors can be brought about by hemodynamic derangements associated with spinal cord injury. Included are factors such as hypotension requiring vasopressor administration, bradycardia requiring pharmacologic and/or procedural intervention, patient positioning restrictions, as well as inability to perform a reliable injury assessment below the level of neurologic injury associated with spinal cord disruption. Cervical SCI may cause profound changes in heart rate and rhythm, blood pressure, and cardiac output. Patients may exhibit hypotension secondary to dysfunction of the sympathetic nervous system and loss of peripheral vascular tone.[17] Patients with high cervical SCI (levels C1-C5) have significantly higher requirements for cardiovascular intervention (i.e., need for of vasoactive agents or assistive device use) than patients with lower injuries (levels C6-C7).[17] Shortly after spinal cord injury (seconds to minutes) there may be a systemic pressor response characterized by widened pulse pressure that results from short-term outflow of sympathetic activity and adrenal hormones.[23] This pressor response is then quickly replaced by neurogenic shock characterized by bradycardia and hypotension.[24] In order to maintain proper systemic tissue perfusion, affected patients commonly require fluid resuscitation, supplemented by administration of vasoactive agents (if patient remains hypotensive despite adequate fluid resuscitation). Because patients with high spinal cord injuries are more susceptible to developing pulmonary edema, it is important to limit the amount of fluid resuscitation while maintaining a systolic blood pressure of 100-110 mmHg.[8]

Ventilatory management strategies for patients with diaphragm dysfunction differ from those used in cases without muscular functional deficits. With injuries involving spinal segments of T1 or higher, the intercostal muscles, important in expanding the anterior-posterior dimension of the thoracic cavity, are flaccid. With higher injuries of the cervical spine, the diaphragm itself may become paralyzed. This results in a paradoxic inward movement of the abdominal wall during inspiration.[25] Pulmonary capacity is further reduced while the patient is supine. Because of the weakened diaphragm, the abdominal contents push cephalad.[26] Initial respiratory management is aimed at providing adequate ventilatory support while reducing ventilator associated complications.

6. Concurrent chest injury

The simultaneous presence of TBI and chest injury involves a distinct set of clinical circumstances and considerations. Life-threatening pulmonary injuries may require aggressive ventilatory approaches, and when considered in the context of TBI, may predispose the patient to both systemic and brain hypoxia. Pericardial tamponade and tension pneumo- and/or hemothorax also represent a life threat by causing hypotension and brain hypoperfusion. In addition, traumatic aortic injury may impose a unique set of hemodynamic restrictions with regards to maintenance of narrow blood pressure and heart rate ranges.[27] For a given mean arterial pressure, any rise in ICP results in a decrease in CPP. In order to maintain adequate cerebral perfusion, CPP should be maintained around 60-70 mmHg.

One special consideration specific to the patient with TBI is the entity of acute lung injury (ALI) associated with isolated brain trauma.[28] This clinico-pathologic entity may not be associated with traumatic pulmonary injury *per se*. Instead, it may be more closely reflective of the global increase in TBI severity (i.e., the presence of a large mass lesion or midline shift on imaging is associated with 5-10 fold increase in risk of ALI).[28]

In addition to ALI, patients with severe brain injury can develop neurogenic pulmonary edema (NPE), which is defined as increased interstitial or alveolar lung water occurring in the absence of cardiac or pulmonary disorders or hypervolemia.[29] The disease process is characterized by alveolar hemorrhage, pulmonary vascular congestion, and the presence of protein rich exudate.[30] Comparatively, the incidence of NPE following severe head injury (20%) is similar to the incidence of NPE in subarachonoid hemorrhage (23%).[9] NPE can present within minutes to hours of the insult and usually resolves by 72 hours. Significant pulmonary edema past this time point suggests another diagnosis. During the injury there is a sympathetic discharge that causes increases in arterial and venous pressures and subsequent vascular damage. This damage is thought to result in vascular extravasation and the development of NPE. In animal models NPE is most reproducible with insults to the nucleus tractus solitarius or the noradrenergic A1 cell group.[31] Interestingly, the exudate seen in NPE has a much higher protein content than that seen in cardiogenic pulmonary edema, supporting a distinct physiologic process.[32]

7. Concurrent abdominal injury

Traumatic abdominal injuries are among the most lethal overall, with intra-abdominal and pelvic hemorrhage continuing to be associated with significant morbidity and mortality. This section will discuss diagnostic and therapeutic approaches needed to effectively manage concurrent abdominal and traumatic brain injuries. Included in the discussion is the management of the abdominal compartment syndrome and the damage control approach to severe abdominal trauma. At times, increasing ICP may be noted in patients with TBI and significant abdominal injury. In highly select cases, the correct diagnosis and surgical decompression of the abdominal compartment syndrome (ACS) may improve intracranial hypertension that is otherwise unresponsive to traditional medical therapy.[33]

It is not uncommon for the brain injured patient to have simultaneous abdominal injury, especially in the setting of blunt polytrauma. In this case, the presence of intra-abdominal hypertension (IAH) can exacerbate elevations in ICP. Thus, the presence of IAH is an independent risk factor for secondary brain injury.[34] The increase in intraabdominal pressure is directly reflected in intrathoracic pressure and central venous pressure. Elevations in central venous and jugular venous pressures result in increased resistance to cerebral outflow, which causes an increase in ICP and decrease in CPP.[35] Animal experiments have demonstrated that IAH of >20 mmHg causes significant increases in ICP and decreases in CPP. Additionally, elevations in CSF lactate and interleukin-6 were also seen, suggesting the associated presence of cerebral ischemia.[36]

Treatment for refractory ICP elevations in the setting of IAH involves several modalities including neuromuscular blockade, vasopressor use to preserve CPP, and abdominal compartment release.[37] In the setting of new onset end-organ dysfunction (i.e., renal failure, worsening pulmonary dysfunction) many physicians would advocate abdominal fascial release (a.k.a., abdominal damage control).[38] Several authors advocate more liberal use of decompressive laparotomy, extending this paradigm to patients with refractory elevations in ICP without intra-abdominal hypertension. In a group of 17 poly-trauma patients with refractory increases in ICP, decompressive laparotomy resulted in significant ICP reductions from 30.0±4.0 to 17.5±3.2 mmHg.[39]

Occasionally, emergent laparotomy and abdominal damage control may be coupled with damage control neurosurgery (DCNS) in the acute setting. Initial neurosurgical interventions include arrest of intracranial bleeding followed by evacuation of hematoma/mass lesion. Therapeutic craniectomy appears beneficial in children with diffuse brain edema.[40] However, DCNS can not be fully recommended in adults until the ICP becomes uncontrolled despite optimal medical therapy.[41, 42]

Stopping non-cranial hemorrhage is critical in the overall management of the multiply injured patient with brain trauma. Continued emphasis on team work and close collaboration between clinical teams is crucial.[43] In the multiply injured patient, an ICP monitor (mostly under local anesthesia or during cranitomy) can be inserted in the emergency room or in the intensive care unit while the patient is being stabilized. At times, ICP monitoring is initiated in tandem with emergency laparotomy, thoracotomy or any other life-saving procedures.[43] Occasionally, a craniotomy concurrent to other operative procedures may be required if the patient has a significant intracranial mass lesion and evidence of critical ICP increases on clinical exam. General surgeons may have to occasionally perform neurosurgery in remote locations for patients with TBI as statistics have shown that early simple interventions have resulted in increased rates of survival between 10-50%.[44, 45] Simpson *et al* have recommended evacuation of an extradural hematoma by the general surgeon in a remote location if the trauma center is >1-2 hours away.[44] Rinker et al advise emergency craniotomy if the GCS is <8, there are lateralizing signs such as a dilated pupil, hemiparesis or development of sustained bradycardia and hypertension.[45] Immediate availability of neurosurgeons may not be essential if a properly trained and credentialed trauma surgeon can appropriately monitor patients for neurologic deterioration and facilitate early transfer to a center capable of full-time operative and postoperative neurosurgical care.[46] In certain extreme situations, the performance of an emergency burr hole may be life saving.[47]

8. Concurrent skeletal injuries

Skeletal injuries are associated with a number of unique therapeutic challenges, especially when associated with significant blood loss and need for emergent skeletal fixation. This section discusses best approaches to deal with brain injured patients who also present with fractures, dislocations, and other musculo-skeletal emergencies. Included in the discussion is the topic of extremity compartment syndrome.

The management of skeletal fractures in brain injured patients continues to be a controversial topic. A comparison of early (<24 hours) versus late fracture fixation demonstrated that early fracture stabilization does not result in increased central nervous system complications.[48] Same study showed that patients undergoing delayed fixation experienced significantly higher pulmonary morbidity.[48] Another study showed that lower extremity fracture fixation within 24 hours did not entail greater risk for adverse outcomes in patients with TBI.[49, 50] The authors did emphasize, however, that avoidance of any undue hypoxia and hypotension is critical.[49, 50] Orthopedic "damage control" strategies have evolved in order to assist in early management of skeletal trauma in multiply injured patients with TBI who may be unable to tolerate traditional operative approaches or may not even be stable enough to leave their intensive care bed.[34, 51]

The clinical syndrome of fat embolism can influence the clinical course in the multiply injured patient, especially following long bone extremity fracture fixation.[52] Although early fracture fixation is thought to minimize the risk of this occurrence, some experimental studies show that intramedullary nailing of femoral fractures and subsequent liberation of bone marrow contents may have a negative influence on the central nervous system function.[52]

An important aspect of orthopedic care in the multiply injured patient with brain trauma is the lack of reliable physical examination. Due to this limitation, extremity compartment syndrome may evade timely diagnosis. The reliance on the traditional early clinical signs and symptoms of compartment syndrome – pain on passive motion that is out of proportion to clinical findings and the presence of paresthesias – has to be substituted with hightened index of clinical suspicion and extremity compartment pressure measurements.[53] Fasciotomies should be performed in a timely fashion when evidence of elevated compartment pressures is present.[54, 55]

9. Concurrent vascular injury

Vascular injuries present a special challenge in the context of simultaneous brain trauma. Specifically, direct managment priority conflicts can be seen with regards to the need for therapeutic anticoagulation and the risk of secondary intracranial hemorrhage. Likewise, the maintenance of cerebral perfusion pressure can pose an increased risk in patients with concurrent traumatic pseudoaneurysms and other injuries that may necessitate strict blood pressure and heart rate control. In addition, high dose vasopressor use to maintain adequate cerebral perfusion may lead to distal extremity ischemic complications up to and including the need for amputation.

With ever improving quality of modern imaging modalities, cerebrovascular injuries are being detected more frequently. Neurologic assessment following blunt cerebrovascular injury can be difficult and distinguishing cerebral ischemia from cerebral infarction is often complex, especially in the setting of altered mental status.[56] The main challenge associated with the diagnosis of blunt carotid or vertebral injury (BCVI) is the relative rarity of BCVI and the need for constant vigilance and high index of suspicion. One of the most important clinical findings associated with BCVI is the presence of an unexplained or new neurologic deficit in the setting of otherwise normal (or unchanged) brain imaging. Trauma practitioners should be familiar with major risk factors for BCVI, both from the injury mechanism standpoint (i.e., cervical seat belt sign, blunt assault to craniofacial area with LeFort III fracture pattern, cervical spine fracture) and from the clinical presentation standpoint (i.e., high-speed motor vehicle crash, flexion-extension neck injury).[57]

10. Missed injuries and diagnostic delays

Important in the context of multiple trauma patient with concomitant brain injury are the concepts of missed injury and delayed diagnosis. Delay in diagnosis occurs when an injury is identified after the usually accepted initial phases of trauma evaluation (i.e., primary, secondary, or tertiary surveys) but before the injury manifests as an overt clinical problem.[58] Missed injury can be defined as a delay in diagnosis that is associated with clinical symptoms and/or is not identified until after discharge from hospital.[58] Although the incidence goal for missed injuries and diagnostic delays should be "zero", this target remains elusive. Major series cite missed injury rates between 0.5% and 65%, with anywhere between 1 and 2.3 missed injuries per patient, depending on population under study, type of study (prospective versus retrospective), and diagnostic definitions (missed injury versus delayed diagnosis).[58] Among missed injuries, over 10% are clinically significant and, of those, 14% to 50% can be associated directly with patient mortality.[1, 58, 59]

The importance of this topic to the brain injured trauma population becomes obvious when one considers the most common contributing factors to missed injury: (a) altered mental status; (b) presence of distracting injury; (c) administration of analgesia and sedation; and (d) overwhelming or multiple simultaneous injuries.[58] Whenever the patient's sensorium is diminished, it becomes more difficult to identify injuries as the patient loses the ability to effectively express complaints related to pain and discomfort. Alterations in pain processing may occur with traumatic brain injury, spinal cord injury, hypoxia, shock, intoxication/substance abuse, and administration of sedation for various reasons (i.e., combative patient). The pain response can be altered after a major injury and the patient may not be able to process pain from all injuries equally. For example, a non-displaced ankle fracture may not be readily evident with a concurrent presence of an open femur fracture. Often direct palpation over a specific injury site will elicit a pain response. Therefore, comprehensive repetitive physical examinations may be required in order to effectively identify the complete injury list in the presence of distracting pain. However, even the most detailed physical examination may fail to detect traumatic injuries in the multiply injured patient with concomitant moderate to severe brain trauma. Moreover, concurrent administration of analgesia and sedation may additionally affect the practitioner's ability to reliably detect various types of injuries, from minor to life threatening.[58] It is important to note that cranio-facial injuries constitute as many as 5%-30% of missed injuries, depending on study cited.[1, 59, 60]

11. Pitfalls and controversies

This section highlights important pitfalls and controversies associated with management of the multiply injured patients with concurrent brain trauma. We emphasize the need for continuous reassessment of competing priorities and need for centralized team coordination. Because many of the topics mentioned are beyond the scope of this chapter, the reader is referred to other sources as referenced herein. Practitioners should always be aware of potential complications related to massive fluid resuscitation, up to and including the abdominal compartment syndrome.[61] On the opposite end of the hemodynamic spectrum, one should always be cognizant of complications related to use of escalating doses of vasoactive agents, including phenomena such as tachyphylaxis [62] and the possibility of skin/limb ischemia due to high-dose vasopressor use.[63] Although the authors encourage the use of advanced hemodynamic monitoring (both invasive and non-invasive), there are many potential complications associated with both errors in hemodynamic data interpretation and iatrogenic injury related to invasive line placement.[64]

Intra-hospital patient transfers (i.e., transport to operating room or imaging suite) carry its own set of complications, with serious adverse outcomes attributed to such transfers in over 30% of critically ill patients.[65] Use of any therapies or diagnostic tests that could potentially contribute to additional complications should always be considered in the context of risk-benefit ratio.[66] For example, although still controversial, evidence suggests that early use of prophylactic anticoagulation is more beneficial than withholding this therapy in the TBI population.[67, 68]

Additional considerations include the effect of sedative agents on both hemodynamic and metabolic aspects of patient management. For example, the use of propofol for sedation may be associated with complications such as hypotension [69], pancreatitis [70], and propofol infusion syndrome.[71] In addition, adjunctive approaches such as therapeutic hypothermia and chemically induced coma are mentioned and referenced for the reader.[72, 73] These

Provider- and Team-related considerations
- Skilled team management, leadership, and effective communication are of critical importance.
- Coordinated care planning, including multi-disciplinary conferences and open dialogue between various clinical specialties, is important to optimizing patient care.
- Trauma teams should work efficiently, utilizing protocolized care as well as well-functioning clinical management / surveillance systems.
- The overall goal of the trauma team is to reconcile conflicting priorities with the overarching goal of maximizing the outcome from the perspective of the "whole patient".

Injury-related considerations
- Knowledge of injury patterns is useful in determining the likelihood of any potential associated non-TBI injuries, especially in the setting of concurrent neurological impairment.
- The very presence of associated injuries in the setting of concurrent brain trauma is associated with significantly increased mortality. Among such associated injuries, those that carry highest mortality usually involve risks of hypotension, hemorrhage and/or hypoxia.
- Familiarity with acceptable physiologic parameter ranges inherent to the management of each injured anatomic area or organ system is important to patient care optimization and reconciliation of potentially conflicting therapeutic priorities.
- Non-conventional measures, including various "damage control" approaches permit the most critical injuries to be given higher priority while adequately temporizing other, less critical injuries.

Patient care-related considerations
- The overarching goal is to prevent secondary physiologic insults that have been shown to adversely affect outcomes.
- Maintenance of adequate cerebral perfusion pressure while minimizing hypotensive and hypoxic events is crucial. It is important to note that while these priorities do not change over time, the nature of inciting events may differ (i.e., hemorrhage causing early hypotension versus sepsis causing late hypotension).
- Intra-hospital patient transfers (i.e., for procedural interventions or imaging studies) carry a significant risk, with nearly one-third of such transfers associated with some sort of adverse event (i.e., hypotension, hypoxia, etc). Therefore, such transfers should be undertaken only if absolutely indicated.
- Lack of reliable physical examination in multiply injured patients with TBI predisposes this group to missed injuries and diagnostic delays. Although modern technolgical advances enable practitioners to partially "compensate" for the lack of adequate bedside assessment, there are no true substitutes for an experienced practitioner with an adequate level of clinical suspicion.

Miscellaneous considerations
- Use of any therapies or diagnostic tests that carry a defined potential for complications should always be considered in the context of careful risk-benefit determination.
Providers should be familiar with potential complications associated with each and every therapeutic agent and procedure. Early recognition of such complications can be life-saving.

Table 1. Important points in management of multiply injured patients with concurrent traumatic brain injury

therapies are still controversial and further research is needed to better define their safety profiles and risk-benefit characteristics, especially in the setting of multiple trauma and competing clinical priorities.

12. The multiply injured patient with TBI – Putting it all together

Management of the multiply injured patient with TBI involves close collaboration of multiple specialties, including critical care, neurosurgery, orthopedic, and trauma experts. Practitioners must always be aware of all competing priorities, including cross-specialty considerations for specific injury patterns and associated pitfalls and complications. Life-threatening injuries should be approached according to the magnitude of the most immediate mortality risk. At times, simultaneous management of multiple injuries may require the initiation of various "damage control" techniques. Complications related to the primary injuries as well as any secondary insults must be recognized and addressed promptly. Early rehabilitation is crucial in order to optimize long-term outcomes in this population. The achievement of these goals requires that trauma teams work efficiently, utilizing protocolized care and well-functioning clinical surveillance systems.[74, 75] The overall goal of the trauma healthcare team is to reconcile any conflicting priorities with the goal of maximizing the outcome from the perspective of the "whole patient".

13. References

[1]   Houshian S, Larsen MS, Holm C. Missed injuries in a level I trauma center. *J Trauma.* Apr 2002;52(4):715-719.
[2]   Mirza A, Ellis T. Initial management of pelvic and femoral fractures in the multiply injured patient. *Crit Care Clin.* Jan 2004;20(1):159-170.
[3]   Dickinson K. The acute management of pelvic ring injuries. In: Kellman JF, Fisher TJ, Tornetta P, Bosse MJ, Harris MB, eds. *Orthopaedic knowledge update: trauma 2.* Rosemont, IL: American Academy of Orthopaedic Surgeons; 2000:229-237.
[4]   Hoff WS, Reilly PM, Rotondo MF, DiGiacomo JC, Schwab CW. The importance of the command-physician in trauma resuscitation. *J Trauma.* Nov 1997;43(5):772-777.
[5]   Ruchholtz S, Waydhas C, Lewan U, et al. A multidisciplinary quality management system for the early treatment of severely injured patients: implementation and results in two trauma centers. *Intensive Care Med.* Oct 2002;28(10):1395-1404.
[6]   Chesnut RM, Marshall LF, Klauber MR, et al. The role of secondary brain injury in determining outcome from severe head injury. *J Trauma.* Feb 1993;34(2):216-222.
[7]   Bullock R, Chesnut RM, Clifton G, et al. Guidelines for the management of severe head injury. Brain Trauma Foundation. *Eur J Emerg Med.* Jun 1996;3(2):109-127.
[8]   Chesnut RM. Management of brain and spine injuries. *Crit Care Clin.* Jan 2004;20(1):25-55.
[9]   Rose J, Valtonen S, Jennett B. Avoidable factors contributing to death after head injury. *Br Med J.* Sep 3 1977;2(6087):615-618.
[10]   Miller JD, Becker DP. Secondary insults to the injured brain. *J R Coll Surg Edinb.* Sep 1982;27(5):292-298.

[11] Leal-Noval SR, Munoz-Gomez M, Arellano-Orden V, et al. Impact of age of transfused blood on cerebral oxygenation in male patients with severe traumatic brain injury. *Crit Care Med.* Apr 2008;36(4):1290-1296.

[12] Leal-Noval SR, Rincon-Ferrari MD, Marin-Niebla A, et al. Transfusion of erythrocyte concentrates produces a variable increment on cerebral oxygenation in patients with severe traumatic brain injury: a preliminary study. *Intensive Care Med.* Nov 2006;32(11):1733-1740.

[13] Smith MJ, Stiefel MF, Magge S, et al. Packed red blood cell transfusion increases local cerebral oxygenation. *Crit Care Med.* May 2005;33(5):1104-1108.

[14] Hariri RJ, Firlick AD, Shepard SR, et al. Traumatic brain injury, hemorrhagic shock, and fluid resuscitation: effects on intracranial pressure and brain compliance. *J Neurosurg.* Sep 1993;79(3):421-427.

[15] Rosner MJ, Daughton S. Cerebral perfusion pressure management in head injury. *J Trauma.* Aug 1990;30(8):933-940; discussion 940-931.

[16] Muizelaar JP. Cerebral ischemia-reperfusion injury after severe head injury and its possible treatment with polyethyleneglycol-superoxide dismutase. *Ann Emerg Med.* Jun 1993;22(6):1014-1021.

[17] Bilello JF, Davis JW, Cunningham MA, Groom TF, Lemaster D, Sue LP. Cervical spinal cord injury and the need for cardiovascular intervention. *Arch Surg.* Oct 2003;138(10):1127-1129.

[18] Stawicki SP, Holmes JH, Kallan MJ, Nance ML. Fatal child cervical spine injuries in motor vehicle collisions: Analysis using unique linked national datasets. *Injury.* Aug 2009;40(8):864-867.

[19] Siegel JH. The effect of associated injuries, blood loss, and oxygen debt on death and disability in blunt traumatic brain injury: the need for early physiologic predictors of severity. *J Neurotrauma.* Aug 1995;12(4):579-590.

[20] Siegel JH, Mason-Gonzalez S, Dischinger P, et al. Safety belt restraints and compartment intrusions in frontal and lateral motor vehicle crashes: mechanisms of injuries, complications, and acute care costs. *J Trauma.* May 1993;34(5):736-758; discussion 758-739.

[21] Siegel JH, Gens DR, Mamantov T, Geisler FH, Goodarzi S, MacKenzie EJ. Effect of associated injuries and blood volume replacement on death, rehabilitation needs, and disability in blunt traumatic brain injury. *Crit Care Med.* Oct 1991;19(10):1252-1265.

[22] Brown R, DiMarco AF, Hoit JD, Garshick E. Respiratory dysfunction and management in spinal cord injury. *Respir Care.* Aug 2006;51(8):853-868;discussion 869-870.

[23] Piepmeier JM, Lehmann KB, Lane JG. Cardiovascular instability following acute cervical spinal cord trauma. *Cent Nerv Syst Trauma.* Fall 1985;2(3):153-160.

[24] Lehmann KG, Lane JG, Piepmeier JM, Batsford WP. Cardiovascular abnormalities accompanying acute spinal cord injury in humans: incidence, time course and severity. *J Am Coll Cardiol.* Jul 1987;10(1):46-52.

[25] Luce JM, Culver BH. Respiratory muscle function in health and disease. *Chest.* Jan 1982;81(1):82-90.

[26] Bergofsky EH. Mechanism for Respiratory Insufficiency after Cervical Cord Injury; a Source of Alveolar Hypoventilation. *Ann Intern Med.* Sep 1964;61:435-447.

[27] Stawicki SP. Trends in nonoperative management of traumatic injuries: a synopsis. *OPUS 12 Scientist.* 2007;1(1):19-35.

[28] Bratton SL, Davis RL. Acute lung injury in isolated traumatic brain injury. *Neurosurgery.* Apr 1997;40(4):707-712; discussion 712.

[29] Ledingham IM, Watt I. Influence of sedation on mortality in critically ill multiple trauma patients. *Lancet.* Jun 4 1983;1(8336):1270.

[30] Miller SM. Management of central nervous system injuries. In: Capan LM, ed. *Trauma Anesthesia and Intensive Care.* Philadelphia: JB Lippincott Co; 1991:321.

[31] Simon RP, Gean-Marton AD, Sander JE. Medullary lesion inducing pulmonary edema: a magnetic resonance imaging study. *Ann Neurol.* Nov 1991;30(5):727-730.

[32] Theodore J, Robin ED. Pathogenesis of neurogenic pulmonary oedema. *Lancet.* Oct 18 1975;2(7938):749-751.

[33] Bloomfield GL, Dalton JM, Sugerman HJ, Ridings PC, DeMaria EJ, Bullock R. Treatment of increasing intracranial pressure secondary to the acute abdominal compartment syndrome in a patient with combined abdominal and head trauma. *J Trauma.* Dec 1995;39(6):1168-1170.

[34] Scalea TM, Boswell SA, Scott JD, Mitchell KA, Kramer ME, Pollak AN. External fixation as a bridge to intramedullary nailing for patients with multiple injuries and with femur fractures: damage control orthopedics. *J Trauma.* Apr 2000;48(4):613-621; discussion 621-613.

[35] Citerio G, Vascotto E, Villa F, Celotti S, Pesenti A. Induced abdominal compartment syndrome increases intracranial pressure in neurotrauma patients: a prospective study. *Crit Care Med.* Jul 2001;29(7):1466-1471.

[36] Marinis A, Argyra E, Lykoudis P, et al. Ischemia as a possible effect of increased intra-abdominal pressure on central nervous system cytokines, lactate and perfusion pressures. *Crit Care.* 2010;14(2):R31.

[37] Cheatham ML. Nonoperative management of intraabdominal hypertension and abdominal compartment syndrome. *World J Surg.* Jun 2009;33(6):1116-1122.

[38] Smith BP, Adams RC, Doraiswamy VA, et al. Review of abdominal damage control and open abdomens: focus on gastrointestinal complications. *J Gastrointestin Liver Dis.* Dec 2010;19(4):425-435.

[39] Joseph DK, Dutton RP, Aarabi B, Scalea TM. Decompressive laparotomy to treat intractable intracranial hypertension after traumatic brain injury. *J Trauma.* Oct 2004;57(4):687-693; discussion 693-685.

[40] Taylor A, Butt W, Rosenfeld J, et al. A randomized trial of very early decompressive craniectomy in children with traumatic brain injury and sustained intracranial hypertension. *Childs Nerv Syst.* Feb 2001;17(3):154-162.

[41] Honeybul S, Ho KM, Lind CR, Gillett GR. Decompressive craniectomy for diffuse cerebral swelling after trauma: long-term outcome and ethical considerations. *J Trauma.* Jul 2011;71(1):128-132.

[42] Soukiasian HJ, Hui T, Avital I, et al. Decompressive craniectomy in trauma patients with severe brain injury. *Am Surg.* Dec 2002;68(12):1066-1071.

[43] Hansen KS, Uggen PE, Brattebo G, Wisborg T. Team-oriented training for damage control surgery in rural trauma: a new paradigm. *J Trauma.* Apr 2008;64(4):949-953; discussion 953-944.

[44] Simpson DA, Heyworth JS, McLean AJ, Gilligan JE, North JB. Extradural haemorrhage: strategies for management in remote places. *Injury.* Sep 1988;19(5):307-312.

[45] Rinker CF, McMurry FG, Groeneweg VR, Bahnson FF, Banks KL, Gannon DM. Emergency craniotomy in a rural Level III trauma center. *J Trauma.* Jun 1998;44(6):984-989; discussion 989-990.

[46] Esposito TJ, Reed RL, 2nd, Gamelli RL, Luchette FA. Neurosurgical coverage: essential, desired, or irrelevant for good patient care and trauma center status. *Ann Surg.* Sep 2005;242(3):364-370; discussion 370-364.

[47] Rosenfeld JV. Damage control neurosurgery. *Injury.* Jul 2004;35(7):655-660.

[48] Starr AJ, Hunt JL, Chason DP, Reinert CM, Walker J. Treatment of femur fracture with associated head injury. *J Orthop Trauma.* Jan 1998;12(1):38-45.

[49] Poole GV, Miller JD, Agnew SG, Griswold JA. Lower extremity fracture fixation in head-injured patients. *J Trauma.* May 1992;32(5):654-659.

[50] Schmeling GJ, Schwab JP. Polytrauma care. The effect of head injuries and timing of skeletal fixation. *Clin Orthop Relat Res.* Sep 1995(318):106-116.

[51] Pape HC, Hildebrand F, Pertschy S, et al. Changes in the management of femoral shaft fractures in polytrauma patients: from early total care to damage control orthopedic surgery. *J Trauma.* Sep 2002;53(3):452-461; discussion 461-452.

[52] Nau T, Aldrian S, Koenig F, Vecsei V. Fixation of femoral fractures in multiple-injury patients with combined chest and head injuries. *ANZ J Surg.* Dec 2003;73(12):1018-1021.

[53] Kosir R, Moore FA, Selby JH, et al. Acute lower extremity compartment syndrome (ALECS) screening protocol in critically ill trauma patients. *J Trauma.* Aug 2007;63(2):268-275.

[54] Branco BC, Inaba K, Barmparas G, et al. Incidence and predictors for the need for fasciotomy after extremity trauma: A 10-year review in a mature level I trauma centre. *Injury.* Jul 31 2010.

[55] Farber A, Tan TW, Hamburg NM, et al. Early fasciotomy in patients with extremity vascular injury is associated with decreased risk of adverse limb outcomes: A review of the National Trauma Data Bank. *Injury.* Jun 28 2011.

[56] Phillips CV, Jacobsen DC, Brayton DF, Bloch JH. Central vessel trauma. *Am Surg.* Aug 1979;45(8):517-530.

[57] Fusco MR, Harrigan MR. Cerebrovascular dissections: a review. Part II: blunt cerebrovascular injury. *Neurosurgery.* Feb 2011;68(2):517-530; discussion 530.

[58] Stawicki SP, Lindsey DE. Missed traumatic injuries: a synopsis. *OPUS 12 Scientist.* 2009;3(2):35-43.

[59] Buduhan G, McRitchie DI. Missed injuries in patients with multiple trauma. *J Trauma.* Oct 2000;49(4):600-605.

[60] Enderson B, Maull KI. Missed injuries: the trauma surgeon's nemesis. *Surg Clin North Am.* 1991;71:399-418.

[61] Balogh Z, McKinley BA, Cocanour CS, et al. Secondary abdominal compartment syndrome is an elusive early complication of traumatic shock resuscitation. *Am J Surg.* Dec 2002;184(6):538-543; discussion 543-534.

[62] Lehmann G, Randall LO. Pharmacological properties of sympathomimetic diamines. *J Pharmacol Exp Ther.* May 1948;93(1):114-125.

[63] Dunser MW, Mayr AJ, Tur A, et al. Ischemic skin lesions as a complication of continuous vasopressin infusion in catecholamine-resistant vasodilatory shock: incidence and risk factors. *Crit Care Med.* May 2003;31(5):1394-1398.

[64] Evans DC, Doraiswamy VA, Prosciak MP, et al. Complications associated with pulmonary artery catheters: a comprehensive clinical review. *Scand J Surg.* 2009;98(4):199-208.

[65] Beckmann U, Gillies DM, Berenholtz SM, Wu AW, Pronovost P. Incidents relating to the intra-hospital transfer of critically ill patients. An analysis of the reports submitted to the Australian Incident Monitoring Study in Intensive Care. *Intensive Care Med.* Aug 2004;30(8):1579-1585.

[66] Stawicki SP, Grossman MD, Cipolla J, et al. Deep venous thrombosis and pulmonary embolism in trauma patients: an overstatement of the problem? *Am Surg.* May 2005;71(5):387-391.

[67] Kim J, Gearhart MM, Zurick A, Zuccarello M, James L, Luchette FA. Preliminary report on the safety of heparin for deep venous thrombosis prophylaxis after severe head injury. *J Trauma.* Jul 2002;53(1):38-42; discussion 43.

[68] Norwood SH, Berne JD, Rowe SA, Villarreal DH, Ledlie JT. Early venous thromboembolism prophylaxis with enoxaparin in patients with blunt traumatic brain injury. *J Trauma.* Nov 2008;65(5):1021-1026; discussion 1026-1027.

[69] Muzi M, Berens RA, Kampine JP, Ebert TJ. Venodilation contributes to propofol-mediated hypotension in humans. *Anesth Analg.* Jun 1992;74(6):877-883.

[70] Leisure GS, O'Flaherty J, Green L, Jones DR. Propofol and postoperative pancreatitis. *Anesthesiology.* Jan 1996;84(1):224-227.

[71] Diedrich DA, Brown DR. Analytic reviews: propofol infusion syndrome in the ICU. *J Intensive Care Med.* Mar-Apr 2011;26(2):59-72.

[72] Clifton GL, Miller ER, Choi SC, et al. Lack of effect of induction of hypothermia after acute brain injury. *N Engl J Med.* Feb 22 2001;344(8):556-563.

[73] Lee MW, Deppe SA, Sipperly ME, Barrette RR, Thompson DR. The efficacy of barbiturate coma in the management of uncontrolled intracranial hypertension following neurosurgical trauma. *J Neurotrauma.* Jun 1994;11(3):325-331.

[74] Gracias VH, Sicoutris CP, Stawicki SP, et al. Critical care nurse practitioners improve compliance with clinical practice guidelines in "semiclosed" surgical intensive care unit. *J Nurs Care Qual.* Oct-Dec 2008;23(4):338-344.

[75] Stawicki SP, Gracias VH, Lorenzo M. Surgical critical care: from old boundaries to new frontiers. *Scand J Surg.* 2007;96(1):17-25.

5

Antioxidant Treatments: Effect on Behaviour, Histopathological and Oxidative Stress in Epilepsy Model

Rivelilson Mendes de Freitas
Federal University of Piaui
Brazil

1. Introduction

The aim of this chapter is to describe several studies which have attempted to measure/detect effects of antioxidant compounds (lipoic acid, ubiquinone, ascorbic acid and alpha-tocopherol) on behavioral alterations, neuronal damage and oxidative stress in hippocampus of rodents in epilepsy model induced by pilocarpine.

Epilepsy can cause an uncomfortable impact on social, educational and emotional development of affected people, especially in childhood and adolescence, but its diagnosis has had great progress over the last years. Nevertheless, among the diagnostic details requiring research, the precise localization and lateralization of epileptogenic focus remains unclear, despite the fact that it has been demonstrated that removal of cerebral cortex region may result in a state free of seizures. Moreover, epilepsy is considered a risk factor for depression and other psychological problems, whereas cognitive impairment may be related to behavioral troubles, particularly of conduct and attention deficit, hyperactivity and psychiatric disorders.

Neurotransmitter systems involved in the experimental model of epilepsy induced by pilocarpine are not fully defined yet. This seizure model in rodents is widely used to study the pathophysiology of convulsive process, since it reproduces behavioral, electroencephalographic (EEG) and neurochemical changes that are similar to those of the temporal lobe epilepsy in humans. The pilocarpine model is used to study the action mechanism of new drugs and antioxidant compounds during the installation and maintenance and/or propagation of epileptogenesis as well as to evaluate effects of new compounds isolated from medicinal plants on behavioral, histopathological, and other parameters relating neurochemical changes with epileptic activity (Costa Júnior et al, 2010).

Histopathological studies using this model have demonstrated neuronal damage in various brain regions. Some specific brain areas revealed typical histopathological changes, mainly hippocampus, striatum and frontal cortex, suggesting the involvement of these different areas during the establishment of the epileptic process. Among those areas, the cellular and structural modifications seen in hippocampus and striatum may be significantly related to the mechanisms of installation and propagation in epileptogenesis of limbic seizures.

The temporal lobe epilepsy is the most common form of epilepsy. It is characterized by spontaneous recurrent seizures that are often blocked by treatment with antiepileptic drugs.

Seizures can be characterized as clinical manifestations resulting from abnormal neuronal discharges, producing an imbalance between the mechanisms of inhibitory and excitatory neurotransmission. The mechanisms of activation, propagation and maintenance of seizures are widely studied but little understood. Many studies have been performed using the pilocarpine model to clarify the effects of new drug modulators on brain mechanisms of seizures and status epilepticus (Santos et al, 2010).

Status epilepticus is clinically defined as prolonged electrical and clinical seizure activity in which the patient does not regain consciousness to a normal alert state between repeated tonic-clonic attacks. The disorder is a neurological emergency associated with a mortality rate of 10-12% and an even greater morbidity. Status epilepticus can lead to permanent pathological damage and altered physiological function in certain brain regions and induces major changes in membrane phospholipids, massive increases in arachidonic acid concentrations, diacylglycerol-mediated activation of protein kinase C, calcium-mediated changes in calmodulin kinase II and possibly generation of free radicals that could play an essential role in mechanism of oxidative stress involved in neuronal damage. Status epilepticus can be characterized by a permanent change in neurotransmitter systems and oxidative stress that it is more facilitated in the brain rather than in other tissues because it contains large quantities of oxidizable lipids and metals (Freitas et al, 2010). Moreover, status epilepticus can produce considerable changes on the enzymatic activity of antioxidants systems according to the brain areas and the phase of the seizure studied.

The role of monoamines, amino acid and oxidative stress in pilocarpine model was investigated in hippocampus, striatum and frontal cortex of adult rats. The status epilepticus was induced by pilocarpine and the results correspond to its acute phase. The data obtained suggest that pilocarpine induced neurotransmitters and oxidative stress changes in brain regions which are similar to those found in human temporal lobe epilepsy (El-Etri et al, 1993, Freitas et al, 2003, Ferreira et al, 2009).

2. Pathophysiology of seizures in epilepsy model induced by pilocarpine

Epilepsies are complex neurobehavioral disorders resulting from increased excitability of neurons in several brain regions involving various neurotransmitters (Rauca et al, 2004). The cholinergic system plays an important role in generating EEG activity as well as regulating the vigilance states. Pilocarpine is a cholinergic agonist with a moderate affinity with M_1 muscarinic receptors and high affinity with M_5 ones. Muscarinic cholinergic agonists have effects on rapid eyes movement (REM) and slow wave sleep, playing a role in REM induction (MacGregor et al, 1997; Perlis et al, 2002). On the other hand, pilocarpine at a high dose (400 mg/kg, i.p.) makes seizures progress to a long-lasting status epilepticus (SE) within 1-2 h and induces behavioral and EEG alterations in rodents, which are similar to human temporal lobe epilepsy (TLE) (Marinho et al, 1998).

Pilocarpine-induced rodent models TLE might provide information regarding histopathological damage and oxidative stress consequences, as well as neurochemical changes associated with seizure activity in hippocampus of young and adult rats (Cavalheiro et al, 1991; Smith and Shibley, 2002, Freitas et al, 2003). TLE can be characterized by a permanent change in neurotransmitter systems and in development of the oxidative stress that is more facilitated in the brain rather than in other tissues because for several reasons, including a high consumption of oxygen, the presence of large quantities of oxidizable lipids and pro-oxidative metals, and its comparatively lower antioxidant capacity

(Frantseva et al, 2000; Naffah-Mazzacoratti et al, 2001). Neuronal cells continuously produce free radicals and reactive oxygen species (ROS) as part of their metabolic processes and during the establishment of convulsive process (Gilbert and Sawas, 1983; Halliwell and Gutteridge, 1999). The free radicals are very reactive and might produce oxidative damage in DNA, proteins and lipids (Peterson et al, 2002), leading to a sequence of outcomes that culminates in neuronal degeneration during the installation of seizures.

ROS can affect the ion transport, proteins and channels, via protein oxidation or via membrane phospholipids peroxidation, resulting in a deleterious change on the ionic homeostasis and the neuronal transmission (Rong et al, 1999; Sah et al, 2002). The ROS increment induces oxidative stress, which is defined as the excessive production of free radicals, such as superoxide (O_2^-), hydroxyl radical (OH·), nitric oxide (NO) and their metabolites (nitrate and nitrite) and others that can dramatically alter the neuronal function. Therefore, some researches have correlated the overproduction of these compounds with seizure-induced neuronal death and status epilepticus (MacGregor et al, 1997; Ferrer et al, 2000).

Several compounds can produce free radical such as H_2O_2, which in high concentration can react with O_2^- (Haber-Weiss reaction) or iron (Fenton reaction) producing highly reactive OH. The conversion of H_2O_2 to H_2O and O_2 is made by catalase and glutathione peroxidase (Michiels et al, 1994; Simonié et al, 2000). The formed OH· radical is likely to react with non-radical molecules, transforming them into secondary free radicals. This reaction occurs during the lipid peroxidation producing hydroperoxides in brain epileptic (Vanhatalo and Riikonen, 1999). Nitric oxide (NO) can be estimated by their metabolites, which are associated with neurodegenerative diseases (Vanhatalo and Riikonen, 2001). Despite the fact that numerous studies clearly indicate the importance of antioxidant enzymatic activities in the epileptic phenomenon, the mechanisms by which these enzymes influence seizures and status epilepticus are not completely understood (Michiels et al, 1994; Simonié et al, 2000).

Status epilepticus is a severe form of continuous seizure attacks and a medical emergency associated with brain damage and significant mortality (Aminoff and Simon, 1980). The common sequels of status epilepticus include continuing recurrent seizures, permanent neurological deficit and brain injury. The status epilepticus can be induced by the administration of pilocarpine or lithium-pilocarpine (Hirsh et al, 1982; Freitas et al, 2004). Pilocarpine administration induces seizures with three distinct phases: [A] an acute period, which lasts 1-2 days and is associated to repetitive seizures and status epilepticus; [B] a seizure-free (silent period) characterized by a progressive return to normal EEG and behavior, which lasts 4 to 44 days; [C] a chronic period characterized by spontaneous recurrent seizures (SRS) that starts 5 to 45 days after pilocarpine administration and persists until the animal dies. In addition, systemic injection of pilocarpine induces status epilepticus in rodents associated to histopathological alterations, which are most prominent in limbic structures (Cavalheiro et al, 1991), such as hippocampus, striatum, frontal cortex and others (Tomé et al, 2010).

Pilocarpine is a muscarinic cholinergic agonist able to elicit seizures and status epilepticus in rodents, characterizing an experimental model frequently used to study SRS (Turski et al, 1983; Freitas et al, 2005). This seizure model resembles several phenomenological features of human temporal lobe epilepsy, including a particular resistance to anticonvulsant medication (Browne and Holmes, 2001). Tissue accumulation of free radicals can occur in many metabolic disorders, such as seizures. Affected patients present a variable degree of neurological dysfunction, including mental retardation, cognitive deficit and cerebral edema. However, the exact mechanisms involved in these alterations remain poorly understood.

It has been described that the impairments in learning, memory and behavior observed in patients with epilepsy are caused, at least in part, by changes in cholinergic system function (Bruce and Baudry, 1995), since there are consistent evidence that high levels of acetylcholine (ACh) in the brain are associated with cognitive dysfunction (Brozek et al, 2000). Cholinergic transmission is mainly terminated after ACh hydrolysis cause by acetylcholinesterase enzyme (AChE).

In the brain, the phenomena of excitotoxicity has been related to an over production of free radicals by the tissue during pilocarpine-induced seizures and status epilepticus (Simonié et al, 2000) and in human epilepsy (Vanhatalo and Riikonen, 1999). The increase in ROS levels can be responsible for this neuropathology and can activate apoptosis processes (Rong et al, 1999). The free radicals in the convulsive process can be neutralized by an elaborate antioxidant defense system consisting of enzymes such as superoxide dismutase, glutathione peroxidase, catalase, and glutathione reductase, and numerous non-enzymatic antioxidants like reduced glutathione (GSH), indicating a neuronal response (Ferrer et al, 2000). Status epilepticus induces ROS production by protein oxidation measured by tyrosine nitration (Rong et al, 1999). It can also be determined by both the end-product of lipid peroxidation, malondialdehyde (MDA) levels (Bruce and Baudry, 1995), and the effectiveness of the antioxidant enzymatic responses (Dal-Pizzol et al, 2000). The hippocampus is the most affected area by pilocarpine-induced seizures. Other authors also characterized the neuropathology associated with this convulsive process in striatum, frontal cortex, thalamus and amygdala (Perlis et al, 2002; Freitas et al, 2004).

Seizures represent one of the most severe in vivo stimulatory stress that the brain is exposed to and generalized status epilepticus represents a very severe form of seizures. The international Classification of seizures has defined it as a condition characterized by an epileptic seizure that is so frequent or so prolonged as to create a fixed and lasting condition (Krug et al, 1981). Major motor status epilepticus can lead to permanent pathological damage and altered physiological function in certain brain regions. The pathophysiological changes seen in complex partial, simple partial and absence status epilepticus are much less clear (Freitas et al, 2005). SE can cause brain damage, but can also result from it, and it has been difficult to separate the two, particularly in humans (Lapin et al, 1998).

Status epilepticus has been widely studied in animal models. In status epilepticus, glutamate, aspartate, serotonin, dopamine and acetylcholine play major roles as excitatory neurotransmitters, and GABA as the dominant inhibitory neurotransmitter (Hort et al, 2000; Costa-Lotufo et al, 2002). However, the relation among brain excitatory and inhibitory neurotransmitters and status epilepticus cannot be perfectly established yet and deserves further studies with the purpose to clarify the pathophysiology of seizures.

The pathophysiology of epilepsy is not yet fully defined. The pilocarpine model of seizures in animals are widely used to study the pathophysiology of convulsive process (Ben-Ari et al, 1980), since it reproduces the behavioral and EEG changes that are similar to humans TLE (Ben-Ari et al, 1981). These models are used to study the involvement of neurotransmitter systems as modulators of epileptogenesis, but also to observe behavioral changes, histopathologic, and other neurochemical parameters related to seizure activity (Marinho et al, 1997; Costa- Lotufo et al, 2002, Freitas et al, 2006).

In general, pilocarpine-induced seizures seem to depend on activation of muscarinic receptor, the enzymatic activity changes in some systems (Simonié et al, 2000; Naffah-

Mazzacoratti et al, 2001; Liu et al, 2002), metabolism of fosfoinositídios (Marinho et al, 1998), as well as on the involvement of other neurotransmitter systems such as noradrenergic, dopamine (Kulkarni and George, 1996), serotonergic, GABAergic (Loup et al. 1999; Costa-Lotufo et al, 2002) and glutamatergic (Massieu et al. 1994; Chamberlain et al, 2000).

3. Behavioral alterations in epilepsy model

Status epilepticus is an emergency situation which requires prompt medical atentem. If it is severe permanent brain damage or death has to be prevented with pretreatment with antioxidant compounds. Status epilepticus often occurs in individuals with a history of seizures, in whom there are neuronal substrates already predisposed towards supporting seizure activity.

The pilocarpine model is an useful animal experimental to investigate the development of acute, silent and chronic phases (Cavalheiro et al, 1991). Immediately after pilocarpine administration, all animals persistently presented behavioral changes, including initial akinesia, ataxic lurching, peripheral cholinergic signs (miosis, piloerection, chromodacryorrhea, diarrhea and masticatory automatisms), stereotyped movements (continuous sniffing, paw licking, rearing and wet dog shakes that persisted for 10-15 min), clonic movements of forelimbs, head bobbing and tremors.

These behavioral changes progressed to motor limbic seizures as previously described by Tursky et al. (1983a). Limbic seizures lasted for 30-50 min evolving to status epilepticus for a period longer than 30 min. During 1 h of acute phase of seizures, no case of fatality was observed between the adult rats. However, during the 24 h observation of this phase, 63% of adult animals died (Cavalheiro et al, 1994; Todorova et al, 2004). Similarly, these results for the behavioral alterations in pilocarpine model were described previously by Marinho et al. (1998).

According to our previous studies (Freitas et al, 2004), few minutes after pilocarpine administration, the animals exhibited stereotyped oral and masticatory movements, hypokinesia, salivation, tremor and partial or generalized limbic seizures. Approximately 30 min after pilocarpine injection, the seizures evolved to status epilepticus lasting 12-18 h. During this period, 40% of animals died due to SE. This acute phase was followed by a silent period varying from 4 to 44 days (mean of 15 days) during which the animals displayed normal behavior. A chronic period of spontaneous and recurrent seizures (SRS) (3-4 seizures/week) was also observed and all animals which survived SE, displayed the chronic phase. During the interictal period, there were no behavioral alterations in the animals.

In epilepsy model, pilocarpine induced the first seizure to occur at 34.93 ± 0.70 min. All the animals that received pilocarpine injection (at a dose 400 mg/kg, i.p.) presented generalized tonic-clonic convulsions with status epilepticus, and 60% survived the seizures (Freitas et al, 2004).

4. Antioxidant compounds effects on behavioral alterations in epilepsy model

The nervous system contains some antioxidant enzymes, including superoxide dismutase and glutathione peroxidase that are expressed in higher quantities than catalase (Shivakumar et al, 1991). This spectrum of enzymatic defense suggests that the brain may efficiently metabolize superoxide, but it may have difficulties in eliminating the hydrogen peroxide produced by this reaction. The accumulation of hydrogen peroxide is of major concern since the brain contains large quantity of iron and copper, which may catalyze the formation of hydroxil radical, which, in turn, can induce lipid peroxidation (Castagne et al, 1999).

The glutathione peroxidase is presented in large amounts during the Central Nervous System (CNS) development, but decreases in aged rats (Nanda et al, 1996). Nevertheless, other scavengers such as ascorbic acid and alpha-tocopherol also decrease the propagation of radical chain reaction. For these reasons, free radicals have been pointed as important molecules involved in the nervous system pathologies such as Huntington disease, Alzheimer, ischaemia and epilepsy (Jenner, 1998).

In epilepsy model induced by pilocarpine administration, we found that superoxide dismutase and catalase activities in the hippocampus are not altered during the acute phase of seizures. On the other hand, according to several authors, the augment of these enzymatic activities could decrease the O_2^- and H_2O_2 levels. Taken together, these results show that during the acute phase, the hippocampus of the adult animals in pilocarpine model after seizures is more vulnerable to oxidative stress.

In addition, high-levels of hydroperoxides were also observed in the same group of animals, which indicated that the lipid peroxidation could be dependent of disability of the antioxidant enzymatic (superoxide dismutase and catalase) activities. As the hydroperoxides are a class of compounds produced as the result of phospholipid peroxidation, its high concentration in the tissue suggests that the hippocampal cells are more vulnerable to damage during the acute period of seizures. Thus, the results described in literature about pilocarpine model suggest that the beneficial effects of antioxidants compounds in reducing the behavioral changes caused by seizures may be partly explained by their ability to remove free radicals, and prevent the formation of hydroperoxides in hippocampus of seized rats.

The need for animal models of epilepsy is driven by the constraints of studying human epileptic brain. Although a great deal has been learned through the study of human epileptic brain tissue throughout the past 100 years, and particularly based in recent experiments with pilocarpine model, our work was aimed at investigating the antioxidant effects of lipoic acid, ubiquinone, ascorbic acid and alpha-tocopherol in adult rats under pilocarpine-induced seizures. Our studies have demonstrated that all animals pretreated with the lipoic acid at the dose (10 or 20 mg/kg) during the first hour of acute phase of seizures induced by pilocarpine injection also manifested behavior alterations, such as peripheral cholinergic signs, tremors, staring spells, facial automatisms, wet dog shakes, rearing and motor seizures, which develop progressively within 1-2 h into a long-lasting status epilepticus. However, these behavioral changes occur at lower rates (Table 1). The findings also suggest that when administered 30 min before pilocarpine, lipoic acid reduces the percentage of animals that seized, increases latency to the first seizure and the survival percentage (Table 1).

Corroborating these data, other antioxidant compound evaluated in pilocarpine model when administered at the dose of 5 mg/kg before pilocarpine, ubiquinone had no effects on seized animals and survival percentage, but increased latency to the first seizure, when compared with the pilocarpine group (Table 1). On the other hand, at a dose of 10 or 20 mg/kg ubiquinone produced a higher reduction of seizures percentage, and a higher increase to that produced by dose of 5 mg/kg in latency to the first seizure and survival rate in pilocarpine model (Table 1).

Drugs	Dose (mg/kg)	Cholinergic Reactions (%)	Latency to first seizure (min)	Seizures (%)	Status epilepticus (%)	Survival rate (%)
Pilocarpine	400	100	35.00 ± 0.70	75	75	40
Ascorbic acid	250	100	80.00 ± 1.30*	33[a]	33[a]	100[a]
	500	100	189.19 ± 1.15*,**	25[a,b]	25[a,b]	100[a,b]
Alpha-tocopherol	200	100	103.00 ± 0.90*	32[a]	32[a]	68[a]
	400	100	158.10 ± 1.05*,**	16[a,b]	16[a,b]	70[a,b]
Ubiquinone	5	100	69.00 ± 0.65*	60[a]	60[a]	60[a]
	10	100	89.00 ± 0.83*,**	35[a,b]	35[a,b]	75[a,b]
Lipoic acid	10	100	106.13 ± 1.05*	00[a]	00[a]	75[a]
	20	100	119.00 ± 1.02*	10[a]	10[a]	90[a]

Rats were acutely treated with the drug doses shown in the table above and 30 min afterwards they received pilocarpine (400 mg/kg). Following, the animals were observed for 24 h for assessment of cholinergic reactions, motor seizures which develop progressively within 1-2 h into a long-lasting status epilepticus and survival rate. Results of latency to first seizure and latency to installation of status epilepticus are expressed in minutes (min) as mean ± S.E.M of the number of experiments shown in the experimental groups and the others in percentages *$p<0.05$, vs pilocarpine. **$p<0.05$ vs lower dose (ANOVA and t-Student Newman Keuls *post hoc* test); [a]$p<0.05$, vs pilocapine. [b]$p<0.05$, vs lower dose (χ^2 test).

Table 1. Effect of pretreatment with antioxidant drugs on behavioral alterations in pilocarpine-induced seizures and lethality in adult rats.

In preclinical practice, the animals pretreated with ascorbic acid (250 mg/kg) in pilocarpine model developed cholinergic reactions, 33% had seizures, 25% built up to status epilepticus and no animal died (Table 1). Ascorbic acid administration, 30 min before pilocarpine injections, increased the latency to the onset of the first seizure in 129% and latency of the status epilepticus in 195% (Table 1). In pilocarpine model, it is also shown that when administered at the smaller dose (200 mg/kg), 30 min before pilocarpine injection, alpha-tocopherol can be decrease by 43% the percentage of animals that seized, increased (194%) latency to the first seizure, and increased survival (41%) (Table 1).

Conversely, a higher dose (500 mg/kg) of the ascorbic acid in pilocarpine model, produced changes in behavior with lower intensity, such as peripheral cholinergic signs (100%), staring spells, facial automatisms, wet dog shakes, rearing and motor seizures (25%) were observed, which progressively developed (1-2 h) into long-lasting status epilepticus (25%), revealing a survival rate of 75% (Table 1). Other studies have revealed that alpha-tocopherol at a dose 400 mg/kg blocks all alterations in behavior, revealing only 16% of motor seizures, which progressively developed (1-2 h) into long-lasting status epilepticus in pilocarpine model and a survival rate of 84% from the seizures (Table 1).

5. Histopathological alterations in epilepsy model

Cholinergic mechanisms play an important role in the activation of limbic seizures, and dopaminergic, serotonergic, GABAergic and glutamatergic systems are responsible for the propagation and/or maintenance of seizures and status epilepticus induced by pilocarpine (Freitas et al, 2004). Previous studies have described a model of limbic seizures followed by brain damage produced by systemic injection of a high dose of pilocarpine in rats. The evidence included temporal correlation among free radical generation, development of seizures and neuroprotective effects of antioxidant drugs against neuronal damage caused by seizures (Kabuto et al, 1998).

Other studies have shown pilocarpine-induced seizures and brain damage in various cerebral regions and a significant hippocampal injury in this epilepsy model (Turski et al, 1991; Curia et al, 2008). The anticonvulsant effect in the absence of anticholinergic drugs subsequent to the seizure onset suggests that muscarinic receptor activation is involved directly in the beginning of seizures by pilocarpine.

However, the oxidative stress might also play an essential role in the production of neuronal damage, which can be justified by neuroprotective actions of antioxidant compounds according to previous studies (Freitas et al, 2004; Xavier et al, 2007; Ayyildiz et al, 2007a). Previous research indicates that anticonvulsant effects of noradrenergic antagonist drugs have a fundamental role in the mechanisms responsible for beginning, severity and duration of seizure. In fact, the reduction of severity and duration of seizures are protective against neurotoxicity caused by seizures induced by chemical convulsants (e.g. pilocarpine, kainic acid and others). These data, in spite of confirming a pivotal role of anticonvulsant drugs in modulating seizure threshold and neuronal death, offer a novel target, which may be used to develop anticonvulsant and neuroprotective agents (Pizzanelli et al, 2009).

There are several indications that free radical plays a role in epileptogenesis. During seizures, the ROS concentration and brain lipid peroxidation increase (Curia et al, 2008). It is currently hypothesized that any pathological process such as status epilepticus, which releases dopamine and glutamate, activates D_2 and NMDA receptors.

This may lead to neuronal necrosis by elevating intracellular calcium and activating potentially destructive calcium-dependent enzymes, augmenting the production of free radicals during seizures induced by pilocarpine (Michotte et al, 1997).

The available experimental data suggest that convulsion generally accelerate brain damage. Limbic status epilepticus causes neuronal necrosis in hippocampus, amygdala, pyriform cortex, entorhinal cortex, thalamus, neocortex, striatum and substantia nigra (Ayyildiz et al, 2007b). The neuronal damage depends on synaptic activation (Vanin et al, 2003), probably via a glutamatergic calcium-medited mechanism (Marinho et al, 1998).

In the epilepsy model induced by a high dose of pilocarpine, we can observe neuronal loss in some brain areas, namely the hippocampus, striatum, amygdala, piriform cortex, entorhinal cortex, lateral septum, thalamus and substantia nigra, suggesting the involvement of these different areas during the establishment of the epileptic process (Honchar et al, 1983; Turski et al, 1983; Clifford et al, 1987; Marinho et al, 1997; Borelli et al, 2002; Freitas et al, 2006).

Among the areas in which neuronal damage occurs, the striatum and fronto-parietal cortex, besides being the most affected areas, may be related in important ways with the mechanism of propagation and/or maintenance (epileptogenesis) limbic seizures (Marinho et al, 1998). Barone and collaborators (1991) demonstrated that through intracerebral administration in the striatum of D_2 dopamine agonists, there was a protection with respect to the development of seizures in adult rats, suggesting the participation of this brain region in limbic seizures.

Histopathological examinations during the acute phase of seizures induced by pilocarpine show extensive hippocampal brain damage, pyriform, entorhinal, frontal, temporal and parietal cortices and in the striatum and amygdaloid nucleus (Marinho et al, 1997).

Cerebral lesions during the acute period are characterized by neuronal loss, gliosis and vacuolation, although there are contradictory data with respect to the severity and relative distribution of brain damage (Mello et al, 1993). Brain necrosis is associated with the occurrence of seizures, although studies have demonstrated that this association is not obligatory, especially in the pilocarpine model (Peredery et al, 1992). The seizures induced by pilocarpine can be blocked by atropine, pointing towards involvement of the cholinergic system. On the other hand, atropine did not act after seizure onset, suggesting that others neurotransmitters and oxidative stress may participate in the maintenance and/or propagation of seizures and brain damage as well (Hirsh et al, 1982). Oxidative stress mediated by free radical produces lipid peroxidation, increases the nitrite content in the hippocampus, striatum and frontal cortex (Freitas et al, 2004) and may play a major role in the neuronal injury development after seizures induced by pilocarpine.

6. Antioxidant compound effects on histopathological alterations in epilepsy model

Hence, it could be expected that antioxidant drugs such as ascorbic acid and alpha-tocopherol, can be used as scavengers of free radicals, reducing brain injury induced by pilocarpine. In previous histopathological analyses, ascorbic acid and alpha-tocopherol antioxidants protected animals against seizures, status epilepticus and brain damage induced by pilocarpine (Figure 1) by decreasing the percentage of seizures, status epilepticus and death in relation to both doses tested.

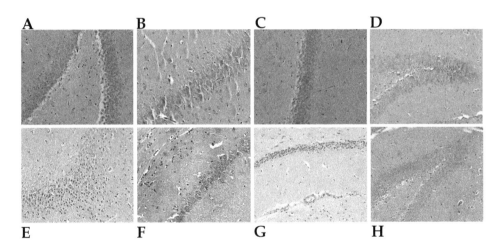

Fig. 1. Histopathological alterations in rat hippocampus treated with pilocarpine, ascorbic acid or their combinations. [A] Control group; [B] Pilocarpine group; [C] ascorbic acid 250 group; [D] ascorbic acid 250 plus Pilocarpine groups was treated with ascorbic acid (250 mg/kg) and 30 min before Pilocarpine; [E] ascorbic acid 500 group; [F] ascorbic acid 500 plus Pilocarpine group was treated with ascorbic acid (500 mg/kg) and 30 min before Pilocarpine. Severity of lesion was expressed as mean ± S.E.M. of scores of damage based in a scale from zero (none) to 100 (total) percent of structural involvement. Brain damage was considered positive if there was at least 50% hippocampal involvement. Hematoxylin & Eosin staining (H&E). Magnification, 100 X. One representative experiment with n=6 is shown.

A variety of epilepsy models reflect the effects of acid ascorbic and alpha-tocopherol and specify their action (Koza et al, 2007; Gaby, 2007). Previously, it had been demonstrated that these compounds reduced the frequency of penicillin-induced epileptiform activity (Ayyildiz et al, 2006; Ayyildiz et al, 2007b). In recent years, many roles of alpha-tocopherol have been discovered, including not only an antioxidant function, but also pro-oxidant, cell signaling, and gene regulatory functions. Some studies have reported that alpha-tocopherol is considered to be the main antioxidant substance in the human body, interfering with the production of hydroxyl radical and also with the oxygen in cell membranes, thereby reducing lipid peroxidation (Barros et al, 2007).

Our results demonstrated that seizure pattern and brain damage observed in pilocarpine-treated animals differ from those pretreated with alpha-tocopherol (400 mg/kg) plus pilocarpine (400 mg/kg). The latter reproduced the syndrome with lower intensity of histopathological changes and mortality rate, in comparison with the alpha-tocopherol (200 mg/kg) plus pilocarpine, corroborating the outcomes obtained by Ribeiro and collaborators (2005) and Ayyildiz and collaborators (2006). The percentage of status epilepticus (75%) that was found further corroborated prior investigations (Clifford et al, 1987; Marinho et al, 1997).

Ascorbic acid is probably the most important water-soluble antioxidant in the brain extracellular fluid, and it is essential in regenerating reduced alpha-tocopherol in membranes (Niki, 1991). Despite the fact that ascorbic acid has an antioxidant role to counter oxidative stress, ascorbic acid also form reactive oxidants, especially in the presence of transition metals. The evidence suggests that ascorbic acid participates in pro-oxidant reactions under certain conditions (Layton et al, 1998).

The outcomes confirm that ascorbic acid (250 or 500 mg/kg) decreased the frequency of pilocarpine-induced seizures, status epilepticus and brain lesions in rats. In addition, ascorbic acid decreases the severity of hippocampal lesions and mortality rate caused by pilocarpine. Yamamoto and collaborators (2002) demonstrated that the injection of ascorbate, 60 min before $FeCl_3$ administration, prevented the occurrence of epileptic discharges. Since there are wide variations of alpha-tocopherol and ascorbic acid doses used in different models of seizure, more detailed investigations are necessary before an ultimate conclusion on the effects of those compounds on pilocarpine-induced seizures can be achieved.

In conclusion, there is an accumulation of free radicals after status epilepticus induced by pilocarpine, and oxidative changes in other parameters during the acute phase. This finding suggests that seizures, status epilepticus and deaths induced by pilocarpine have a large participation in brain oxidative stress, which is closely related to the mechanism of propagation and/or maintenance of the epileptic focus by pilocarpine. These results suggest that free radicals as well as the muscarinic receptor activation seem to be involved in the genesis of seizures and brain damage obtained with pilocarpine. On the other hand, the muscarinic activation seems to play a major role in the neuronal damage produced by pilocarpine. Antioxidant compounds can exert neuroprotective function during acute phase of seizures, thereby decreasing the severity of hippocampal lesions. All these outcomes indicate the promising therapeutic potential of ascorbic acid and alpha-tocopherol in treatments for neurodegenerative diseases.

Brain tissue examinations of the animals pretreated with ascorbic acid (250 or 500 mg/Kg; Figure 1), alpha-tocopherol (200 or 400 mg/kg Figure 2), lipoic acid (10 or 20 mg/kg, Figure 3) or ubiquinone (5 or 10 mg/kg; Figure 4), did not reveal hippocampal and striatal histopathological changes. Then again, pilocarpine-treated animals presented neuronal loss, gliosis, and typical vacuolar degeneration in hippocampus and striatum regions. Histopathological damage in hippocampus was observed in 50, 33, 33 and 17% of the animals co-administered with ascorbic acid (250 or 500 mg/kg) or alpha-tocopherol (200 or 400 mg/kg), and that 30 min after pretreatment received pilocarpine (400 mg/kg), respectively (Table 2). In addition, the analyses of histopathological damage in hippocampus of rats pretreated with lipoic acid (10 or 20 mg/kg) or ubiquinone (5 or 10 mg/kg), and that 30 min after pretreatment received pilocarpine (400 mg/kg) revealed a reduction of 52, 68, 52 and 100% in the number of animals with neuronal damage, respectively (Table 2).

Drugs	Dose (mg/kg)	Rats with lesion (%)	Severity of lesion (%)	Number of animals with lesion per group
Pilocarpine	400	83	59.92 ± 0.23	5
Ascorbic acid	250	00	00	0
	500	00	00	0
Ascorbic acid plus P400	250	50[a]	20.00 ± 0.32[a]	3
	500	33[a,b]	17.66 ± 0.33[a,b]	2
Alpha-tocopherol	200	00	00	0
	400	00	00	0
Alpha-tocopherol plus P400	200	33[a]	13.66 ± 0.33[a]	2
	400	17[a,b]	5.97	1
Ubiquinone	5	00	00	0
	10	00	00	0
Ubiquinone plus P400	5	33[a]	12.00 ± 0.25[a]	2
	10	00	00	0
Lipoic acid	10	00	00	0
	20	00	00	0
Lipoic acid plus P400	10	33[a]	11.96 ± 0.12[a]	2
	20	17[a,b]	5.97	1

Pilocarpine was administered in a single dose (400 mg/kg, P400, n=6), ascorbic acid groups with ascorbic acid (250 or 500 mg/kg), alpha-tocopherol (200 or 400 mg/kg, n=6), ubiquinone (5 or 10 mg/kg, n=6) and lipoic acid group with lipoic acid (10 or 20 mg/kg; n=6). The ascorbic plus P400 groups were treated with ascorbic acid (250 or 500 mg/kg, n=6) and 30 min before P400. The alpha-tocopherol plus P400 group was treated with alpha-tocopherol (200 or 400 mg/kg) and 30 min before P400. The ubiquinone plus P400 group was treated with ubiquinone (5 or 10 mg/kg) and 30 min before P400. The lipoic acid plus P400 group was treated with lipoic acid (10 or 20 mg/kg) and 30 min before P400. Severity of lesion was expressed as mean ± S.E.M. of scores of damage based on a scale from zero (none) to 100 (total) percent of structural involvement. Brain damage was defined as present if there was at least 50% hippocampal involvement. Results for % rats with brain lesion and % severity of lesion are expressed as percentages of the number of animals inside in parenthesis. [a]$p<0.05$ compared with P400 group (χ^2 test). [b]$p<0.05$ compared with ascorbic acid 250 plus P400 group or alpha-tocopherol 200 mg/kg plus P400 group or ubiquinone 5 mg/kg plus P400 group or lipoic acid 10 mg/kg plus P400 group (χ^2 test).

Table 2. Histopathological alterations in hippocampus of rats pretreated with antioxidant compounds after 24 h of phase acute of pilocarpine-induced seizures.

Histopathological damage in striatum was observed only in 33, 17, 17 and 17% of the animals co-administered with ascorbic acid (250 or 500 mg/kg), ubiquinone (5 mg/kg) and lipoic acid (10 mg/kg) and that 30 min after pretreatment received pilocarpine (400 mg/kg), respectively (Table 2). Moreover, the analyses of histopathological damage in striatum of rats pretreated with lipoic acid (20 mg/kg), alpha-tocopherol (200 or 400 mg/kg) or ubiquinone (10 mg/kg), and that 30 min after pretreatment received pilocarpine (400 mg/kg) revealed no neuronal damage (Table 2).

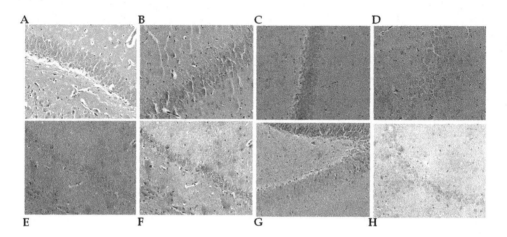

Fig. 2. Histopathological alterations in rat hippocampus treated with pilocarpine, atropine, alpha-tocopherol or their combinations. [A] Control group; [B] Pilocarpine group; [C] alpha-tocopherol 200 group; [D] alpha-tocopherol 200 plus Pilocarpine group was treated with alpha-tocopherol (200 mg/kg) and 30 min before P400; [E] alpha-tocopherol 400 group; [F] alpha-tocopherol 400 plus Pilocarpine group was treated with alpha-tocopherol (400 mg/kg) and 30 min before Pilocarpine. Severity of lesion was expressed as mean ± S.E.M. of scores of damage based in a scale from zero (none) to 100 (total) percent of structural involvement. Brain damage was considered positive if there was at least 50% hippocampal involvement. Hematoxylin & Eosin staining (H&E). Magnification, 100 X. One representative experiment with n=6 is shown.

7. Oxidative stress in epilepsy model

The lipid peroxidation level in the brain homogenates are increased in this model. During the acute phase of seizures induced by pilocarpine, increases in lipid peroxidation level, nitrite concentration and GSH content in striatum, frontal cortex and hippocampus have been verified in the same way (Freitas et al, 2004). The improved review demonstrates that status epilepticus induces different changes in superoxide dismutase activity according to the brain region, as that enzymatic activity remained unaltered in striatum and hippocampus but increased in frontal cortex. After the first hour of acute phase of seizures an increase is detected in several regions (striatum, hippocampus and frontal cortex). In addition, catalase activity was increased in striatum, hippocampus and frontal cortex in this epilepsy model (Freitas et al, 2003).

Drugs	Dose (mg/kg)	Rats with lesion (%)	Severity of lesion (%)	Number of animals with lesion per group
Pilocarpine	400	67	55.39 ± 0.52	4
Ascorbic acid	250	00	00	0
	500	00	00	0
Ascorbic acid plus P400	250	33[a]	25.42 ± 0.25[a]	2
	500	17[a,b]	13.46	1
Alpha-tocopherol	200	00	00	0
	400	00	00	0
Alpha-tocopherol plus P400	200	00	00	0
	400	00	00	0
Ubiquinone	5	00	00	0
	10	00	00	0
Ubiquinone plus P400	5	17[a]	14.31	1
	10	00	00	0
Lipoic acid	10	00	00	0
	20	00	00	0
Lipoic acid plus P400	10	17[a]	12.96 ± 0.22[a]	1
	20	00	00	0

Pilocarpine was administered in a single dose (400 mg/kg, P400, n=6), ascorbic acid groups with ascorbic acid (250 or 500 mg/kg), alpha-tocopherol (200 or 400 mg/kg, n=6), ubiquinone (5 or 10 mg/kg, n=6) and lipoic acid group with lipoic acid (10 or 20 mg/kg; n=6). The ascorbic plus P400 groups were treated with ascorbic acid (250 or 500 mg/kg, n=6) and 30 min before P400. The alpha-tocopherol plus P400 group was treated with alpha-tocopherol (200 or 400 mg/kg) and 30 min before P400. The ubiquinone plus P400 group was treated with ubiquinone (5 or 10 mg/kg) and 30 min before P400. The lipoic acid plus P400 group was treated with lipoic acid (10 or 20 mg/kg) and 30 min before P400. Severity of lesion was expressed as mean ± S.E.M. of scores of damage based on a scale from zero (none) to 100 (total) percent of structural involvement. Brain damage was defined as present if there was at least 50% straital involvement. Results for % rats with brain lesion and % severity of lesion are expressed as percentages of the number of animals inside in parenthesis. [a]$p<0.05$ compared with P400 group (χ^2 test). [b]$p<0.05$ compared with ascorbic acid 250 plus P400 group or alpha-tocopherol 200 mg/kg plus P400 group or ubiquinone 5 mg/kg plus P400 group or lipoic acid 10 mg/kg plus P400 group (χ^2 test).

Table 3. Histopathological alterations in striatum of rats pretreated with antioxidant compounds after 24 h of phase acute of pilocarpine-induced seizures.

Lipid peroxidation in a tissue is an index of irreversible biological damage of the cell membrane phospholipid, which in turn leads to inhibition of most of the sulphydryl and some nonsulphydryl enzymes (Gilbert and Sawas, 1983). Lipid peroxidation level increase and reduce, whereas glutathione decrease can be induced by many chemicals (e.g. kainic acid and pilocarpine) and by many tissue injuries, and has been suggested as a possible mechanism for the neurotoxic effects of epileptic activity (Sah et al, 2002). Our findings demonstrated that lipid peroxidation levels increase after the first hour and during 24 h of the acute phase of seizures induced by pilocarpine in hippocampus, striatum and frontal cortex.

In normal conditions, there is a steady state balance between the production of ROS and their destruction by cellular antioxidant system. It is demonstrated that nitrite content in striatum and frontal cortex is augmented after seizures and status epilepticus in adult rats, suggesting a possible increase in ROS level, which can be involved in neuronal damage induced status epilepticus. Other studies have shown that nitrite and nitrate levels were not elevated in patients with cryptogenic west syndrome (Vanhatalo and Riikonen, 2001), but it is tempting to speculate that the seizure activity per se did not account for the whole increment observed in nitrite and nitrate levels, and other mechanisms may be associated with this parameter in this epilepsy model, as well as neuronal degeneration observed in human beings. However, new studies using antioxidants drugs during status epilepticus induced by pilocarpine can indicate whether lipid peroxidation, nitrite and glutathione reduced (GSH) concentrations are involved in the pathophysiology of status epilepticus in this model.

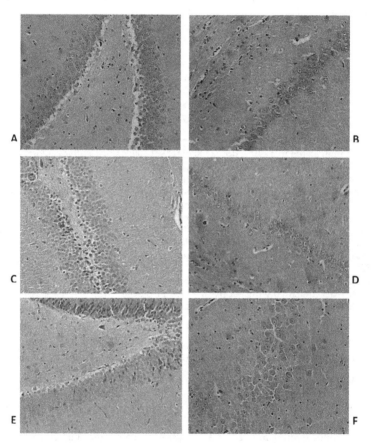

Fig. 3. Histopathological alterations in rat hippocampus pretreated with lipoic acid prior to pilocarpine-induced seizures. Severity of lesion was expressed as a mean ± S.E.M. of scores of damage based in a scale from zero (none) to 100 (total) percentage of hippocampus involvement. Brain damage was considered positive if there was at least 50% hippocampal involvement showed by Hematoxylin & Eosin staining (HE). Pictures (100 X) shown are from one representative experiment of n=8. [A]: Control group; [B]: Pilocarpine group; [C]: lipoic acid 10 group; [D]: lipoic acid 10 plus pilocarpine group; [E]: lipoic acid 20 group; [F]: lipoic acid 20 plus pilocarpine group.

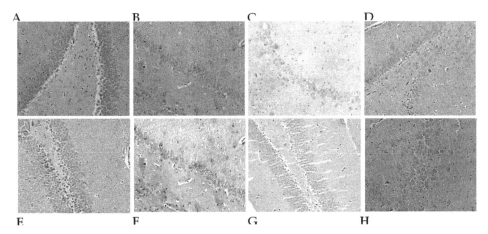

Fig. 4. Histopathological alterations in rat hippocampus pretreated with ubiquinone prior to pilocarpine-induced seizures. Severity of lesion was expressed as a mean ± S.E.M. of scores of damage based in a scale from zero (none) to 100 (total) percentage of hippocampus involvement. Brain damage was considered positive if there was at least 50% hippocampal involvement showed by Hematoxylin & Eosin staining (HE). Pictures (100 X) shown are from one representative experiment of n=8. [A]: Control group; [B]: Pilocarpine group; [C]: Ubiquinone 5 group; [D]: Ubiquinone 10 group; [E]: Ubiquinone 20 group; [F]: Ubiquinone 5 plus P400 group [G]: Ubiquinone 10 plus P400; [H]: Ubiquinone 20 plus P400.

Although there were no selective brain regions particularly vulnerable to oxidative stress, there were some regional variations in the amount of oxidative damage observed. In the regions studied, there were nearly equal elevations in lipid oxidative, nitrite content and GSH markers that persisted during the acute phase of seizures.

All living organisms can suffer oxidative damage, yet the animal brain is often said to be especially sensitive (Gilbert and Sawas, 1983; Bruce and Baudry, 1995). The experimental data demonstrate that pilocarpine administration and its resulting status epilepticus produce significant alterations in hippocampus, striatum and frontal cortex. We recorded alterations in superoxide dismutase activity in frontal cortex during the seizures, however, no alterations were observed in striatal superoxide dismutase activity of rats under the same conditions. It is likely that the unaltered superoxide dismutase activity in striatum might not be related to the mechanisms involved in installation and propagation of seizures and status epilepticus induced by pilocarpine, which produces several changes in parameters related to generation and elimination of oxygen free radicals in adult rats (Sawas and Gilbert, 1985). An increase in free radical formation can be accompanied by an immediate compensatory increase of free radical scavenging enzymatic (superoxide dismutase and catalase) activities and this action was observed during status epilepticus in brain regions. Nevertheless, a similar compensatory mechanism of scavenging was observed in catalase activity after status epilepticus, suggesting that the enzymatic function of different systems can be modified either during the acute phase of seizures or according to cerebral area investigated. Literature reports the involvement of catalase activity in hippocampus, striatum and frontal cortex after status epilepticus. An increase in catalase activity in these brain areas can be related to a long-term compensatory mechanism including modulation activity of enzymes from the ROS catabolism.

Moreover, the catalase activity might be one of the mechanisms capable to avoid the development of neurotoxic effects mediated by SE, indicating that basal-oxygen radical production can damage the cell and that its control is necessary (McCord, 1989; Naffah-Mazzacoratti, 2001).

Evidences for the role of free radicals in seizures has been found by using exogenously administered enzymatic and non-enzymatic antioxidants for protection against seizures and status epilepticus-induced neuronal damage (Kulkarni and George, 1996; Freitas et al, 2005). A steady state level of O_2^- and H_2O_2 is always present within cells as a result of a normal metabolism. Superoxide dismutase and catalase are responsible for degradation of O_2^- and H_2O_2, respectively. The balance between antioxidants enzymes, superoxide dismutase and catalase can be important during seizures and status epilepticus induced by pilocarpine. The present data indicate that pilocarpine treatment and its resulting status epilepticus induce neurochemical changes such as an increase in nitrite content and lipid peroxidation level, a decrease in GSH content as well as an activation of brain antioxidant mechanisms. The anatomic distribution of alterations observed in the enzymatic activities (superoxide dismutase and catalase) can suggest that the frontal cortex can be extensively involved in the propagation of epileptic activity and further studies should be carried out to ascertain that the catabolism of nitrite, ROS and GSH can be involved in the pathogenesis of status epilepticus.

The pilocarpine model is essential to investigate the mechanisms for initiation and propagation of seizures and status epilepticus. Additionally, it may be assumed that the increased generation of nitrite and lipid peroxidation levels after status epilepticus is not primary caused by an exhaustion of both the enzymatic and non-enzymatic defense systems measured. Adaptative mechanisms, as the induction of catalase activity, may be taken into consideration to counteract oxidative stress mediated by status epilepticus. However, the relation among brain structures, antioxidant systems, lipid peroxidation, nitrite concentration and status epilepticus cannot be perfectly established and deserves further investigation.

8. Antioxidant compound effects on oxidative stress in epilepsy model

Neurochemical alterations are observed in pilocarpine-induced seizures (Freitas et al, 2005), whose physiopathology is still poorly understood. However, there is data in literature suggesting that elevated reactive oxygen species concentrations and/or its metabolites are potentially neurotoxic (Freitas et al, 2004). We have demonstrated that lipoic acid reduces brain oxidative metabolism (Militão et al, 2010) and cannot inhibit Na^+, K^+-ATPase activity in rat hippocampus.

Animal models are useful to better understand the pathophysiology of seizures. In this context, the antioxidants compound effects in pilocarpine model were recently investigated (Mudd et al, 2001), revealing that they might produce a decrease in nitrite levels in rat hippocampus (Koçak et al, 2000; Augoustides-Savvopoulou et al, 2003). Animals exposed to lipoic acid treatment presented no differences in physical growth and brain, suggesting that lipoic acid ameliorates metabolic parameters in pilocarpine model (Mesulam et al, 2002).

By using this model, we investigated the effect of lipoic acid on spatial navigation tasks in the Morris water maze. Results have shown that seized rats did not present performance impairment neither in the acquisition phase nor on the time spent in target quadrant and in platform location nor in the latency to cross over the platform location in the reference memory task session . However, lipoic acid significantly impaired working memory performance, since there was a significant effect with the 9-day interaction group and significant differences after days 2 and 5.

The biological effects of free radicals are controlled in vivo by a wide range of antioxidants, such as alpha-tocopherol, ascorbic acid, vitamin A, and glutathione reduced (Halliwell and Gutteridge, 1990; Ayyildiz et al, 2006). Acid ascorbic and alpha-tocopherol have many functions in the brain and in the neuronal microenvironment. They work as neuromodulators as well as antioxidant/free radical scavengers (Koza et al, 2007; Devi et al, 2008). It has been suggested that ascorbic acid and alpha-tocopherol have neuroprotective properties in some experimental models of excitotoxic neurological disorders, including seizure activity induced by pilocarpine (Gaby, 2007; Barros et al., 2007).

Systemic injection of pilocarpine, a cholinergic muscarinic agonist, induces status epilepticus in rodents, which is associated to histopathological and neurochemical changes as well as oxidative stress (Turski et al, 1983; Cavalheiro et al, 1994; Freitas et al, 2005). Elevated free radical products were observed during the status epilepticus. Free radicals are highly reactive chemical compounds due to the tendency of electrons to pair, which are normally associated with oxidative damage (Castagne et al, 1999).

Free radicals can be generated in the brain by several mechanisms such as inefficiency of the electron-carrying components of the mitochondrial transport chain, monoamines degradation, xanthine oxidase reaction or by metabolism of arachidonic acid. Nevertheless, the free radicals produced could be metabolized especially by antioxidant enzymes such as superoxide dismutases, catalase and glutathione peroxidase (Hussain et al, 1995; Meister, 1995; Frantseva et al, 2000; Ferreira et al, 2009). Then, the resulting free radicals are very likely to react with non-radical molecules and transform them into secondary free radicals, which are normally observed during the lipid peroxidation producing hydroperoxides (MacDonald et al, 1989). The lipid peroxidation and nitrite are increased in hippocampus rats during pilocarpine-induced seizures (Freitas, 2009; Militão et al, 2010). Thus, it is worthwhile assessing the role of antioxidant compounds in the prevention of these neurochemical alterations on oxidative stress during seizures.

The excitotoxicity has been shown to be related to over-production of free radicals in hippocampus of adult rats. The excessive release of excitatory amino acids such as glutamate may kill neurons via excessive activation of their receptors facilitating the installation and/or propagation of seizures (MacDonald et al., 1989; Cavalheiro et al., 1994; Meldrum, 1994).

Depending on neuronal maturity, the glutamate may induce either apoptotic or necrotic types of death (Ferrer et al, 1995) by impairing the Ca^{2+} homeostasis and inducting the oxidative stress (Leite et al, 1990; Murphy and Baraban, 1990). Based on this fact, it is important to evaluate the role of ubiquinone on oxidative stress in rat hippocampus during seizures since ubiquinone is a powerful antioxidant that prevents oxidative damage caused by free radicals, including oxidation of lipids within the mitochondrial membrane (Geromel et al., 2002).

Several antioxidant compounds, such as acid ascorbic (Xavier et al, 2007), lipoic acid (Freitas, 2009) and alpha-tocopherol (Barros et al, 2007) can protect the brain against oxidative stress in rat hippocampus caused by pilocarpine-induced seizures. Studies have suggested that ubiquinone (UQ) serves as an antioxidant by activating and increasing expression of mitochondrial uncoupling proteins which have antiapoptotic and antioxidant properties (Shults and Haas, 2005; Chaturvedi and Beal, 2008). Ubiquinol, a reduced form of ubiquinone, decreases lipid peroxidation directly by acting as a chain-breaking antioxidant

and indirectly by recycling alpha-tocopherol. Thus, it is important to investigate the neuroprotective effect of ubiquinone against hippocampal damage caused by oxidative stress observed during seizures.
In addition to preventing lipid peroxidation, UQ, as an effective antioxidant, also reacts with ROS (James et al., 2004). This study implies that ubiquinone may alter the oxidative stress in rat hippocampus caused by the seizures. To further attest this hypothesis, this study was aimed at evaluating the effects of ubiquinone on superoxide dismutase, catalase and glutathione peroxidase activities as well as in hydroperoxide concentration in the rat hippocampus during acute phase of seizures induced by pilocarpine.
The pilocarpine model could prove to be useful to delineate and understand the development of behavioral and neurochemical changes associated with temporal lobe epilepsy. Pilocarpine status may provide a model for studying the basic mechanisms responsible for refractory status epilepticus, amino acids and oxidative stress in humans and evaluating new drugs. The pilocarpine model may prove useful in the study of status epilepticus for number of reasons. First, these seizures accurately model human generalized epilepsy as it is seen from the anticonvulsant profile drugs. Secondly, the serve and refractory nature of this model indicates that it should be valuable in the development of new anticonvulsant agents. Finally, the prolonged and uniform degree of status epilepticus is useful for metabolic, neurochemical and neuroanatomical studies of the sequelae of prolonged seizure activity.

9. Acknowledgments

This work was supported by a research grant from the Brazilian National Research Council (CNPq). R.M.F. is fellow from CNPq. The technical assistance of Stênio Gardel Maia is gratefully acknowledged.

10. References

Aminoff, M.J. & Simon, R.P. (1980). Status epilepticus. Causes, clinical features and consequences in 98 patients, *The American Journal of Medicine* 12: 657-666.

Ayyildiz, M., Yildirim, M., & Agar, E. (2006). The effects of vitamin E on penicilin-induced epileptiform activity in rats, *Experimental Brain Research* 174: 109-113.

Ayyildiz, M., Coskun, S., Yildirim, M. & Agar, E. (2007a). The involvement of nitric oxide in the anticonvulsant effects of α-tocopherol on penicillin-induced epileptiform activity in rats, *Epilepsy Research* 73: 166-172.

Ayyildiz, M., Coskun, S., Yildirim, M. & Agar E. (2007b). The effects of ascorbic acid on penicillin-induced epileptiform activity in rats, *Epilepsia* 48: 1388-1395.

Augoustides-Savvopoulou, P., Luka, Z., Karyda, S., Stabler, S.P., Allen, R.H., Patsiaoura, K., Wagner, C. & Mudd, S.H. (2003). Glycine N-methyltransferase deficiency: a new patient with a novel mutation, *Journal of Inherited Metabolic Disease* 26: 745–759

Barone, P., Palma, V., Debartolomeis, A., Tedeschi, E., Muscettola, G. & Campanella, G. 1991. Dopamine D_1 and D_2 receptors mediate opposite functions in seizures induced by lithium-pilocarpine, *European Journal of Pharmacology* 95: 157-162.

Barros, D.O., Xavier, S.M.L., Barbosa, C.O., Silva, R.F., Maia, F.D., Oliveira, A.A. & Freitas, R.M. (2007). Effects of the vitamin E in catalase activities in hippocampus after status epilepticus induced by pilocarpine in Wistar rats, *Neuroscience Letters* 416: 227-230.

Ben-Ari, Y., Tremblay, E. & Ottersen, O.P. (1980). Injections of kainic acid into the amygdaloid complex of the rat: an electrographic, clinical and histological study in relation to the pathology of epilepsy, *Neuroscience* 5: 515-528.

Ben-Ari, Y., Tremblay, E., Riche, D., Ghilini, G. & Naquet, R. (1981). Electrographic, clinical and pathological alterations following systemic administration of kainic acid, bicuculdeoxyglucose or pentylenetetrazole: metabolite mapping using the deoxyglucose method with special reference to the pathology of epilepsy, *Neuroscience* 6: 1361-1391.

Borelli, E. & Bozzi, Y. (2002). Dopamine D_2 receptor signaling controls neuronal cell death induced by muscarinic and glutamtergic drugs, *Molecular and Cellular Neuroscience* 19: 263-271.

Brozek, G., Hort, J., Komarek, V., Langmeier, M. & Mares, P. (2000). Interstrain differences in cognitive functions in rats in relation to status epilepticus, *Behavioural Brain Research* 112: 77–83.

Browne, T.R. & Holmes, G.L. (2001). Epilepsy, *New Jersey Med.* 344: 1145–1451.

Bruce, A.J. & Baudry, M. (1995). Oxygen free radicals in rat limbic structures after kainate-induced seizures, *Free Radical Biology and Medicine* 18: 993-1002.

Castagne, V., Gastschi, M., Lefevre, K., Posada, A. & Clarke, P.G.H. (1999). Relationship between neuronal death and cellular redox status, focus on the developing nervous system, *Progress in Neurobiology* 59: 397–423.

Cavalheiro, E.A., Leite, J.P., Bortolotto, Z.A., Turski, W.A., Ikonomidou, C. & Turski, L. (1991). Long-term effects of pilocarpine in rats: structural damage of the brain triggers kindling and spontaneous recurrent seizures, *Epilepsia* 32: 778-782.

Cavalheiro, E.A., Fernandes, M.J., Turski, L. & Naffah-Mazzacoratti, M.G. (1994). Spontaneous recurrent seizures in rats: amino acid and monoamine determination in the hippocampus, *Epilepsia* 35: 1-11.

Chamberlain, M., Johnson, M.P. & Kelly G.M. (2000). Blockade of pilocarpine-induced cerebellar phosphoinositide hydrolysis with metabotropic glutamate antagonists: evidence for an indirect control of granulle cell glutamate release by muscarinic agonists, *Neuroscience Letters* 285: 71-75.

Chaturvedi, R.K. & Beal, M.F. (2008). Mitochondrial approaches for neuroprotection, *Annals of the New York Academy of Sciences* 1147: 395–412.

Clifford, D.B., Olney, J.W., Maniotis, A., Collins, R.C. & Zorumski, C.F. (1987). The functional anatomy and pathology of lithium-pilocarpine and high-dose pilocarpine seizures, *Neuroscience* 23: 953-968.

Costa Junior, J.S., Feitosa, C.M., Cito, A.M.G.L., Freitas, R.M., Henriques, J.A.P. & Saffi, J. (2010). Evaluation of Effects of Ethanolic Extract from *Platonia insignis* Mart. on Pilocarpine-induced Seizures, *Journal of Biological Sciences* 10: 747-753.

Costa-Lotufo, L.V., Fonteles, M.M.F., Lima, I.S.P., Oliveira, A.A., Nascimento, V.S., Bruin, V.M.S. & Viana, G.S.B. (2002). Attenuating effects of melatonin on pilocarpine-induced seizures in rats, *Comparative Biochemistry and Physiology Part C* 131: 521-529.

Curia, G., Longo, D., Biagini, G., Jones, R.S.G. & Avoli, M. (2008). The pilocarpine model of temporal lobe epilepsy, *Journal of Neuroscience Methods* 172: 143-157.

Dal-Pizzol, F., Klant, F., Vianna, M.M., Schroder, N., Quevedo, J., Benfato, M.S., Moreira, J.C. & Walz, R. (2000). Lipid peroxidation in hippocampus early and late after status epilepticus induced by pilocarpina of kainic acid in Wistar rats, Neuroscience Letters 291: 179-182.

Devi, P.U., Manocha, A. & Vohora, D. (2008). Seizures, antiepileptics, antioxidants and oxidative stress: an insight for researchers, *Expert Opinion on Pharmacotherapy* 9: 3169-3177.

El-Etri, M.M., Ennis, M., Jiang, M. & Shipley, M.T. (1993). Pilocarpine-induced convulsions in rats: evidence for muscarinic receptor-mediated activation of locus coeruleus and norepinephrine release in cholinolytic seizure development, *Experimental Neurology* 121: 24- 39.

Ferrer, I., Martin, F., Reiriz, J., Perez-Navarro, E., Alberch, J., Macaya, A. & Planas, A.M. (1995). Both apoptosis and necrosis occur following intrastriatal administration of excitotoxins, *Acta Neuropathologica* 90: 504–510.

Ferrer, I., Lopez, E., Blanco, R., Rivera, R., Krupinski, J. & Marti, E. (2000). Differential c-Fos and caspase expression following kainic acid excitotoxicity, *Acta Neuropathologica* 99: 245-256.

Ferreira, P.M.P., Militão, G.C.G. & Freitas, R.M. (2009). Lipoic acid effects on lipid peroxidation level, superoxide dismutase activity and monoamines concentration in rat hippocampus, *Neuroscience letters* 464: 131-134.

Frantseva, M.V., Perez, V.J.L., Hwang, P.A. & Carlen, P.L. (2000). Free radical production correlates with cell death in an in vitro model of epilepsy, *European Journal of Neuroscience* 12: 1431–1439.

Freitas, R.M., Sousa, F.C.F., Vasconcelos, S.M.M., Viana, G.S.B. & Fonteles, M.M.F. (2003). Acute alterations of neurotransmitters levels in striatum of young rat after pilocarpine-induced status epilepticus, *Arquivos de Neuropsiquiatria* 61: 430-433.

Freitas, R.M., Sousa, F.C.F., Vasconcelos, S.M.M., Viana, G.S.B. & Fonteles, M.M.F. (2004). Pilocarpine-induced seizures in adult rats: lipid peroxidation level, nitrite formation, GABAergic and glutamatergic receptor alterations in the hippocampus, striatum and frontal cortex, *Pharmacology Biochemistry and Behavior* 78: 327-332.

Freitas, R.M., Aguiar, L.M.V., Vasconcelos, S.M.M., Sousa, F.C.F., Viana, G.S.B. & Fonteles, M.M.F. (2005). Modifications in muscarinic, dopaminergic and serotonergic receptors concentrations in the hippocampus and striatum of epileptic rats, *Life Sciences* 78: 253-258.

Freitas, R.M., Sousa, F.C.F., Viana, G.S.B. & Fonteles, M.M.F. (2006). Acetylcholinesterase activities in hippocampus, frontal cortex and striatum of Wistar rats after pilocarpine-induced status epilepticus, *Neuroscience Letters* 399: 76-78.

Freitas, R.M. (2009). The evaluation of effects of lipoic acid on the lipid peroxidation, nitrite formation and antioxidant enzymes in the hippocampus of rats after pilocarpine-induced seizures, *Neuroscience letters* 455: 140–144.

Freitas, R.M., Jordan, J. & Feng D. (2010). Lipoic acid effects on monoaminergic system after pilocarpine-induced seizures, *Neuroscience Letters* 477: 129-133.

Gaby, A.R. (2007). Natural approaches to epilepsy, *Alternative Medicine Review* 12: 9-24.

Geromel, V., Rotig, A., Munnich, A. & Rustin, P. (2002). Coenzyme Q10 depletion is comparatively less detrimental to human cultured skin fibroblasts than respiratory chain complex deficiencies, *Free Radical Research* 36: 375–379.

Gilbert, J.C. & Sawas, A.H. (1983). ATPase activities and lipid peroxidation in rat cerebral cortex synaptosomes, *Archives internationales de pharmacodynamie et de thérapie* 263: 189-196.

Halliwell, B. & Gutteridge, J.M.C. (1990). The antioxidants of human extracellular fluids, *Archives of Biochemistry and Biophysics* 280: 1-8.

Halliwell, B. & Gutteridge, J.M.C. (1999). Free radicals in biology and medicine, Oxford Science Publications, London.

Hirsh, E., Baran, T.Z. & Snead, O.C. (1982). Ontogenic study of lithium-pilocarpine induced status epilepticus in rats, *Brain Research* 583: 120-126.

Honchar, M.P., Olney, J.W. & Sherman, W.R. (1983). Systemic cholinergic agents induce seizures and brain damage in lithium-treated rats, *Science* 220: 323-325.

Hort, J., Brozek, G., Komárek, V., Langmeier, M. & Mares, P. (2000). Interstrain differences in cognitive functions in rats in relation to status epilepticus, *Behavioral Brain Research* 112: 77-83.

Hussain, S., Slikker, W. & Ali, S.F. (1995). Age-related changes in antioxidant enzymes, superoxide dismutase, catalase, glutathione peroxidase and glutathione in different regions of mouse brain, *International Journal of Developmental Neuroscience* 13: 811-817.

James, A.M., Smith, R.A. & Murphy, M.P. (2004). Antioxidant and prooxidant properties of mitochondrial coenzyme Q, *Archives of Biochemistry and Biophysics* 423: 47-56.

Jenner, P. (1998). Oxidative mechanisms in nigral cell death in Parkinson's disease, *Movement Disorders* 13: 24-34.

Kabuto, H, Yokoi, I. & Ogawa, N. (1998). Melatonin inhibits iron-induced epileptic discharges in rats by suppressing peroxidation, Epilepsia 30: 237-243.

Koçak, G., Aktan, F., Canbolat, O., Ozogul, C., Elbeg, S., Yildizoglu-Ari, N. & Karasu, C. (2000) Alpha-lipoic acid treatment ameliorates metabolic parameters, blood pressure, vascular reactivity and morphology of vessels already damaged by streptozotocin-diabetes, *Diabetes, Nutrition & Metabolism* 13: 308-318.

Kozan, R., Ayyildiz, M., Bas, O., Kaplan, S. & Agar, E. (2007). The influence of ethanol intake and its withdrawal on the anticonvulsant effect of α-tocopherol in the penicillin-induced pileptiform activity in rats, *Neurotoxicology* 28: 463-470.

Krug, M.; Brodemann, R. & Ott, T. (1981). Identical responses of the two hippocampal theta generators to physiological and pharmacological activation, *Brain Research Bulletin* 6: 5-11.

Kulkarni, S.K. & George, B. (1996). Protective effects of GABAergic drugs and other anticovulsivants in lithium-pilocarpine-induced status epilepticus, *Methods & Findings in Experimental & Clinical Pharmacology* 18: 335-340.

Lapin, I.P., Mirzaev, S.M., Ryzov, I.V. & Oxenkrug, G.F. (1998). Anticonvulsant activity of melatonin against seizures induced by quinolinate, kainite, glutamate, NMDA, and pentylenetetrazole in mice, *Journal of Pineal Research* 24: 215-218.

Layton, M.E., Samson, F.E. & Pazdernik, T.L. (1998). Kainic acid causes redox changes in cerebral cortex extracellular fluid: NMDA receptor activity increases ascorbic acid whereas seizure activity increases uric acid, *Neuropharmacology* 37: 149-157.

Leite, J.P., Bortolotto, Z.A. & Cavalheiro, E.A., 1990. Spontaneous recurrent seizures in rats: an experimental model of partial epilepsy, *Neuroscience & Biobehavioral Reviews* 14: 511-517.

Liu, K.J.; Liu, S.; Morrow, D. & Peterson S.L. (2002). Hydroethidine detection of superoxide production during the lithium-pilocarpine model of status epilepticus, *Epilepsy Research* 49: 226-238.

Loup, F., Fritschy, J.M., Kiener, T. & Bouilleret, V. (1999). GABAergic neurons and GABA$_A$-receptors in temporal lobe epilepsy, *Neurochemistry International* 34: 435-445.

MacDonald, J.F., Mody, I. & Salter, M.W. (1989). Regulation of N-metyl-D-aspartate receptor revealed by intracellular dialysis of murine neurones in culture, *The Journal of Physiology* 414: 17-34.

MacGregor, D.G., Graham, D.I. & Stone, T.W. (1997). The attenuation of kainate-induced neurotoxicity by chlormethiazole and its enhancement by dizocilpine, muscimol, and adenosine receptor agonists, *Experimental Neurology* 148: 110-123.

Marinho, M.M.F., Sousa, F.C.F., Bruin, V.M.S., Aguiar, L.M.V., Pinho, R.S.N. & Viana, G.S.B. (1997). Inhibitory action of a calcium channel blocker (nimodipine) on seizures and brain damage induced by pilocarpine and lithium-pilocarpine in rats, *Neuroscience Letters* 235: 13-16.

Marinho, M.M.F., Sousa, F.C.F., Bruin, V.M.S., Vale, M.R. & Viana, G.S.B. (1998). Effects of lithium, alone or associated with pilocarpine, on muscarinic and dopaminergic receptors and on phosphoinositide metabolism in rat hippocampus and striatum, *Neurochemisty International* 33: 299-306.

Massieu, L., Rivera, A. & Tapia, R. (1994). Convulsions and inhibition of glutamate decarboxylase by pyridoxal phosphate-γ-glutamyl hydrazone in the developing rat, *Neurochemical Research* 19: 183-187.

McCord, J.M. (1989). Superoxide radical: controversies, contradiction and paradoxes, Proceedings of the Society for Experimental Biology and Medicine 209: 112-117.

Meister, A. (1995). Glutathione biosynthesis and its inhibition, *Methods in Enzymology* 252: 26-30.

Meldrum, B.S. (1994). The role of glutamate in epilepsy and other CNS disorders, *Neurology* 44: 14-23.

Mello, L.E.A.M., Cavalheiro, E.A., Tan, A.M., Kupfer, W. R., Pretorius, J.K., Babb, T.L. & Finch, D.M. (1993). Circuit Mechanisms of Seizures in the Pilocarpine Model of Chronic Epilepsy: Cell Loss and Mossy Fiber Sprouting, *Epilepsia* 34: 985-995.

Mesulam, M-M., Guillozet, A., Shaw, P., Levey, A., Duysen, E.G. & Lockridge, O. (2002) Acetylcholinesterase knockouts establish central cholinergic pathways and can use butyrylcholinesterase to hydrolyze acetylcholine, *Neuroscience* 170: 627-639.

Michiels, C., Raes, M., Toussaint, O. & Remacle, J. (1994). Importance of Se-glutathione peroxidase, catalase, and Cu/Zn-SOD for cell survival against oxidative stress, *Free Radical Biology & Medicine* 17: 235-248.

Michotte, Y., Ebinger, G., Manil, J., Khan, G.M. & Smolders, I. (1997). NMDA receptor-mediated pilocarpine-induced seizures: characterization in freely moving rats by microdialysis, *British Journal of Pharmacology* 121: 1171-1179.

Militão, G.C.G., Ferreira, P.M.P. & Freitas, R.M. (2010) Effects of lipoic acid on oxidative stress in rat striatum after pilocarpine-induced seizures, *Neurochemistry International* 56: 16-20.

Mudd, S.H., Levy, H.L. & Kraus, J.P. (2001). Disorders of trans sulfuration. In: Scriver CR, Beaudet AL, Sly WS, Valle D (eds) The metabolic and molecular bases of inherited disease, 8 th edn. McGraw-Hill, New York, pp 2007-2056.

Murphy, T.H. & Baraban, J.M. (1990). Glutamate toxicity in immature cortical neurons precedes development of glutamate receptor current, *Developmental Brain Research* 57: 146–150.

Naffah-Mazzacoratti, M.G., Cavalheiro, E.A., Ferreira, E.C., Abdalla, D.S.P., Amado, D. & Bellissimo, M.I. (2001). Pilocarpine-induced status epilepticus increases glutamate release in rat hippocampal synaptosomes, *Epilepsy Research* 46: 121-128.

Nanda, D., Tolputt, J. & Collard, K.J. (1996). Changes in brain glutathione levels during postnatal development in the rat, *Developmental Brain Research*. 94: 238–241.

Niki, E. (1991). Action of ascorbic acid as a scavenger of active and stable oxygen radicals, *The American Journal of Clinical Nutrition* 54: S1119-S1124

Peredery, O., Blomme, M.A. & Parker, G. (1992). Absence of maternal behaviour in rats with lithium/pilocarpine seizure induced brain damage: support of macleans triune brain theory, *Physiology and Behavior*, 52: 665-671.

Perlis, M.L., Smith, M.T., Orff, H.J., Andrews, P.J., Gillin, J.C. & Giles, D.E. (2002). The effects of an orally administered cholinergic agonist on REM sleep in major depression, *Biological Psychiatry* 51: 457-462.

Peterson, S.L., Morrow, D., Liu, S. & Liu, K.J. (2002). Hydroethidine detection of superoxide during lithium-pilocarpine model of status epilepticus, *Epilepsy Research* 49: 226-238.

Pizzanelli, C., Lazzeri, G., Fulceri, F., Giorgi, F.S., Pasquali, L., Cifelli, G., Murri, L. & Fornai, F. (2009). Lack of alpha 1b-adrenergic receptor protects against epileptic seizures, *Epilepsia* 50: 59-64.

Rauca, C., Wiswedel, I., Zerbe, R., Keilhoff, G. & Krug, M. (2004). The role of superoxide dismutase and α-tocopherol in the development of seizures and kindling induced by pentylenetetrazol - influence of the radical scavenger a-phenyl-N-tert-butyl nitrone, *Brain Research* 1009: 203-212.

Ribeiro MCP, Avila DS, Scheneider CYM, Hermes, F.S., Furian, A.F., Oliveira, M.S., Rubin, M.A., Lehmann, M., Krieglstein, J. & Mello, C.F. (2005). α-tocopherol protects against pentylenetetrazol- and methylmalonate-induced convulsions, *Epilepsy Research* 66: 185-194.

Rong, Y., Doctrow, S.R., Tocco, G. & Baudry, M. (1999). EUK-134, a synthetic superoxide dismutase and catalase mimetic, prevents oxidative stress and attenuates kainate-induced neuropathology, *Proceedings of the National Academy of Sciences*, 96: 9897-9902.

Sah, R., Galeffi, F., Ahfens, R., Jordan, G. & Schartz-Bloom, R.D.J. (2002). Modulation of the GABA(A)-gated chloride channel by reactive oxygen species, *Journal of Neurochemistry* 80: 383 - 391.

Santos, I.M.S., Freitas, R.L.M., Silva, E.P., Feitosa, C.M., Saldanha, G.B., Souza, G.F., Tomé, A.R., Feng D. & Freitas, R.M. (2010). Effects of ubiquinone on hydroperoxide concentration and antioxidant enzymatic activities in the rat hippocampus during pilocarpine-induced seizures, *Brain Research* 1315: 33-40.

Sawas, A.H. & Gilbert, J.C. (1985). Lipid peroxidation as a possible mechanism for the neurotoxic and nephrotoxic effects of a combination of lithium carbonate and haloperidol, *Archives internationales de pharmacodynamie et de thérapie* 276: 301-312.

Shivakumar, B.R., Ananndatheerthavarada, H.K. & Ravindranath, V. (1991). Free radical scavenging system in developing rat brain, *International Journal of Developmental Neuroscience* 9: 181-185.

Shults, C.W. & Haas, R., 2005. Clinical trials of coenzyme Q10 in neurological disorders, *Biofactors* 25: 117-126.

Simonié, A., Laginja, J., Varljen, J., Zupan, G. & Erakovié, V. (2000) Lithium plus pilocarpine induced status epilepticus – biochemical changes, *Neuroscience Research* 36: 157-166.

Smith, B.N. & Shibley, H. (2002). Pilocarpine-induced status epilepticus results in mossy fiber sproutng and spontaneous seizures in C57BL/6 and CD-1 mice, *Epilepsy Research* 49: 109-120.

Todorova, V.K., Harms, S.A., Kaufmam, Y., Luo, S., Luo, K.Q., Babb, K. & Klimberg, V.S. (2004). Effect of dietary glutamine on tumor glutathione levels and apoptosis-related proteins in DMBA-induced breast cancer of rats, *Breast Cancer Research and Treatment* 88: 247-256.

Tomé, A.R., Ferreira, P.M.P. & Freitas, R.M. (2010). Inhibitory action of antioxidant (ascorbic acid or α-tocopherol) on seizures and brain damage induced by pilocarpine in rats, *Arquivos de Neuropsiquiatria* 68: 355-361.

Turski, W.A., Cavalheiro, E.A., Schwarz, M., Czuczwar, S.J., Kleironk, Z. & Turski, L. (1983). Limbic seizures produced by pilocarpine in rats: behavioural, eletroencephalographic and neuropathological study, *Behavioral Brain Research* 9: 315-336.

Turski, L., Cavalheiro, E.A., Leite, J.P., Bortolotto, Z.A., Turski, W.A. & Ikonomidou, C. (1991). Long-term effects of pilocarpine in rats: structural damage of the brain triggers kindling and spontaneous recurrent seizures, *Epilepsia* 32: 778-782.

Vanhatalo, S. & Riikonen, R. (1999). Markedly elevated nitrate/nitrite levels in the cerebrospinal fluid of children with progressive encephalopathy with edema, hypsarrhythmia and optic atrophy (PEHO syndrome), *Epilepsia* 40: 210-212.

Vanhatalo, S. & Riikonen, R. (2001). Nitric oxide metabolites, nitrates and nitrites in the cerebrospinal fluid in children with west syndrome, *Epilepsy Research* 46: 3-13.

Vanin, A., Vitskova, G., Narkevich, V. & Bashkatova, V. (2003). The influence of anticonvulsant and antioxidant drugs on nitric oxide level and lipid peroxidation in the rat brain during penthylenetetrazole-induce epileptiform model seizures, *Prog Neuro-Psychopaharm Biol Psychiatry* 27: 487-492.

Xavier, S.M.L., Barbosa, C.O., Barros, D.O., Silva, R.F., Oliveira, A.A. & Freitas, R.M. (2007). Vitamin C antioxidant in hippocampus of adult Wistar rats after seizures and status epilepticus induced by pilocarpine, *Neuroscience Letters* 420: 76-79.

Yamamoto, N., Kabuto, H., Matsumoto, S., Ogawa, N. & Yokoi, I. (2002). α-tocopheryl-L-ascorbate-2-O-phosphate diester, a hydroxyl radical scavenger, prevents the occurrence of epileptic foci in a rat model of post-traumatic epilepsy, *Pathophysiology* 8: 205-214.

6

Traumatic Brain Injury – Acute Care

Angela N. Hays and Abhay K. Varma
Medical University of South Carolina
USA

1. Introduction

Traumatic brain injury (TBI) is a spectrum of pathological changes in the brain that result from application of external mechanical force(s) leading to temporary or permanent impairment of neurological function. TBI is a global health problem. In 1990, 9.5 million individuals worldwide sustained a TBI severe enough to warrant medical attention or result in death (Corrigan, Selassie, & Orman 2010). In the United States, the annual incidence of TBI is 506.4 per 100,000 population (Langlois JA 2006), in Europe it is 235 per 100,000 population (Tagliaferri et al. 2006), and in Asia it is reported to range from 160 (Gururaj G 2004) to 344 (Chiu et al. 1997) per 100,000 population (incidence rate from United States is inclusive of emergency department visits, hospital discharges and deaths, incidence rates from Europe and Asia are inclusive of hospital discharges and deaths only). Severe TBI has long term consequences for the individual and the society. In the United States, it is estimated that annually 43.1% (124,000) of the individuals discharged after acute hospitalization for TBI (Selassie et al. 2008) develop long term disability. The prevalence of individuals in the United States with disability secondary to TBI is estimated to be 3.2 million (Zaloshnja et al. 2008). The total life time cost of treating TBI cases in the United States, including loss of productivity, is estimated to be $ 60.4 billion for the year 2000 (Corrigan, Selassie, & Orman 2010).The enormous economic and social burden imposed by TBI demands aggressive measures to prevent and treat TBI.

Technological developments and better understanding of brain physiology have resulted in a dramatic improvement in mortality related to TBI. Mortality rates declined precipitously between 1970 and 1990, likely related to the routine use of computed tomography (CT) scans and intracranial pressure (ICP) monitoring, as well as improvement in trauma resuscitation generally. However, despite more recent advances in neuromonitoring and neuroimaging, mortality has remained steady at approximately 35% since the 1990s (Stein et al. 2010). The reasons for this lack of progress are multifactorial; no doubt the increase in severe TBI among the elderly is a contributing factor (Colantonio et al. 2008). Nevertheless, the field of neurotrauma has suffered from the lack of well organized multicenter, randomized clinical trials designed to assess the efficacy of the newer techniques and interventions for the management of TBI. Efforts to design and conduct clinical trials in TBI have been challenging for many reasons including the heterogeneity of the disease, barriers to recruitment, and lack of standardized management protocols across centers (Narayan et al. 2002). This chapter presents an overview of the pathophysiology and basic principals of management of TBI, and the challenges facing the scientific community in dealing with this debilitating disorder.

2. Mechanism

TBI results from the application of external force to cranium and its contents. The severity of injury is determined by the nature, magnitude and duration of load applied to cranium and the force vector (rotational, translational or angular) (Gennarelli 1993). Force applied to cranium can be static (delivered over more than 200 milliseconds) or dynamic (delivered over less than 200 milliseconds). Static loading is a less common cause of TBI in clinical situations, and usually leads to focal brain damage. Dynamic loading is a more common cause of TBI, and produces more complex and widespread brain damage. Dynamic loading itself results from direct blow to the cranium (contact load), or rapid acceleration or deceleration of the cranium (inertial load) that causes differential motion of the brain relative to the skull. Inertial loading can cause translational movement (linear motion of brain in the skull), rotational movement (shearing motion of different layers of brain in relation to one another), and angular movement (a combination of translational and rotational movements). In most clinical situations, severe TBI is initiated by impact to the head of a solid object at a high velocity, leading to brain damage by a combination of contact and inertial loading (Graham, Adams, & Gennarelli 1988).

Traumatic brain injury can be focal or diffuse. Focal injury manifests as fractures, contusion or hematoma with mass effect. Contact loading, wherein a significant force is applied to cranium, can cause fracture at the site of impact with underlying contusion or epidural/subdural hematoma. If contact loading also produces translational acceleration or deceleration of the brain within the cranium, it can also cause focal damage by compression of brain under the site of impact (coup contusion) or remote from it (counter coup contusion). Diffuse brain injury results from rotational or angular acceleration or deceleration of the brain; the presentation can vary from transient loss of consciousness (concussion) to diffuse axonal injury (DAI) with prolonged coma. With increasing magnitude of inertial force progressively deeper structures in the brain suffer DAI (Adams et al. 1989). In clinical situations focal lesions and DAI frequently coexist (Skandsen et al. 2010).

3. Pathophysiology

TBI is not a static event, but a constantly evolving dynamic process. The initial insult leads to instant brain damage known as primary brain injury. Primary brain injury triggers a cascade of events that cause brain edema, intracranial hypertension, and consequent ischemia, categorized as secondary brain damage (Enriquez & Bullock 2004). In diffuse injury the primary insult is at the cellular level and initiates events that lead to release of excitatory neurotransmitters, loss of ionic homeostasis, disruption of ATP production, toxicity from free radical production, loss of auto regulation and breakdown of blood brain barrier (BBB). These pathological changes lead to secondary injury. Similar secondary changes also occur in the region surrounding an area of contusion or traumatic hematoma, with a zone of ischemia and swelling developing around the focal injury. Tissue in this "ischemic penumbra" is at risk of dying but also salvageable (Schroder et al. 1995; Leker & Shohami 2002). Treatment of acute TBI is directed at minimizing secondary brain damage that follows focal as well as diffuse TBI.

A good understanding of cellular and biochemical changes that follow brain trauma is required for the optimal management of brain injury, and for directing future research aimed at design of new therapies and protocols. A detailed discussion of these changes is beyond the scope of this chapter; however, a brief summary is presented. Following trauma, the excitatory amino acid glutamate is released from the presynaptic neurons and activates both post synaptic neurons and glial cells. Under physiological conditions both glial cells and postsynaptic neurons actively remove glutamate from the synaptic space. Following trauma the high levels of glutamate activate receptors in the cell membranes of postsynaptic neurons and glial cells, resulting in Ca^{2+} influx into the cell with consequent free radical formation and increased oxidative stress. Calcium ions also accumulate in the mitochondria leading to mitochondrial membrane damage and disruption of energy cycle. These events eventually trigger necrosis and apoptosis in the cells (Enriquez & Bullock 2004; Shohami et al. 1997).

TBI disrupts the BBB that allows fluid to move from intravascular compartment to extravascular compartment in the brain with resultant brain swelling and intracranial hypertension, which in turn leads to fall in cerebral perfusion thus further exacerbating brain ischemia. Aquaporins, matrix metalloproteinases and vasoactive inflammatory agents are potential mediators of BBB breakdown following trauma (Donkin & Vink 2010). A porous BBB allows infiltration of inflammatory cells into damaged brain. These cells (neutrophils and macrophages) release free radicals and cytokines into the brain tissue accentuating the damage (Soares et al. 1995).

4. Initial management at the scene of injury

Pre-hospital management is a critical step in the overall care of acute brain injury. Early institution of optimal care will minimize secondary injury while the patient is transported to a tertiary care facility. About half the deaths following TBI occur within first 2 hours of the injury (Badjatia, Carney et al. 2008) thereby signifying the importance of optimal pre-hospital care.

Pillars of pre-hospital care are restoring and maintaining airway, breathing and circulation (ABC) (Dewall 2010). The cervical spine must be immobilized as the patient is resuscitated, and spine precautions should be maintained till the patient is transferred to a trauma center. Intubation is indicated to secure the airway if the Glasgow Coma Scale (GCS) is less than 9, if the patient is hypoxic (SpO_2 < 90%) despite supplemental oxygen, or if the patient is unable to maintain a patent airway (Gabriel et al. 2002). The SpO_2 should be kept above 95%, while maintaining eucapnea with an end tidal carbon dioxide ($EtCO_2$) of 35 to 40 mm Hg (Badjatia, Carney et al. 2008). Hypotension accelerates secondary injury, and must be promptly recognized and treated. Systolic blood pressure below 90 mm Hg has been shown to increase mortality by two fold in TBI (Chesnut et al. 1993). Intravenous access should be promptly established, and normal saline is a reasonable choice for pre hospital fluid resuscitation (Dewall 2010). Intravenous dextrose should be administered only if blood glucose is less than 70 mg/dl (Badjatia, Carney et al. 2008). Persistent hypotension should prompt search for extracranial injury or spinal cord injury. Neurogenic hypotension presents with bradycardia and hypotension as opposed to hypovolemic shock that is characterized by tachycardia and hypotension.

Glasgow coma scale (GCS) and pupillary response should be documented after the ABCs of resuscitation are complete, and if more than one provider is available, this can be done while the ABCs are being secured. Assessment of the GCS and pupillary response in pre-hospital setting allows the emergency medical personnel to communicate to the receiving hospital the neurological status of the patient, screen for cerebral herniation and trend the

neurological status (Badjatia, Carney et al. 2008). A quick secondary survey for extracranial injuries should be performed prior to transport (Dewall 2010).
Timely transport of these patients to tertiary care center is critical to a favorable outcome. Patients with severe TBI (GCS < 9) should be transported directly to a facility equipped with an immediately available CT scanner, prompt neurosurgical care and the ability to monitor intracranial pressure and treat intracranial hypertension (Badjatia, Carney et al. 2008), even if it is not the closest hospital (Hartl et al. 2006). Mortality can increase by 50%, if a severe TBI patient is not directly transported to such a facility (Hartl et al. 2006). Mode of transport (by road or air) should be chosen to minimize the transit time (Dewall 2010), as mortality following acute subdural hematoma has been shown to be directly linked to time to surgical intervention (Seelig et al. 1981).

5. Medical management

5.1 Principles of intensive care

Management of the patient with traumatic brain injury is directed predominantly at minimizing and preventing secondary brain injury, which can result from intracranial or systemic causes. Although the mechanisms of secondary brain injury are incompletely understood, inadequate cerebral perfusion and oxygenation are integral factors. Systemic hypoxia and hypotension are significantly associated with increased morbidity and mortality. This effect was demonstrated in a data set from the Traumatic Coma Data Bank, in which a single episode of systemic hypotension was associated with double the risk of death (Chesnut et al. 1993; Bratton et al. 2007). This observation serves to demonstrate that good basic critical care is paramount. Current guidelines recommend a systolic blood pressure greater than 90 mmHg as a resuscitation end-point (Bratton et al. 2007). Adequate fluid resuscitation is important, but vasopressors should be used if fluids are insufficient to maintain adequate systemic blood pressures. Intubation and mechanical ventilation are necessary for patients presenting with severe brain injuries in order to ensure adequate oxygenation and ventilation, and to minimize the risk of aspiration (Valadka & Robertson 2007). Admission to a dedicated neuroscience critical care unit, when available, may also result in improved outcomes (Patel et al. 2005).
Ventilator management in patients with severe TBI presents some unique challenges because of the effect of $PaCO_2$ on cerebrovascular autoregulation. Hyperventilation has long been recognized as an effective means for treating acutely elevated intracranial pressure. Hyperventilation results in a systemic respiratory alkalosis, which in turn lowers the pH of the cerebrospinal fluid. In patients with intact cerebral autoregulation, this change in pH results in constriction of cerebral arterioles, thereby decreasing the cerebral blood volume and lowering the intracranial pressure. As a result of this phenomenon, routine hyperventilation of TBI patients has been advocated in the past. However, experimental evidence has demonstrated that the vasoconstrictive effect is relatively short-lived, (Muizelaar et al. 1988) and there is concern that continued hyperventilation could potentiate cerebral ischemia (Bratton et al. 2007). Furthermore, subsequent efforts to correct an iatrogenic respiratory alkalosis sometimes precipitate rebound increases in intracranial pressure (Valadka & Robertson 2007). For these reasons, hyperventilation is usually employed only as a temporizing measure in patients suffering an acute neurological decline. The relationship between $PaCO_2$ and cerebral blood flow becomes particularly problematic in TBI patients with co-morbid lung injury. Acute lung injury (ALI) and acute respiratory distress syndrome (ARDS) are not uncommon in the neurological critical care unit. Since the

publication of the ARDSnet trial in 2000, the mainstay of therapy for patients with ALI and ARDS has been lung-protective ventilation, which minimizes barotrauma to the lungs by employing lower tidal volumes (The Acute Respiratory Distress Syndrome Network 2000). This strategy results in a moderate degree of hypercapnea and hypoxemia. While lung-protective ventilation significantly improved mortality in the study population, the relative hypercarbia and hypoxemia may have deleterious effects in a patient who is at risk for cerebral edema, ischemia, or vasospasm. Randomized trials in TBI patients with ARDS are lacking. Monitoring of cerebral perfusion and oxygenation, which is discussed in subsequent sections, is particularly crucial in this scenario (Young et al. 2010).

Because of the brain's role in regulating metabolism, patients with severe traumatic brain injury demonstrate a number of metabolic derangements which ultimately result in systemic catabolism (Cook, Peppard, & Magnuson 2008). Adequate nutritional support is essential to forestall adverse consequences, including protein loss and immunocompromise (Sacks et al. 1995). Early institution of nutritional support has a significant impact on mortality and decreases the rate of hospital-acquired infections (Hartl et al. 2008; Taylor et al. 1999). Patients with severe TBI will require replacement of approximately 140% of their resting energy expenditure, though this requirement will be decreased somewhat in the setting of pharmacological paralysis or deep sedation. Protein requirements are estimated at about 1.5-2 grams/kg of protein (Cook, Peppard, & Magnuson 2008). Close monitoring is essential to ensure adequate supplementation and avoid complications such as hyperglycemia. Early hyperglycemia has been associated with poor outcome in TBI patients (Liu-DeRyke et al. 2009), but intensive glycemic control may exacerbate metabolic stress in some patients (Vespa et al. 2006). Although the optimal glucose range for TBI patients has yet to be determined, our institution has chosen 140-180 mg/dL as a reasonable target range.

Because of their increased sympathetic tone, severity of illness, and degree of immobility, TBI patients are at high risk of complications of critical illness including infection and thromboembolism. Long-term use of prophylactic antibiotics is discouraged, though there is some evidence that brief treatment at the time of endotracheal intubation reduces the incidence of ventilator-associated pneumonia (Sirvent et al. 1997). Fevers are common in patients with traumatic brain injury, and may represent an underlying infection, hypothalamic dysfunction, or other non-infectious cause. Hyperpyrexia must be investigated exhaustively in order to rule out the possibility of an infectious etiology; however, any fever in a patient with neurological injury must be treated aggressively. Increased temperature results in increased cerebral blood flow, which can exacerbate intracranial hypertension and reduce intracranial compliance (Segatore 1992). Furthermore, animal studies have indicated that hyperthermia can increase infarct size and potentiate cellular damage (Dietrich et al. 1996; Dietrich & Bramlett 2007). For these reasons, aggressive treatment of fever in brain-injured patients is warranted. First-line treatments generally include antipyretics such as acetaminophen; cooling blankets, fans, and chilled fluids have also been employed (Johnston et al. 2006). Control of shivering is also important, as shivering can increase metabolic demand and impede efforts to maintain normothermia (Badjatia, Strongilis et al. 2008).

Prevention of thromboembolic events is a major consideration in patients with severe TBI, especially in poly-trauma patients. Mechanical prophylaxis with graduated compression stockings and/or pneumatic compression devices is recommended, though these interventions may be contraindicated in the presence of significant injury to the lower extremities (Bratton et al. 2007). Pharmacological prophylaxis with unfractionated (UH) or low-molecular weight heparin (LMWH) has been the subject of some debate. There is concern that use of pharmacological interventions could result in exacerbation of cerebral contusions, intracranial hemorrhage, and systemic bleeding. Evidence in a neurosurgical population indicates that pharmacological prophylaxis used in conjunction with mechanical devices is more effective than mechanical measures alone (Nurmohamed et al. 1996; Agnelli et al. 1998). Recent observational evidence suggests that initiation of prophylactic treatment with LMWH within 48 hours of injury or neurosurgical intervention is effective and associated with an acceptably low risk of complications (Norwood et al. 2008; Dudley et al. 2010). Unfortunately, the most effective agent and dosing strategy is yet to be determined.

5.2 Cerebral edema, intracranial hypertension and cerebral perfusion pressure

The components of the intracranial compartment under normal circumstances consist of brain tissue, cerebrospinal fluid, and blood. Because the intracranial contents are contained within the rigid confines of the skull, any increase in volume—in the form of cerebral edema or a pathological mass lesion—must be met with a compensatory decrease in one of the other components, or the ICP will rise. Elevated ICP can result in cerebral ischemia, an important cause of secondary brain injury, by reducing cerebral perfusion pressure (CPP):

$$CPP = MAP - ICP$$

Where MAP is the mean arterial pressure.

There is a considerable amount of debate regarding the relative importance of CPP and ICP thresholds. On one hand, observational data indicates that ICP > 20 mmHg is an independent predictor of morbidity and mortality (Helmy, Vizcaychipi, & Gupta 2007; Valadka & Robertson 2007; Robertson et al. 1999; Hiler et al. 2006; Czosnyka et al. 2005); however, good outcomes are possible even in the setting of exceptionally high ICPs, provided that cerebral perfusion is maintained. As a consequence, some centers advocate a CPP guided strategy, where as other clinical protocols focus predominantly on ICP and minimization of cerebral edema (Eker et al. 1998). Guidelines recommend ICP monitoring in patients with a Glasgow Coma Score (GCS) ≤ 8 who have abnormalities visible on computed tomography (CT). In the absence of CT abnormalities, ICP monitoring is indicated in comatose patients meeting 2 of the following criteria: age > 40 years, presence of motor posturing on exam, and/or SBP < 90 mmHg(Bratton et al. 2007). ICP values in excess of 20 mmHg are considered pathological, though it is important to note that herniation can occur at lower ICPs, especially in the presence of intracranial mass lesions (Bratton et al. 2007).

The situation is complicated by the fact that the relationship between ICP and CPP is affected by the integrity of cerebrovascular autoregulatory mechanisms. When cerebral autoregulation is intact, a fall in CPP is met with reflex cerebral vasodilation. This can precipitate an increase in ICP, thereby further diminishing cerebral perfusion (Robertson 2001). In this setting, efforts to augment CPP artificially may abort a destructive cycle and arrest ongoing secondary brain injury. However, if CPP falls outside of the range of normal autoregulation, or if cerebral autoregulation is impaired, this relationship is reversed: ICP will rise in a linear fashion with increasing CPP, and artificial augmentation of cerebral blood flow may result in worsening cerebral edema and hyperemia. Initially, observational data using historical controls lead to the conclusion that CPP should be maintained at > 70 mmHg. However, in a retrospective analysis of the Selfotel trial, Juul *et al.* found that there was no outcome benefit obtained by maintaining CPP > 60; interestingly, ICP ≥ 20 was the most powerful predictor of outcome (Juul et al. 2000). The only randomized trial to date addressing the question of CPP vs. ICP was published by Robertson, *et al.* in 1999. In this trial, the CPP in one group was maintained at > 70 mmHg; in the other group, the ICP was maintained at ≤ 20 mmHg and CPPs as low as 50 mmHg were permitted. The investigators found no significant difference in outcome, but the CPP-targeted strategy carried five times the risk of ARDS (Robertson et al. 1999). An increasing appreciation of the role of cerebrovascular autoregulation in secondary brain injury has led some investigators to incorporate assessment of autoregulatory function into clinical protocols. The most readily available measure is the pressure reactivity index (PRx), which is a moving correlation coefficient calculated from measurements of ICP and MAP (Czosnyka et al. 1998). Centers that employ this measurement have reported that patients with intact autoregulation (PRx is low) have improved outcomes when managed according to a CPP guided paradigm, whereas those with impaired autoregulation (PRx is elevated) benefit from an ICP targeted strategy (Howells et al. 2005). Clearly, this observation warrants additional study.

Interventions to control intracranial hypertension generally act to decrease the volume of one component of the intracranial compartment: blood, brain, or CSF. First line interventions include patient positioning, adequate sedation and analgesia, and maintenance of normothermia. The head of the bed should be elevated and any obstructions to jugular venous outflow, such as cervical collars, should be minimized. Adequate sedation and analgesia serve to minimize ventilator dyssynchrony, lower intrathoracic and intraabdominal pressure, and decrease agitation (Helmy, Vizcaychipi, & Gupta 2007). Treating systemic fever can mitigate the associated CNS hyperemia prevent shivering and rigors, which often result in increased ICP. If an external ventricular drain is present, diversion of cerebrospinal fluid can be helpful as well.

Use of hyperosmolar substances is the mainstay of therapy for cerebral edema, with or without associated intracranial hypertension (Bhardwaj 2007). Infusion of a hyperosmolar substance serves to generate an osmotic gradient across the blood-brain-barrier, which reduces cerebral edema by drawing water out of the brain tissue. Mannitol and hypertonic saline (HTS) are the most commonly used agents in clinical practice. Mannitol is generally given as a bolus in doses ranging from 0.25-1.5 grams/kg. Hypertonic saline can be administered as a bolus or as a continuous infusion. For continuous use, concentrations ranging from 2% to 7.5% have been reported; boluses of 23.4% NaCl can be used in the setting of acute neurological decline. Use of either agent can result in rapid improvement in ICP; therefore, selection of the appropriate treatment will depend upon the clinical scenario. Mannitol can easily be infused through a peripheral intravenous line, whereas concentrations of HTS > 2% require central access. Mannitol acts as an osmotic diuretic, and can result in intravascular volume depletion, hypokalemia, and hypotension. There is concern that repeated dosing can result in renal impairment, especially if the drug is not adequately cleared by the kidneys; this can be monitored by calculating the osmolal gap. Hypertonic saline, on the other hand, acts as a volume expander and has been shown to be an effective means of reducing ICP even in patients who did not respond to mannitol (Ogden, Mayer, & E. Sander Connolly 2005; Vialet et al. 2003; Schwarz et al. 2002). Potential adverse events include congestive heart failure and hyperoncotic hemolysis; rapid administration of concentrated solutions may also result in transient hypotension. Either agent has the potential to accumulate in brain tissue in the presence of disruption of the blood-brain-barrier, Also, continued exposure to a hypertonic environment induces the generation of idiogenic osmoles within brain tissue, possibly setting the stage for rebound intracranial hypertension when the serum osmolarity begins to fall (Diringer & Zazulia 2004). Consequently, close monitoring of the patients' ICP, CPP, serum sodium, and serum osmolarity is required. Despite the lack of convincing evidence, general consensus it that driving the serum sodium above 160 mEq/L is rarely beneficial, and most clinicians try to maintain the serum osmolarity below 320 mOsm/L (Hays et al. 2011).

When intracranial hypertension persists despite maximal osmotherapy, ICP may be controlled by interventions designed to decrease the cerebral blood volume. This can be accomplished by suppressing brain metabolism, either by inducing a pharmacological coma or with therapeutic hypothermia. Induction of a pharmacological coma is usually accomplished using barbiturates, such as pentobarbital. Barbiturates have been shown experimentally to mitigate the development of brain edema (Mishina & Yabuki 1994), decrease cerebral metabolism, and lower cerebral blood flow (Kassell, Hitchon et al. 1980). Early experimental data suggested a neuroprotective effect in models of focal cerebral ischemia (Smith et al. 1974); however, subsequent small-scale clinical trials were disappointing (Ward et al. 1985; Kassell, Peerless et al. 1980). Studies in brain injured patients indicate that barbiturates may be less effective than mannitol as an initial intervention, but nevertheless are useful in patients who have failed maximal osmotherapy (Eisenberg et al. 1988; Schwartz et al. 1984; Marshall et al. 2010). Pentobarbital has a number of undesireable side-effects including systemic hypotension, decreased gastric motility, and bone marrow suppression (Meyer et al. 2010). In addition, continuous infusion of pentobarbital results in delayed drug clearance, which can delay detection of neurological improvement or decline. Continuous electroencephalography allows the clinician to titrate to burst-suppression, thereby ensuring that the minimum effective dose is employed. Several other agents, including propofol and midazolam, can be used to suppress CNS metabolism and induce burst-suppression, though they do not appear to be as effective as barbiturates in the treatment of intracranial hypertension (Meyer et al. 2010; Stewart et al. 1994). Unfortunately, no comparative trials are available.

Induced hypothermia has been investigated as a neuroprotective strategy in many disease states, and is currently the standard of care for comatose patients following cardiac arrest (Bernard & Buist 2003; Mild therapeutic hypothermia to improve the neurologic outcome after cardiac arrest 2002; Bernard et al. 2002). Moderate hypothermia has been shown to decrease the cerebral metabolic rate considerably (Rosomoff & Holaday 1954). In models of ischemia, it serves to decrease the concentrations of lactate and excitotoxic neurotransmitters (Illievich et al. 1994). Although clinical trials have failed to demonstrate an outcome benefit for early hypothermia in traumatic brain injury (Clifton et al. 2001), there is ample evidence that moderate hypothermia is an effective intervention for intracranial hypertension (Meyer et al. 2010). Most investigators used a target temperature between 33-35ºC, which can be achieved using a variety of cooling methods (Marion et al. 1993; Marion et al. 1997; Liu et al. 2006; Qiu et al. 2007; Jiang, Yu, & Zhu 2000; Shiozaki et al. 1993). Complications of moderate hypothermia include an increased susceptibility to infection, cardiac arrhythmias, coagulopathy, and electrolyte disturbances. Iatrogenic hypothermia can also mask a fever, and potentially delay the diagnosis of an underlying infection; for that reason, the authors advocate following the white blood cell count and obtaining periodic cultures in all hypothermic patients. Shivering is often encountered during the induction and rewarming phases, and this can counteract the beneficial effects of hypothermia on ICP and cerebral metabolic rate. Pharmacological paralysis is often used to prevent shivering, but other interventions including magnesium, dexmedetomidine, and meperidine have also been used successfully (Weant et al. 2010). Many of these complications of systemic hypothermia may be mitigated by the use of selective brain cooling devices, which are employed at some institutions (Qiu et al. 2006; Liu et al. 2006).

The duration of hypothermia therapy can vary widely depending upon the clinical needs of the individual patient; reports in the literature range from 24 hours to 14 days (McIntyre et al. 2003). The rewarming phase of therapy is critical due to the risk of mitochondrial injury, vascular dysregulation, and rebound increases in ICP (Jiang, Yu, & Zhu 2000; Jiang & Yang 2007; Povlishock & Wei 2009). Although the optimum rewarming rate has yet to be determined, most authors advocate rates of approximately 0.5-1º/hour (Bernard & Buist 2003; Bernard et al. 2002; Alzaga, Cerdan, & Varon 2006). At our institution, cooling is generally performed for a minimum of 48 hours. If the patient's ICP remains well-controlled during that period, rewarming is initiated at a rate of approximately 0.5º/hr. In the event of recurrent intracranial hypertension, rewarming is halted for an additional 12-24 hours before repeating the attempt.

5.3 Advanced neuromonitoring

In an effort to elucidate the mechanisms of secondary brain injury in severe TBI and improve outcomes from this highly morbid condition, a number of technologies have been developed to provide information regarding brain function, oxygenation, and perfusion. Neurophysiologic techniques such as electroencephalography have been used intermittently in brain injured patients for decades; however, recent evidence suggests that continuous monitoring may provide considerable benefit. Similarly, recent technological advances have enabled the bedside assessment of cerebral perfusion and oxygenation at the bedside. These techniques will be discussed briefly in the following sections.

5.3.1 Continuous electroencephalography

Electroencephalography (EEG) is used for a variety of indications in brain injured patients. Continuous electroencephalography (cEEG) can be employed for the diagnosis and treatment of seizures, in order to titrate barbiturate therapy, as an indicator of cerebral ischemia, and to provide information regarding prognosis. Seizures are a well known complication of TBI, and can contribute to ongoing secondary brain injury (Claassen et al. 2004; Vespa et al. 1999). The incidence of electrographic seizures in severely head injured patients has been reported at 22-33%, with more than half of these events being clinically silent (Vespa et al. 1999; Ronne-Engstrom & Winkler 2006). Moreover, investigators utilizing intracortical electroencephalography report recording several seizures which were occult on simultaneous scalp EEG (Waziri et al. 2009). Seizures are both more likely and more difficult to detect in comatose patients, suggesting that these patients are most likely to benefit from continuous EEG (cEEG) monitoring (Claassen et al. 2004). Early post-traumatic seizures have been associated with adverse physiological events, including elevation of intracranial pressure and an increase in the lactate to pyruvate ratio (Vespa et al. 2007). There is no clear association between isolated post-traumatic seizures and increased mortality; however, case series suggest that post-traumatic status epilepticus carries a high risk of death (Vespa et al. 1999; Bratton et al. 2007). Although most investigators advocate treatment of early post-traumatic seizures as a means for reducing secondary brain injury, it remains to be determined if this intervention improves patient outcome.

5.3.2 Cerebral blood flow and brain tissue oxygenation

The recognition of cerebral ischemia as a major contributing factor to secondary brain injury has generated considerable interest in measurement of cerebral perfusion in head injured patients. A number of imaging techniques, including transcranial Doppler ultrasound, xenon-enhanced CT, CT perfusion imaging, perfusion weighted MRI, and positron emitted tomography are available to evaluate cerebral perfusion. Using these techniques, investigators have demonstrated that cerebral blood flow following head trauma follows three distinct hemodynamic phases: initial hypoperfusion, accompanied by reduced cerebral metabolic rate of oxygen ($CMRO_2$); subsequent hyperemia, without an associated increase in $CMRO_2$, which may be associated with intracranial hypertension; followed by a period in which cerebral blood flow (CBF) may be reduced secondary to vasospasm (Martin et al. 1997). However, the physiological and pathophysiological significance of these phases has been debated, and significant regional variation of cerebral perfusion is present (Wintermark et al. 2004). As discussed previously, cerebral perfusion can be significantly affected by systemic factors that impact the MAP and the CPP; the magnitude of this effect is dependent upon the individual's autoregulatory status (Czosnyka et al. 1998; Howells et al. 2005). Furthermore, the reports of the incidence and significance of cerebral vasospasm after trauma are variable, and likely are affected by the mechanism of injury (Martin et al. 1997; Zubkov et al. 2000). MR, CT, and PET based imaging techniques provide information regarding cerebral perfusion over large regions of the brain parenchyma, but for the most part the data obtained is useful only for a single time point. Transcranial Doppler can be performed for extended periods of time, but it is limited to the evaluation of the large vessels surrounding the Circle of Willis, and image quality is highly operator-dependent. More recently, parenchymal monitors have been used to provide a continuous measurement of cerebral blood flow in a specific, small region of tissue using thermal diffusion. This device is placed in the perilesional white matter via a burr hole in the skull. Use of CBF monitoring is currently employed in some centers and may provide a method for continuous assessment of cerebrovascular autoregulation in the future (Rosenthal et al. 2011).

In addition to CBF, brain oxygenation is often used as an indicator of cerebral ischemia. For decades, brain oxygenation could be assessed only indirectly, by intermittent sampling of the jugular venous blood. However, in the 1990s, a fiber-optic catheter which permitted continuous assessment of jugular venous oxygen saturation ($SjvO_2$) became available (Ritter et al. 1996). $SjvO_2$ provides a global measure of cerebral oxygenation and can permit early detection of cerebral ischemia. Studies have shown that jugular venous desaturations (< 50%) are correlated with poor outcome, especially if prolonged and/or recurrent (Gopinath et al. 1994). However, cerebral metabolism in TBI demonstrates regional heterogeneity, and a global measure such as $SjvO_2$ may not permit detection of focal regions of ischemia (Valadka et al. 2000). More recently, intraparenchymal monitors have become available for the purpose of monitoring local brain tissue oxygen tension ($PbrO_2$). These monitors are typically inserted in normal-appearing brain tissue adjacent to a focal lesion, or in the right frontal region in the setting of diffuse axonal injury. As with $SjvO_2$ monitoring, episodes of desaturation detected by $PbrO_2$ monitoring have been shown to correlate with increased mortality (Stiefel et al. 2005). The critical value appears to be approximately 15 mmHg, though some clinicians prefer a treatment threshold of 20 mmHg (Bratton et al. 2007). Various investigators have studied the relationships between $PbrO_2$ and more conventional clinical parameters. In particular, positive correlations have been described between $PbrO_2$ and various determinants of oxygen supply to the CNS, including FiO_2, PaO_2, CPP, and hemoglobin concentration (Stiefel et al. 2005). However, studies using PET imaging and monitoring of the arteriovenous oxygen tension difference have provided evidence that barriers to local oxygen diffusion, rather than determinants of oxygen supply, are significant determinants of $PbrO_2$ (Rosenthal et al. 2008; Bratton et al. 2007).

A drop in cerebral oxygenation (as measured by $PbrO_2$ or $SjvO_2$) should prompt an investigation for an underlying cause, such subclinical seizures; an expanding mass lesion; suboptimal CPP; or systemic derangements such as hypotension or worsening lung function. The two monitoring methods are often complementary. For instance, $PbrO_2$ is more sensitive to changes in the arterial oxygen content, and would be more likely to signal the expansion of a nearby contusion (Valadka et al. 2000). Cerebral oxygen desaturation can be successfully treated using measures designed to augment oxygen delivery, such as optimizing the CPP, increasing the fraction of inspired oxygen (FiO_2), and transfusion of red blood cells depending upon the patient's specific clinical characteristics; however, these interventions carry some risk. Normobaric hyperoxia has been shown to improve $PbrO_2$ as well as some other markers of brain metabolism, but prolonged use exposes the patient to the risk of oxygen toxicity (Tisdall et al. 2008). Similarly, the optimal transfusion threshold for brain injured patients has yet to be determined, and injudicious use of blood products carries the risk of transfusion related lung injury, as well as other potential complications. A recent trial of 70 patients reported that a group of patients with severe TBI who received $PbrO_2$ guided therapy (goal > 20 mmHg) demonstrated improved mortality and better functional outcomes than those managed using traditional ICP (< 20 mmHg) and CPP goals (> 60 mmHg)(Spiotta et al. 2010). However, this trial relied on historical controls, and the authors did not report on the incidence of ARDS or other medical complications in either cohort. A multicenter randomized controlled trial addressing the use of $PbrO_2$ monitoring in severe TBI is currently underway.

6. Surgical management

Surgical intervention is indicated in TBI for control of intracranial hypertension or restoring integrity of structures covering the brain as in compound injuries. High ICP, following TBI, can result from a focal intracranial hematoma or diffuse brain swelling. "Moderate" sized contusion hematomas can present the surgeon with a dilemma about whether to operate or observe the patient. Presence of alcohol or drugs on board can further compound the situation. Close clinical observation, ICP monitoring, and a follow-up head CT scan can help to guide the therapy, but ultimately surgeon's experience and clinical judgment plays a crucial role in decision making.

Evidence based guidelines are available to help with decision-making (Bullock et al. 2006, 2006; Bullock et al. 2006, 2006, 2006). Any mass lesion with progressive neurological decline referable to the lesion should be operated upon. A supratentorial lesion with a midline shift of 5 mm or more and effacement of the basal cisterns, and a posterior fossa lesion with compression or distortion of fourth ventricle or effacement of basal cisterns or obstructive hydrocephalus in patients with GCS of 8 or less should be evacuated. Epidural hematomas (EDH) larger than 30 cm³ and subdural hematomas greater than 10mm in thickness or causing more than 5 mm of midline shift should be evacuated, independent of the GCS. An EDH less than 30 cm³, *and* less than 15mm in maximal thickness, *and* with less than 5 mm midline shift, in a patient with a GCS of 9 or more *without* a focal deficit, can be managed non-surgically with close monitoring and repeat CT scans. Frontal or temporal lobe contusions greater than 20 cm³ associated with midline shift of 5 mm or more, in patients with GCS of 6 to 8 or any parenchymal lesion greater than 50 cm³ should be operated upon. An open (compound) cranial fracture depressed greater than the thickness of cranium should be operated upon to prevent infection. An open (compound) depressed fracture *may* be treated non surgically if it is not depressed more than 1 cm, there is no dural penetration, no intracranial mass lesion, no frontal sinus involvement, no pneumocephalus, no cosmetic deformity, and no wound contamination or infection.

Decompressive craniectomy (DC) is being increasingly used for patients with severe diffuse TBI and medically refractory intracranial hypertension (Ahmad & Bullock 2011). DC is effective in reducing the ICP and increasing the survival, but has not been shown to improve long term neurological outcome(Li, Timofeev et al. 2010). In fact, there is strong evidence to suggest that DC in patients with severe TBI (GCS 3-8) with medically refractory intracranial hypertension is associated with a worse neurological outcome at 6 months after injury compared to similar patients who were treated with controlled ventilation, mannitol, hypertonic saline, external ventricular drainage, mild hypothermia and barbiturates(Cooper et al. 2011). DC for treatment of medically refractory intracranial hypertension, in severe diffuse TBI, is discouraged till parameters other than ICP control are available, to gauge the success of therapy (Marion 2011).This procedure can still be an effective therapy in very select group of patients such as those undergoing craniotomy for intracranial hematoma (particularly SDH) with significant brain swelling. Unwarranted use of DC may prove counterproductive in terms of neurological recovery in patients with severe TBI.

7. Future directions

7.1 Microdialysis

Microdialysis is an invasive monitoring technique which allows sampling of the extracellular fluid within the brain parenchyma in order to test for a variety of substances. Although a wide variety of substances can be analyzed successfully, glucose, lactate, pyruvate, glycerol, and glutamate are the most commonly employed. Glycerol is monitored primarily as a marker of membrane breakdown, whereas glucose, lactate, pyruvate, and the lactate/pyruvate ratio are used as markers of cerebral energy metabolism. The lactate/pyruvate ratio, in particular, is often employed as an indicator of the brain redox state and an early sign of focal ischemia. Microdialysis probes are usually placed in the frontal white matter in patients with diffuse brain injury, or in the pericontusional tissue in patients with focal radiographic abnormalities (Bellander et al. 2004). Although cerebral microdialysis has been widely used in animal studies for more than 30 years, its use in clinical practice is limited primarily to large academic centers where it is generally used in conjunction with other monitoring devices to provide an early indicator of evolving secondary brain injury. For instance, in cases of cerebral ischemia, the lacate/pyruvate ratio increases markedly, whereas the glucose level declines to near zero. These findings have been shown to correlate with $SjVO_2$ and $PbrO_2$ measurements, as well as the oxygen extraction fraction as measured by PET (Robertson et al. 1995; Valadka et al. 1998; Hutchinson et al. 2002). When used in conjunction with CPP and ICP monitoring, microdialysis may have a role in early detection of focal (as opposed to global) pathological processes, such as vasospasm or expanding contusions (Valadka & Robertson 2007; Hillered, Vespa, & Hovda 2005).

The data acquired by centers that utilize microdialysis routinely provides considerable insight into the pathophysiology of secondary brain injury in this population. For instance, Vespa et al. have reported persistently low glucose levels in cerebral microdialysate in the first 50 hours following brain injury in patients with poor outcome, which was unrelated to cerebral ischemia (Vespa et al. 2003). This may reflect a disorder of energy metabolism related to ongoing brain injury in patients with severe TBI. Work from the same group has demonstrated that intensive insulin therapy, as practiced in many surgical ICUs, often results in evidence of metabolic stress in patients with TBI (Vespa et al. 2006). Investigators studying the relationship between CPP on cerebral glucose metabolism have noted significant increases in the lactate/pyruvate ratio at CPPs less than 50mmHg which were confined to perilesional tissue. This work would seem to support the contention that susceptibility to ischemic insult is greater in a region of "tissue at risk" adjacent to contused brain (Nordstrom et al. 2003). Data on hyperventilated patients have been conflicting, with some studies reporting no effect (Letarte et al. 1999). In contrast, another study demonstrated that increased glutamate and lactate/pyruvate ratio could be demonstrated in TBI patients hyperventilated within 36 hours of injury, though these changes were seen much less commonly at later time points (Marion et al. 2002). This observation reinforces the hypothesis that sustained hyperventilation is particularly detrimental in the early stages following TBI.

Microdialysis data has also been used to investigate the physiological effects of various therapeutic interventions. Hyperbaric oxygen therapy has been shown to result in a reproducible decrease in lactate and lactate/pyruvate ratio, which was accompanied by improvements in cerebral blood flow, $CMRO_2$, and ICP (Rockswold et al. 2010). Similarly, microdialysis has been used to investigate the effect of barbiturates and propofol on cerebral energy metabolism. Thiopental coma was shown to reduce lactate in a small number of TBI patients, suggesting reduced anaerobic metabolism (Goodman et al. 1996). In contrast, propofol was not shown to have any significant effect on lactate, pyruvate, or glucose concentrations even when titrated to burst suppression (Johnston et al. 2003). Although both studies involved small numbers of patients, this would seem to suggest that barbiturates are more effective for the prevention of secondary brain injury.

7.2 Biomarkers

One of the major goals of ongoing research in TBI is the identification of reliable biomarkers. The ideal biomarker would enable early diagnosis of underlying brain injury, provide an early indicator of secondary brain injury, and enable clinicians to monitor the patient's response to therapy. Conceivably, use of a variety of biomarkers specific to different tissue types or mechanisms of injury may help to guide therapy and provide insight into ongoing pathophysiology. Over the past 40 years, a variety of candidate molecules have been evaluated in both clinical settings and in animal models. Perhaps the most widely studied is S100B, a calcium-binding protein that is found in astrocytes. S100B has a half-life of < 60 min in serum; consequently, elevated levels are unlikely to persist for more than 24 hours in the absence of severe TBI (Berger 2006). This protein can be quantified in the serum and in the CSF; the peak serum levels appear to occur roughly 48 hours after the peak CSF concentration is reached (Petzold et al. 2003). Elevated levels of S100B have been shown to correlate with poor outcome, contusion volume, and (inversely) with certain quality of life measures (Raabe et al. 1998; Woertgen, Rothoerl, & Brawanski 2002). Unfortunately, the time course of S100B release, the dynamics of transport across the blood-brain-barrier, and the patho- physiological implications of elevated S100B levels remain to be determined (Kleindienst et al. 2010). Other candidate biomarkers associated with outcome in TBI patients include neuron specific enlace, a cytoplasm protein found in neuronal tissue, and glial fibrillary acidic protein (GFAP), an intermediate filament protein found in astrocytes (Vos et al. 2004) GFAP, in particular, has been shown to correlate with CT findings and with outcome in trauma patients (Lumpkins et al. 2008; Nylen et al. 2006). Although no large scale studies are available, some investigators suggest that GFAP may prove to be more sensitive than neuron-specific enolase (NSE) or S100B, due to the lack of extracerebral sources (Honda et al. 2010).

Whereas NSE, S100B, and GFAP are markers of cellular breakdown, certain other candidate biomarkers serve as indicators of ongoing pathophysiological processes. For instance, diffuse axonal injury is characterized pathologically by axonal degradation, which is associated with the breakdown of axonal microtubules. This results in the release of microtubule-associated protein tau, which is cleaved into fragments which are known as cleaved-tau (C-tau) (Li, Li et al. 2010). The presence of C-tau in the CSF has been found to be a sensitive indicator of diffuse axonal injury, and levels correlate inversely with clinical improvement (Zemlan et al. 1999). Other putative biomarkers have the potential to allow investigators to differentiate between cell death related to apoptosis as opposed to necrosis. The alpha-II spectrin protein, for example, is a component of the axonal cytoskeleton which is cleaved by enzymes involved in both cellular necrosis (caspase-3) and apoptosis (calpain 1 and 2). Western blot analysis of the alpha-II spectrin breakdown products present in a given sample can therefore provide insight into the predominant mechanism of cellular loss (Li, Li et al. 2010). Preliminary studies using alpha-II spectrin breakdown products in humans have demonstrated that necrosis, mediated by calpain, is the predominant mechanism involved in acute DAI, suggesting that calpain inhibitors may be a potential therapeutic target (Brophy et al. 2009).

7.3 Pharmacotherapy

A major factor contributing to intractable intracranial hypertension following severe TBI is cerebral edema. Both cytotoxic and vasogenic edema contribute to post traumatic cerebral edema (Barzo et al. 1997). Therapeutic interventions directed at mediators of cerebral edema offer potential treatment options for TBI. Aquaporins (AQPs) are integral membrane proteins that form pores in membranes of mammalian cells, and play an important role in development and resolution of cerebral edema (Pasantes-Morales & Cruz-Rangel 2010). AQPs modulation offers a potential therapeutic intervention to prevent or treat brain swelling (Manley et al. 2000; Papadopoulos & Verkman 2008; Taya et al. 2008). Matrix metalloproteinases (MMPs) are zinc dependent endopeptidases involved in the process of tissue remodeling following brain injury from stroke or trauma. MMPs are upregulated following TBI, causing disruption of BBB and cerebral edema in the early phase, followed by neurogenesis and neurovascular remodeling in the later stages of recovery. Thus selective therapeutic blocking of the detrimental effects in the early phase offers the possibility of preventing cerebral edema without disrupting the later reparative phase (Donkin & Vink 2010). A group of neuropeptides released from sensory neurons have been implicated in neurogenic inflammation. Neurogenic inflammation that includes vasodilation, plasma extravasation and neuronal hypersensitivity, has been shown to play a role in the development of post traumatic cerebral edema. Therapeutic inhibition of neurogenic inflammation offers another potential target to prevent cerebral edema after TBI (Donkin & Vink 2010). Progesterone is another agent with potential therapeutic role in the management of TBI. Progesterone receptors are distributed throughout the central nervous system, and the steroid has neuroprotective properties. Progesterone decreases brain edema, attenuates free radicals and reduces neuronal loss in TBI animal model. There is class II evidence to suggest it may improve neurologic outcome in patients with TBI (Junpeng, Huang, & Qin 2011).

8. Conclusion

TBI is a serious disorder with significant morbidity, mortality and economic implications. It is a dynamic process, and timely intervention can prevent progression of neurological decline. Foundation of acute care is built upon prompt resuscitation and transport from the site of accident to a tertiary care facility, appropriate imaging, and intensive monitoring focused on minimization and prevention of secondary damage. Considerable progress has been made in understanding the physiology of ICP and treatment of intracranial hypertension, but control of ICP does not always translate into good neurological outcome. Better understanding of pathophysiology, identification of newer parameters of brain function, and development of innovative therapeutic modalities is required to improve the outcome from TBI.

9. References

Adams, J. H., Doyle, D., Ford, I., Gennarelli, T. A., Graham, D. I., & McLellan, D. R. (1989). Diffuse axonal injury in head injury: definition, diagnosis and grading, *Histopathology*, Vol.15, No. 1, (Jul 1989), pp. 49-59, ISSN 0309-0167

Agnelli, G., Piovella, F., Buoncristiani, P., Severi, P., Pini, M., D'Angelo, A., Beltrametti, C., Damiani, M., Andrioli, G. C., Pugliese, R., Iorio, A., & Brambilla, G. (1998). Enoxaparin plus compression stockings compared with compression stockings alone in the prevention of venous thromboembolism after elective neurosurgery, *N Engl J Med*, Vol.339, No. 2, (Jul 9 1998), pp. 80-85, ISSN 0028-4793 (Print)

Ahmad, F. U., & Bullock, R. (2011). Decompressive craniectomy for severe head injury, *World Neurosurg*, Vol.75, No. 3-4, (Mar-Apr 2011), pp. 451-453, ISSN 1878-8750

Alzaga, A. G., Cerdan, M., & Varon, J. (2006). Therapeutic hypothermia, *Resuscitation*, Vol.70, No. 3, (Sep 2006), pp. 369-380, ISSN 0300-9572

Badjatia, N., Carney, N., Crocco, T. J., Fallat, M. E., Hennes, H. M., Jagoda, A. S., Jernigan, S., Letarte, P. B., Lerner, E. B., Moriarty, T. M., Pons, P. T., Sasser, S., Scalea, T., Schleien, C. L., & Wright, D. W. (2008). Guidelines for prehospital management of traumatic brain injury 2nd edition, *Prehosp Emerg Care*, Vol.12 Suppl 1, No., 2008), pp. S1-52, ISSN 1545-0066

Badjatia, N., Strongilis, E., Gordon, E., Prescutti, M., Fernandez, L., Fernandez, A., Buitrago, M., Schmidt, J. M., Ostapkovich, N. D., & Mayer, S. A. (2008). Metabolic impact of shivering during therapeutic temperature modulation: the Bedside Shivering Assessment Scale, *Stroke*, Vol.39, No. 12, (Dec 2008), pp. 3242-3247, ISSN 1524-4628

Barzo, P., Marmarou, A., Fatouros, P., Hayasaki, K., & Corwin, F. (1997). Contribution of vasogenic and cellular edema to traumatic brain swelling measured by diffusion-weighted imaging, *J Neurosurg*, Vol.87, No. 6, (Dec 1997), pp. 900-907, ISSN 0022-3085

Bellander, B. M., Cantais, E., Enblad, P., Hutchinson, P., Nordstrom, C. H., Robertson, C., Sahuquillo, J., Smith, M., Stocchetti, N., Ungerstedt, U., Unterberg, A., & Olsen, N. V. (2004). Consensus meeting on microdialysis in neurointensive care, *Intensive Care Med*, Vol.30, No. 12, (Dec 2004), pp. 2166-2169, ISSN 0342-4642

Berger, R. P. (2006). The use of serum biomarkers to predict outcome after traumatic brain injury in adults and children, *J Head Trauma Rehabil*, Vol.21, No. 4, (Jul-Aug 2006), pp. 315-333, ISSN 0885-9701

Bernard, S. A., & Buist, M. (2003). Induced hypothermia in critical care medicine: a review, *Crit Care Med*, Vol.31, No. 7, (Jul 2003), pp. 2041-2051, ISSN 0090-3493 (Print)

Bernard, S. A., Gray, T. W., Buist, M. D., Jones, B. M., Silvester, W., Gutteridge, G., & Smith, K. (2002). Treatment of comatose survivors of out-of-hospital cardiac arrest with induced hypothermia, *N Engl J Med*, Vol.346, No. 8, (Feb 21 2002), pp. 557-563, ISSN 1533-4406

Bhardwaj, Anish. (2007). Osmotherapy in neurocritical care, *Current Neurology and Neuroscience Reports*, Vol.7, No., 2007), pp. 513-521

Bratton, S. L., Chestnut, R. M., Ghajar, J., McConnell Hammond, F. F., Harris, O. A., Hartl, R., Manley, G. T., Nemecek, A., Newell, D. W., Rosenthal, G., Schouten, J., Shutter, L., Timmons, S. D., Ullman, J. S., Videtta, W., Wilberger, J. E., & Wright, D. W. (2007). Guidelines for the management of severe traumatic brain injury. I. Blood pressure and oxygenation, *J Neurotrauma*, Vol.24 Suppl 1, No., 2007), pp. S7-13, ISSN 0897-7151

Bratton, S. L., Chestnut, R. M., Ghajar, J., McConnell Hammond, F. F., Harris, O. A., Hartl, R., Manley, G. T., Nemecek, A., Newell, D. W., Rosenthal, G., Schouten, J., Shutter, L., Timmons, S. D., Ullman, J. S., Videtta, W., Wilberger, J. E., & Wright, D. W. (2007). Guidelines for the management of severe traumatic brain injury. V. Deep vein thrombosis prophylaxis, *J Neurotrauma*, Vol.24 Suppl 1, No., 2007), pp. S32-36, ISSN 0897-7151

Bratton, S. L., Chestnut, R. M., Ghajar, J., McConnell Hammond, F. F., Harris, O. A., Hartl, R., Manley, G. T., Nemecek, A., Newell, D. W., Rosenthal, G., Schouten, J., Shutter, L., Timmons, S. D., Ullman, J. S., Videtta, W., Wilberger, J. E., & Wright, D. W. (2007). Guidelines for the management of severe traumatic brain injury. VI. Indications for intracranial pressure monitoring, *J Neurotrauma*, Vol.24 Suppl 1, No., 2007), pp. S37-44, ISSN 0897-7151

Bratton, S. L., Chestnut, R. M., Ghajar, J., McConnell Hammond, F. F., Harris, O. A., Hartl, R., Manley, G. T., Nemecek, A., Newell, D. W., Rosenthal, G., Schouten, J., Shutter, L., Timmons, S. D., Ullman, J. S., Videtta, W., Wilberger, J. E., & Wright, D. W. (2007). Guidelines for the management of severe traumatic brain injury. VIII. Intracranial pressure thresholds, *J Neurotrauma*, Vol.24 Suppl 1, No., 2007), pp. S55-58, ISSN 0897-7151

Bratton, S. L., Chestnut, R. M., Ghajar, J., McConnell Hammond, F. F., Harris, O. A., Hartl, R., Manley, G. T., Nemecek, A., Newell, D. W., Rosenthal, G., Schouten, J., Shutter, L., Timmons, S. D., Ullman, J. S., Videtta, W., Wilberger, J. E., & Wright, D. W. (2007). Guidelines for the management of severe traumatic brain injury. X. Brain oxygen monitoring and thresholds, *J Neurotrauma*, Vol.24 Suppl 1, No., 2007), pp. S65-70, ISSN 0897-7151

Bratton, S. L., Chestnut, R. M., Ghajar, J., McConnell Hammond, F. F., Harris, O. A., Hartl, R., Manley, G. T., Nemecek, A., Newell, D. W., Rosenthal, G., Schouten, J., Shutter, L., Timmons, S. D., Ullman, J. S., Videtta, W., Wilberger, J. E., & Wright, D. W. (2007). Guidelines for the management of severe traumatic brain injury. XIII. Antiseizure prophylaxis, *J Neurotrauma*, Vol.24 Suppl 1, No., 2007), pp. S83-86, ISSN 0897-7151

Bratton, S. L., Chestnut, R. M., Ghajar, J., McConnell Hammond, F. F., Harris, O. A., Hartl, R., Manley, G. T., Nemecek, A., Newell, D. W., Rosenthal, G., Schouten, J., Shutter, L., Timmons, S. D., Ullman, J. S., Videtta, W., Wilberger, J. E., & Wright, D. W. (2007). Guidelines for the management of severe traumatic brain injury. XIV. Hyperventilation, *J Neurotrauma*, Vol.24 Suppl 1, No., 2007), pp. S87-90, ISSN 0897-7151

Bratton, S. L., Chestnut, R. M., Ghajar, J., McConnell Hammond, F. F., Harris, O. A., Hartl, R., Manley, G. T., Nemecek, A., Newell, D. W., Rosenthal, G., Schouten, J., Shutter, L., Timmons, S. D., Ullman, J. S., Videtta, W., Wilberger, J. E., & Wright, D. W. (2007). Guidelines for the management of severe traumatic brain injury. XV. Steroids, *J Neurotrauma*, Vol.24 Suppl 1, No., 2007), pp. S91-95, ISSN 0897-7151

Brophy, G. M., Pineda, J. A., Papa, L., Lewis, S. B., Valadka, A. B., Hannay, H. J., Heaton, S. C., Demery, J. A., Liu, M. C., Tepas, J. J., 3rd, Gabrielli, A., Robicsek, S., Wang, K. K., Robertson, C. S., & Hayes, R. L. (2009). alphaII-Spectrin breakdown product cerebrospinal fluid exposure metrics suggest differences in cellular injury mechanisms after severe traumatic brain injury, *J Neurotrauma*, Vol.26, No. 4, (Apr 2009), pp. 471-479, ISSN 1557-9042

Bullock, M. R., Chesnut, R., Ghajar, J., Gordon, D., Hartl, R., Newell, D. W., Servadei, F., Walters, B. C., & Wilberger, J. (2006). Surgical management of depressed cranial fractures, *Neurosurgery*, Vol.58, No. 3 Suppl, (Mar 2006), pp. S56-60; discussion Si-iv, ISSN 1524-4040

Bullock, M. R., Chesnut, R., Ghajar, J., Gordon, D., Hartl, R., Newell, D. W., Servadei, F., Walters, B. C., & Wilberger, J. (2006). Surgical management of posterior fossa mass lesions, *Neurosurgery*, Vol.58, No. 3 Suppl, (Mar 2006), pp. S47-55; discussion Si-iv, ISSN 1524-4040

Bullock, M. R., Chesnut, R., Ghajar, J., Gordon, D., Hartl, R., Newell, D. W., Servadei, F., Walters, B. C., & Wilberger, J. (2006). Surgical management of traumatic parenchymal lesions, *Neurosurgery*, Vol.58, No. 3 Suppl, (Mar 2006), pp. S25-46; discussion Si-iv, ISSN 1524-4040

Bullock, M. R., Chesnut, R., Ghajar, J., Gordon, D., Hartl, R., Newell, D. W., Servadei, F., Walters, B. C., & Wilberger, J. E. (2006). Surgical management of acute epidural hematomas, *Neurosurgery*, Vol.58, No. 3 Suppl, (Mar 2006), pp. S7-15; discussion Si-iv, ISSN 1524-4040

Bullock, M. R., Chesnut, R., Ghajar, J., Gordon, D., Hartl, R., Newell, D. W., Servadei, F., Walters, B. C., & Wilberger, J. E. (2006). Surgical management of acute subdural hematomas, *Neurosurgery*, Vol.58, No. 3 Suppl, (Mar 2006), pp. S16-24; discussion Si-iv, ISSN 1524-4040

Chesnut, R. M., Marshall, L. F., Klauber, M. R., Blunt, B. A., Baldwin, N., Eisenberg, H. M., Jane, J. A., Marmarou, A., & Foulkes, M. A. (1993). The role of secondary brain injury in determining outcome from severe head injury, *J Trauma*, Vol.34, No. 2, (Feb 1993), pp. 216-222, ISSN 0022-5282

Chiu, W. T., Yeh, K. H., Li, Y. C., Gan, Y. H., Chen, H. Y., & Hung, C. C. (1997). Traumatic brain injury registry in Taiwan, *Neurol Res*, Vol.19, No. 3, (Jun 1997), pp. 261-264, ISSN 0161-6412

Claassen, J., Mayer, S. A., Kowalski, R. G., Emerson, R. G., & Hirsch, L. J. (2004). Detection of electrographic seizures with continuous EEG monitoring in critically ill patients, *Neurology*, Vol.62, No. 10, (May 25 2004), pp. 1743-1748, ISSN 1526-632X

Clifton, G. L., Miller, E. R., Choi, S. C., Levin, H. S., McCauley, S., Smith, K. R., Jr., Muizelaar, J. P., Wagner, F. C., Jr., Marion, D. W., Luerssen, T. G., Chesnut, R. M., & Schwartz, M. (2001). Lack of effect of induction of hypothermia after acute brain injury, *N Engl J Med*, Vol.344, No. 8, (Feb 22 2001), pp. 556-563, ISSN 0028-4793

Colantonio, A., Escobar, M. D., Chipman, M., McLellan, B., Austin, P. C., Mirabella, G., & Ratcliff, G. (2008). Predictors of postacute mortality following traumatic brain injury in a seriously injured population, *J Trauma*, Vol.64, No. 4, (Apr 2008), pp. 876-882, ISSN 1529-8809

Cook, A. M., Peppard, A., & Magnuson, B. (2008). Nutrition considerations in traumatic brain injury, *Nutr Clin Pract*, Vol.23, No. 6, (Dec-2009 Jan 2008), pp. 608-620, ISSN 0884-5336

Cooper, D. J., Rosenfeld, J. V., Murray, L., Arabi, Y. M., Davies, A. R., D'Urso, P., Kossmann, T., Ponsford, J., Seppelt, I., Reilly, P., & Wolfe, R. (2011). Decompressive craniectomy in diffuse traumatic brain injury, *N Engl J Med*, Vol.364, No. 16, (Apr 21 2011), pp. 1493-1502, ISSN 1533-4406

Corrigan, J. D., Selassie, A. W., & Orman, J. A. (2010). The epidemiology of traumatic brain injury, *J Head Trauma Rehabil*, Vol.25, No. 2, (Mar-Apr 2010), pp. 72-80, ISSN 1550-509X

Czosnyka, M., Balestreri, M., Steiner, L., Smielewski, P., Hutchinson, P. J., Matta, B., & Pickard, J. D. (2005). Age, intracranial pressure, autoregulation, and outcome after brain trauma, *J Neurosurg*, Vol.102, No. 3, (Mar 2005), pp. 450-454, ISSN 0022-3085

Czosnyka, M., Smielewski, P., Kirkpatrick, P., Piechnik, S., Laing, R., & Pickard, J. D. (1998). Continuous monitoring of cerebrovascular pressure-reactivity in head injury, *Acta Neurochir Suppl*, Vol.71, No., 1998), pp. 74-77, ISSN 0065-1419 (Print)

Dewall, J. (2010). The ABCs of TBI. Evidence-based guidelines for adult traumatic brain injury care, *JEMS*, Vol.35, No. 4, (Apr 2010), pp. 54-61; quiz 63, ISSN 0197-2510

Dietrich, W. D., Alonso, O., Halley, M., & Busto, R. (1996). Delayed posttraumatic brain hyperthermia worsens outcome after fluid percussion brain injury: a light and electron microscopic study in rats, *Neurosurgery*, Vol.38, No. 3, (Mar 1996), pp. 533-541; discussion 541, ISSN 0148-396X

Dietrich, W. D., & Bramlett, H. M. (2007). Hyperthermia and central nervous system injury, *Prog Brain Res*, Vol.162, No., 2007), pp. 201-217, ISSN 0079-6123

Diringer, M. N., & Zazulia, A. R. (2004). Osmotic therapy: fact and fiction, *Neurocrit Care*, Vol.1, No. 2, 2004), pp. 219-233, ISSN 1541-6933

Donkin, J. J., & Vink, R. (2010). Mechanisms of cerebral edema in traumatic brain injury: therapeutic developments, *Curr Opin Neurol*, Vol.23, No. 3, (Jun 2010), pp. 293-299, ISSN 1473-6551

Dudley, R. R., Aziz, I., Bonnici, A., Saluja, R. S., Lamoureux, J., Kalmovitch, B., Gursahaney, A., Razek, T., Maleki, M., & Marcoux, J. (2010). Early venous thromboembolic event prophylaxis in traumatic brain injury with low-molecular-weight heparin: risks and benefits, *J Neurotrauma*, Vol.27, No. 12, (Dec 2010), pp. 2165-2172, ISSN 1557-9042

Eisenberg, H. M., Frankowski, R. F., Contant, C. F., Marshall, L. F., & Walker, M. D. (1988). High-dose barbiturate control of elevated intracranial pressure in patients with severe head injury, *J Neurosurg*, Vol.69, No. 1, (Jul 1988), pp. 15-23, ISSN 0022-3085

Eker, C., Asgeirsson, B., Grande, P. O., Schalen, W., & Nordstrom, C. H. (1998). Improved outcome after severe head injury with a new therapy based on principles for brain volume regulation and preserved microcirculation, *Crit Care Med*, Vol.26, No. 11, (Nov 1998), pp. 1881-1886, ISSN 0090-3493

Enriquez, P., & Bullock, R. (2004). Molecular and cellular mechanisms in the pathophysiology of severe head injury, *Curr Pharm Des*, Vol.10, No. 18, 2004), pp. 2131-2143, ISSN 1381-6128

Gabriel, E. J., Ghajar, J., Jagoda, A., Pons, P. T., Scalea, T., & Walters, B. C. (2002). Guidelines for prehospital management of traumatic brain injury, *J Neurotrauma*, Vol.19, No. 1, (Jan 2002), pp. 111-174, ISSN 0897-7151 (Print)

Gennarelli, T. A. (1993). Mechanisms of brain injury, *J Emerg Med*, Vol.11 Suppl 1, No., 1993), pp. 5-11, ISSN 0736-4679

Goodman, J. C., Valadka, A. B., Gopinath, S. P., Cormio, M., & Robertson, C. S. (1996). Lactate and excitatory amino acids measured by microdialysis are decreased by pentobarbital coma in head-injured patients, *J Neurotrauma*, Vol.13, No. 10, (Oct 1996), pp. 549-556, ISSN 0897-7151

Gopinath, S. P., Robertson, C. S., Contant, C. F., Hayes, C., Feldman, Z., Narayan, R. K., & Grossman, R. G. (1994). Jugular venous desaturation and outcome after head injury, *J Neurol Neurosurg Psychiatry*, Vol.57, No. 6, (Jun 1994), pp. 717-723, ISSN 0022-3050

Graham, D. I., Adams, J. H., & Gennarelli, T. A. (1988). Mechanisms of non-penetrating head injury, *Prog Clin Biol Res*, Vol.264, No., 1988), pp. 159-168, ISSN 0361-7742 (Print)

Gururaj G, Sastry Koeluri V, Chandramouli B, Subbakrishna D. 2004. Neurotrauma Registry in the NIMHANS. Bangalore, India: National Institute of Mental Health and Neurosciences.

Hartl, R., Gerber, L. M., Iacono, L., Ni, Q., Lyons, K., & Ghajar, J. (2006). Direct transport within an organized state trauma system reduces mortality in patients with severe traumatic brain injury, *J Trauma*, Vol.60, No. 6, (Jun 2006), pp. 1250-1256; discussion 1256, ISSN 0022-5282

Hartl, R., Gerber, L. M., Ni, Q., & Ghajar, J. (2008). Effect of early nutrition on deaths due to severe traumatic brain injury, *J Neurosurg*, Vol.109, No. 1, (Jul 2008), pp. 50-56, ISSN 0022-3085

Hays, A. N., Lazaridis, C., Neyens, R., Nicholas, J., Gay, S., & Chalela, J. A. (2011). Osmotherapy: use among neurointensivists, *Neurocrit Care*, Vol.14, No. 2, (Apr 2011), pp. 222-228, ISSN 1556-0961

Helmy, A., Vizcaychipi, M., & Gupta, A. K. (2007). Traumatic brain injury: intensive care management, Br J Anaesth, Vol.99, No. 1, (Jul 2007), pp. 32-42, ISSN 0007-0912

Hiler, M., Czosnyka, M., Hutchinson, P., Balestreri, M., Smielewski, P., Matta, B., & Pickard, J. D. (2006). Predictive value of initial computerized tomography scan, intracranial pressure, and state of autoregulation in patients with traumatic brain injury, J Neurosurg, Vol.104, No. 5, (May 2006), pp. 731-737, ISSN 0022-3085 (Print)

Hillered, L., Vespa, P. M., & Hovda, D. A. (2005). Translational neurochemical research in acute human brain injury: the current status and potential future for cerebral microdialysis, J Neurotrauma, Vol.22, No. 1, (Jan 2005), pp. 3-41, ISSN 0897-7151

Honda, M., Tsuruta, R., Kaneko, T., Kasaoka, S., Yagi, T., Todani, M., Fujita, M., Izumi, T., & Maekawa, T. (2010). Serum glial fibrillary acidic protein is a highly specific biomarker for traumatic brain injury in humans compared with S-100B and neuron-specific enolase, J Trauma, Vol.69, No. 1, (Jul 2010), pp. 104-109, ISSN 1529-8809

Howells, T., Elf, K., Jones, P. A., Ronne-Engstrom, E., Piper, I., Nilsson, P., Andrews, P., & Enblad, P. (2005). Pressure reactivity as a guide in the treatment of cerebral perfusion pressure in patients with brain trauma, J Neurosurg, Vol.102, No. 2, (Feb 2005), pp. 311-317, ISSN 0022-3085

Hutchinson, P. J., Gupta, A. K., Fryer, T. F., Al-Rawi, P. G., Chatfield, D. A., Coles, J. P., O'Connell, M. T., Kett-White, R., Minhas, P. S., Aigbirhio, F. I., Clark, J. C., Kirkpatrick, P. J., Menon, D. K., & Pickard, J. D. (2002). Correlation between cerebral blood flow, substrate delivery, and metabolism in head injury: a combined microdialysis and triple oxygen positron emission tomography study, J Cereb Blood Flow Metab, Vol.22, No. 6, (Jun 2002), pp. 735-745, ISSN 0271-678X

Illievich, U. M., Zornow, M. H., Choi, K. T., Scheller, M. S., & Strnat, M. A. (1994). Effects of hypothermic metabolic suppression on hippocampal glutamate concentrations after transient global cerebral ischemia, Anesth Analg, Vol.78, No. 5, (May 1994), pp. 905-911, ISSN 0003-2999

Jiang, J. Y., & Yang, X. F. (2007). Current status of cerebral protection with mild-to-moderate hypothermia after traumatic brain injury, Curr Opin Crit Care, Vol.13, No. 2, (Apr 2007), pp. 153-155, ISSN 1070-5295

Jiang, J., Yu, M., & Zhu, C. (2000). Effect of long-term mild hypothermia therapy in patients with severe traumatic brain injury: 1-year follow-up review of 87 cases, J Neurosurg, Vol.93, No. 4, (Oct 2000), pp. 546-549, ISSN 0022-3085

Johnston, A. J., Steiner, L. A., Chatfield, D. A., Coleman, M. R., Coles, J. P., Al-Rawi, P. G., Menon, D. K., & Gupta, A. K. (2003). Effects of propofol on cerebral oxygenation and metabolism after head injury, Br J Anaesth, Vol.91, No. 6, (Dec 2003), pp. 781-786, ISSN 0007-0912

Johnston, N. J., King, A. T., Protheroe, R., & Childs, C. (2006). Body temperature management after severe traumatic brain injury: methods and protocols used in the United Kingdom and Ireland, Resuscitation, Vol.70, No. 2, (Aug 2006), pp. 254-262, ISSN 0300-9572

Junpeng, M., Huang, S., & Qin, S. (2011). Progesterone for acute traumatic brain injury, Cochrane Database Syst Rev, No. 1, 2011), p. CD008409, ISSN 1469-493X

Juul, N., Morris, G. F., Marshall, S. B., & Marshall, L. F. (2000). Intracranial hypertension and cerebral perfusion pressure: influence on neurological deterioration and outcome in severe head injury. The Executive Committee of the International Selfotel Trial, *J Neurosurg*, Vol.92, No. 1, (Jan 2000), pp. 1-6, ISSN 0022-3085

Kassell, N. F., Hitchon, P. W., Gerk, M. K., Sokoll, M. D., & Hill, T. R. (1980). Alterations in cerebral blood flow, oxygen metabolism, and electrical activity produced by high dose sodium thiopental, *Neurosurgery*, Vol.7, No. 6, (Dec 1980), pp. 598-603, ISSN 0148-396X

Kassell, N. F., Peerless, S. J., Drake, C. G., Boarini, D. J., & Adams, H. P. (1980). Treatment of ischemic deficits from cerebral vasospasm with high dose barbiturate therapy, *Neurosurgery*, Vol.7, No. 6, (Dec 1980), pp. 593-597, ISSN 0148-396X

Kleindienst, A., Meissner, S., Eyupoglu, I. Y., Parsch, H., Schmidt, C., & Buchfelder, M. (2010). Dynamics of S100B release into serum and cerebrospinal fluid following acute brain injury, *Acta Neurochir Suppl*, Vol.106, No., 2010), pp. 247-250, ISSN 0065-1419

Langlois JA, Rutland-Brown W, Thomas KE. 2006. Traumatic Brain Injury in the United States: Emergency Department Visits, Hospitalization and Deaths. Atlanta, GA: Centers for Disease Control and Prevention, National Center for Injury Control and Prevention.

Leker, R. R., & Shohami, E. (2002). Cerebral ischemia and trauma-different etiologies yet similar mechanisms: neuroprotective opportunities, *Brain Res Brain Res Rev*, Vol.39, No. 1, (Jun 2002), pp. 55-73

Letarte, P. B., Puccio, A. M., Brown, S. D., & Marion, D. W. (1999). Effect of hypocapnea on CBF and extracellular intermediates of secondary brain injury, *Acta Neurochir Suppl*, Vol.75, No., 1999), pp. 45-47, ISSN 0065-1419

Li, J., Li, X. Y., Feng, D. F., & Pan, D. C. (2010). Biomarkers associated with diffuse traumatic axonal injury: exploring pathogenesis, early diagnosis, and prognosis, *J Trauma*, Vol.69, No. 6, (Dec 2010), pp. 1610-1618, ISSN 1529-8809

Li, L. M., Timofeev, I., Czosnyka, M., & Hutchinson, P. J. (2010). Review article: the surgical approach to the management of increased intracranial pressure after traumatic brain injury, *Anesth Analg*, Vol.111, No. 3, (Sep 2010), pp. 736-748, ISSN 1526-7598

Liu-DeRyke, X., Collingridge, D. S., Orme, J., Roller, D., Zurasky, J., & Rhoney, D. H. (2009). Clinical impact of early hyperglycemia during acute phase of traumatic brain

Liu, W. G., Qiu, W. S., Zhang, Y., Wang, W. M., Lu, F., & Yang, X. F. (2006). Effects of selective brain cooling in patients with severe traumatic brain injury: a preliminary study, *J Int Med Res*, Vol.34, No. 1, (Jan-Feb 2006), pp. 58-64, ISSN 0300-0605

Lumpkins, K. M., Bochicchio, G. V., Keledjian, K., Simard, J. M., McCunn, M., & Scalea, T. (2008). Glial fibrillary acidic protein is highly correlated with brain injury, *J Trauma*, Vol.65, No. 4, (Oct 2008), pp. 778-782; discussion 782-774, ISSN 1529-8809

Manley, G. T., Fujimura, M., Ma, T., Noshita, N., Filiz, F., Bollen, A. W., Chan, P., & Verkman, A. S. (2000). Aquaporin-4 deletion in mice reduces brain edema after acute water intoxication and ischemic stroke, *Nat Med*, Vol.6, No. 2, (Feb 2000), pp. 159-163, ISSN 1078-8956

Marion, D. W. (2011). Decompressive craniectomy in diffuse traumatic brain injury, *Lancet Neurol*, Vol.10, No. 6, (Jun 2011), pp. 497-498, ISSN 1474-4465

Marion, D. W., Obrist, W. D., Carlier, P. M., Penrod, L. E., & Darby, J. M. (1993). The use of moderate therapeutic hypothermia for patients with severe head injuries: a preliminary report, *J Neurosurg*, Vol.79, No. 3, (Sep 1993), pp. 354-362, ISSN 0022-3085

Marion, D. W., Penrod, L. E., Kelsey, S. F., Obrist, W. D., Kochanek, P. M., Palmer, A. M., Wisniewski, S. R., & DeKosky, S. T. (1997). Treatment of traumatic brain injury with moderate hypothermia, *N Engl J Med*, Vol.336, No. 8, (Feb 20 1997), pp. 540-546, ISSN 0028-4793

Marion, D. W., Puccio, A., Wisniewski, S. R., Kochanek, P., Dixon, C. E., Bullian, L., & Carlier, P. (2002). Effect of hyperventilation on extracellular concentrations of glutamate, lactate, pyruvate, and local cerebral blood flow in patients with severe traumatic brain injury, *Crit Care Med*, Vol.30, No. 12, (Dec 2002), pp. 2619-2625, ISSN 0090-3493

Marshall, G. T., James, R. F., Landman, M. P., O'Neill, P. J., Cotton, B. A., Hansen, E. N., Morris, J. A., Jr., & May, A. K. (2010). Pentobarbital coma for refractory intra-cranial hypertension after severe traumatic brain injury: mortality predictions and one-year outcomes in 55 patients, *J Trauma*, Vol.69, No. 2, (Aug 2010), pp. 275-283, ISSN 1529-8809

Martin, N. A., Patwardhan, R. V., Alexander, M. J., Africk, C. Z., Lee, J. H., Shalmon, E., Hovda, D. A., & Becker, D. P. (1997). Characterization of cerebral hemodynamic phases following severe head trauma: hypoperfusion, hyperemia, and vasospasm, *J Neurosurg*, Vol.87, No. 1, (Jul 1997), pp. 9-19, ISSN 0022-3085

McIntyre, L. A., Fergusson, D. A., Hebert, P. C., Moher, D., & Hutchison, J. S. (2003). Prolonged therapeutic hypothermia after traumatic brain injury in adults: a systematic review, *JAMA*, Vol.289, No. 22, (Jun 11 2003), pp. 2992-2999, ISSN 1538-3598

Meyer, M. J., Megyesi, J., Meythaler, J., Murie-Fernandez, M., Aubut, J. A., Foley, N., Salter, K., Bayley, M., Marshall, S., & Teasell, R. (2010). Acute management of acquired brain injury part I: an evidence-based review of non-pharmacological interventions, *Brain Inj*, Vol.24, No. 5, 2010), pp. 694-705, ISSN 1362-301X

Meyer, M. J., Megyesi, J., Meythaler, J., Murie-Fernandez, M., Aubut, J. A., Foley, N., Salter, K., Bayley, M., Marshall, S., & Teasell, R. (2010). Acute management of acquired brain injury part II: an evidence-based review of pharmacological interventions, *Brain Inj*, Vol.24, No. 5, 2010), pp. 706-721, ISSN 1362-301X (Electronic)

Mild therapeutic hypothermia to improve the neurologic outcome after cardiac arrest. (2002). *N Engl J Med*, Vol.346, No. 8, (Feb 21 2002), pp. 549-556, ISSN 1533-4406

Mishina, H., & Yabuki, A. (1994). Relationship of cerebral blood flow, cerebral metabolism, and electroencephalography to outcome in acute experimental compression ischemia--barbiturate effects on delayed brain swelling, *Neurol Med Chir (Tokyo)*, Vol.34, No. 6, (Jun 1994), pp. 345-352, ISSN 0470-8105

Muizelaar, J. P., van der Poel, H. G., Li, Z. C., Kontos, H. A., & Levasseur, J. E. (1988). Pial arteriolar vessel diameter and CO2 reactivity during prolonged hyperventilation in the rabbit, *J Neurosurg*, Vol.69, No. 6, (Dec 1988), pp. 923-927, ISSN 0022-3085

Narayan, R. K., Michel, M. E., Ansell, B., Baethmann, A., Biegon, A., Bracken, M. B., Bullock, M. R., Choi, S. C., Clifton, G. L., Contant, C. F., Coplin, W. M., Dietrich, W. D., Ghajar, J., Grady, S. M., Grossman, R. G., Hall, E. D., Heetderks, W., Hovda, D. A., Jallo, J., Katz, R. L., Knoller, N., Kochanek, P. M., Maas, A. I., Majde, J., Marion, D. W., Marmarou, A., Marshall, L. F., McIntosh, T. K., Miller, E., Mohberg, N.,

Muizelaar, J. P., Pitts, L. H., Quinn, P., Riesenfeld, G., Robertson, C. S., Strauss, K. I., Teasdale, G., Temkin, N., Tuma, R., Wade, C., Walker, M. D., Weinrich, M., Whyte, J., Wilberger, J., Young, A. B., & Yurkewicz, L. (2002). Clinical trials in head injury, *J Neurotrauma*, Vol.19, No. 5, (May 2002), pp. 503-557, ISSN 0897-7151

Nordstrom, C. H., Reinstrup, P., Xu, W., Gardenfors, A., & Ungerstedt, U. (2003). Assessment of the lower limit for cerebral perfusion pressure in severe head injuries by bedside monitoring of regional energy metabolism, *Anesthesiology*, Vol.98, No. 4, (Apr 2003), pp. 809-814, ISSN 0003-3022

Norwood, S. H., Berne, J. D., Rowe, S. A., Villarreal, D. H., & Ledlie, J. T. (2008). Early venous thromboembolism prophylaxis with enoxaparin in patients with blunt traumatic brain injury, *J Trauma*, Vol.65, No. 5, (Nov 2008), pp. 1021-1026; discussion 1026-1027, ISSN 1529-8809

Nurmohamed, M. T., van Riel, A. M., Henkens, C. M., Koopman, M. M., Que, G. T., d'Azemar, P., Buller, H. R., ten Cate, J. W., Hoek, J. A., van der Meer, J., van der Heul, C., Turpie, A. G., Haley, S., Sicurella, A., & Gent, M. (1996). Low molecular weight heparin and compression stockings in the prevention of venous thromboembolism in neurosurgery, *Thromb Haemost*, Vol.75, No. 2, (Feb 1996), pp. 233-238, ISSN 0340-6245

Nylen, K., Ost, M., Csajbok, L. Z., Nilsson, I., Blennow, K., Nellgard, B., & Rosengren, L. (2006). Increased serum-GFAP in patients with severe traumatic brain injury is related to outcome, *J Neurol Sci*, Vol.240, No. 1-2, (Jan 15 2006), pp. 85-91, ISSN 0022-510X

Ogden, Alfred T., Mayer, Stephan A., & E. Sander Connolly, Jr. (2005). Hyperosmolar agents in neurosurgical practice: the evolving role of hypertonic saline *Neurosurgery*, Vol.57, No. 2, 2005), pp. 207-215

Papadopoulos, M. C., & Verkman, A. S. (2008). Potential utility of aquaporin modulators for therapy of brain disorders, *Prog Brain Res*, Vol.170, No., 2008), pp. 589-601, ISSN 1875-7855

Pasantes-Morales, H., & Cruz-Rangel, S. (2010). Brain volume regulation: osmolytes and aquaporin perspectives, *Neuroscience*, Vol.168, No. 4, (Jul 28 2010), pp. 871-884, ISSN 1873-7544

Patel, H. C., Bouamra, O., Woodford, M., King, A. T., Yates, D. W., & Lecky, F. E. (2005). Trends in head injury outcome from 1989 to 2003 and the effect of neurosurgical care: an observational study, *Lancet*, Vol.366, No. 9496, (Oct 29-Nov 4 2005), pp. 1538-1544, ISSN 1474-547X

Petzold, A., Keir, G., Lim, D., Smith, M., & Thompson, E. J. (2003). Cerebrospinal fluid (CSF) and serum S100B: release and wash-out pattern, *Brain Res Bull*, Vol.61, No. 3, (Aug 15 2003), pp. 281-285, ISSN 0361-9230

Povlishock, J. T., & Wei, E. P. (2009). Posthypothermic rewarming considerations following traumatic brain injury, *J Neurotrauma*, Vol.26, No. 3, (Mar 2009), pp. 333-340, ISSN 1557-9042

Qiu, W., Shen, H., Zhang, Y., Wang, W., Liu, W., Jiang, Q., Luo, M., & Manou, M. (2006). Noninvasive selective brain cooling by head and neck cooling is protective in severe traumatic brain injury, *J Clin Neurosci*, Vol.13, No. 10, (Dec 2006), pp. 995-1000, ISSN 0967-5868

Qiu, W., Zhang, Y., Sheng, H., Zhang, J., Wang, W., Liu, W., Chen, K., Zhou, J., & Xu, Z. (2007). Effects of therapeutic mild hypothermia on patients with severe traumatic brain injury after craniotomy, *J Crit Care*, Vol.22, No. 3, (Sep 2007), pp. 229-235, ISSN 0883-9441

Raabe, A., Grolms, C., Keller, M., Dohnert, J., Sorge, O., & Seifert, V. (1998). Correlation of computed tomography findings and serum brain damage markers following severe head injury, *Acta Neurochir (Wien)*, Vol.140, No. 8, 1998), pp. 787-791; discussion 791-782, ISSN 0001-6268

Ritter, A. M., Gopinath, S. P., Contant, C., Narayan, R. K., & Robertson, C. S. (1996). Evaluation of a regional oxygen saturation catheter for monitoring SjvO2 in head injured patients, *J Clin Monit*, Vol.12, No. 4, (Jul 1996), pp. 285-291, ISSN 0748-1977

Robertson, C. S. (2001). Management of cerebral perfusion pressure after traumatic brain injury, *Anesthesiology*, Vol.95, No. 6, (Dec 2001), pp. 1513-1517, ISSN 0003-3022

Robertson, C. S., Gopinath, S. P., Goodman, J. C., Contant, C. F., Valadka, A. B., & Narayan, R. K. (1995). SjvO2 monitoring in head-injured patients, *J Neurotrauma*, Vol.12, No. 5, (Oct 1995), pp. 891-896, ISSN 0897-7151

Robertson, C. S., Valadka, A. B., Hannay, H. J., Contant, C. F., Gopinath, S. P., Cormio, M., Uzura, M., & Grossman, R. G. (1999). Prevention of secondary ischemic insults after severe head injury, *Crit Care Med*, Vol.27, No. 10, (Oct 1999), pp. 2086-2095, ISSN 0090-3493

Rockswold, S. B., Rockswold, G. L., Zaun, D. A., Zhang, X., Cerra, C. E., Bergman, T. A., & Liu, J. (2010). A prospective, randomized clinical trial to compare the effect of hyperbaric to normobaric hyperoxia on cerebral metabolism, intracranial pressure, and oxygen toxicity in severe traumatic brain injury, *J Neurosurg*, Vol.112, No. 5, (May 2010), pp. 1080-1094, ISSN 1933-0693

Ronne-Engstrom, E., & Winkler, T. (2006). Continuous EEG monitoring in patients with traumatic brain injury reveals a high incidence of epileptiform activity, *Acta Neurol Scand*, Vol.114, No. 1, (Jul 2006), pp. 47-53, ISSN 0001-6314

Rosenthal, G., Hemphill, J. C., 3rd, Sorani, M., Martin, C., Morabito, D., Obrist, W. D., & Manley, G. T. (2008). Brain tissue oxygen tension is more indicative of oxygen diffusion than oxygen delivery and metabolism in patients with traumatic brain injury, *Crit Care Med*, Vol.36, No. 6, (Jun 2008), pp. 1917-1924, ISSN 1530-0293

Rosenthal, G., Sanchez-Mejia, R. O., Phan, N., Hemphill, J. C., 3rd, Martin, C., & Manley, G. T. (2011). Incorporating a parenchymal thermal diffusion cerebral blood flow probe in bedside assessment of cerebral autoregulation and vasoreactivity in patients with severe traumatic brain injury, *J Neurosurg*, Vol.114, No. 1, (Jan 2011), pp. 62-70, ISSN 1933-0693

Rosomoff, H. L., & Holaday, D. A. (1954). Cerebral blood flow and cerebral oxygen consumption during hypothermia, *Am J Physiol*, Vol.179, No. 1, (Oct 1954), pp. 85-88, ISSN 0002-9513

Sacks, G. S., Brown, R. O., Teague, D., Dickerson, R. N., Tolley, E. A., & Kudsk, K. A. (1995). Early nutrition support modifies immune function in patients sustaining severe head injury, *JPEN J Parenter Enteral Nutr*, Vol.19, No. 5, (Sep-Oct 1995), pp. 387-392, ISSN 0148-6071

Schroder, M. L., Muizelaar, J. P., Bullock, M. R., Salvant, J. B., & Povlishock, J. T. (1995). Focal ischemia due to traumatic contusions documented by stable xenon-CT and ultrastructural studies, *J Neurosurg*, Vol.82, No. 6, (Jun 1995), pp. 966-971, ISSN 0022-3085

Schwartz, M. L., Tator, C. H., Rowed, D. W., Reid, S. R., Meguro, K., & Andrews, D. F. (1984). The University of Toronto head injury treatment study: a prospective, randomized comparison of pentobarbital and mannitol, *Can J Neurol Sci*, Vol.11, No. 4, (Nov 1984), pp. 434-440, ISSN 0317-1671

Schwarz, S., Georgiadis, D., Aschoff, A., & Schwab, S. (2002). Effects of hypertonic (10%) saline in patients with raised intracranial pressure after stroke, *Stroke*, Vol.33, No. 1, (Jan 2002), pp. 136-140, ISSN 1524-4628

Seelig, J. M., Becker, D. P., Miller, J. D., Greenberg, R. P., Ward, J. D., & Choi, S. C. (1981). Traumatic acute subdural hematoma: major mortality reduction in comatose patients treated within four hours, *N Engl J Med*, Vol.304, No. 25, (Jun 18 1981), pp. 1511-1518, ISSN 0028-4793

Segatore, M. (1992). Fever after traumatic brain injury, *J Neurosci Nurs*, Vol.24, No. 2, (Apr 1992), pp. 104-109, ISSN 0888-0395

Selassie, A. W., Zaloshnja, E., Langlois, J. A., Miller, T., Jones, P., & Steiner, C. (2008). Incidence of long-term disability following traumatic brain injury hospitalization, United States, 2003, *J Head Trauma Rehabil*, Vol.23, No. 2, (Mar-Apr 2008), pp. 123-131, ISSN 0885-9701

Shiozaki, T., Sugimoto, H., Taneda, M., Yoshida, H., Iwai, A., Yoshioka, T., & Sugimoto, T. (1993). Effect of mild hypothermia on uncontrollable intracranial hypertension after severe head injury, *J Neurosurg*, Vol.79, No. 3, (Sep 1993), pp. 363-368, ISSN 0022-3085

Shohami, E., Beit-Yannai, E., Horowitz, M., & Kohen, R. (1997). Oxidative stress in closed-head injury: brain antioxidant capacity as an indicator of functional outcome, *J Cereb Blood Flow Metab*, Vol.17, No. 10, (Oct 1997), pp. 1007-1019, ISSN 0271-678X

Sirvent, J. M., Torres, A., El-Ebiary, M., Castro, P., de Batlle, J., & Bonet, A. (1997). Protective effect of intravenously administered cefuroxime against nosocomial pneumonia in patients with structural coma, *Am J Respir Crit Care Med*, Vol.155, No. 5, (May 1997), pp. 1729-1734, ISSN 1073-449X

Skandsen, T., Kvistad, K. A., Solheim, O., Strand, I. H., Folvik, M., & Vik, A. (2010). Prevalence and impact of diffuse axonal injury in patients with moderate and severe head injury: a cohort study of early magnetic resonance imaging findings and 1-year outcome, *J Neurosurg*, Vol.113, No. 3, (Sep 2010), pp. 556-563, ISSN 1933-0693

Smith, A. L., Hoff, J. T., Nielsen, S. L., & Larson, C. P. (1974). Barbiturate protection in acute focal cerebral ischemia, *Stroke*, Vol.5, No. 1, (Jan-Feb 1974), pp. 1-7, ISSN 0039-2499

Soares, H. D., Hicks, R. R., Smith, D., & McIntosh, T. K. (1995). Inflammatory leukocytic recruitment and diffuse neuronal degeneration are separate pathological processes resulting from traumatic brain injury, *J Neurosci*, Vol.15, No. 12, (Dec 1995), pp. 8223-8233, ISSN 0270-6474

Spiotta, A. M., Stiefel, M. F., Gracias, V. H., Garuffe, A. M., Kofke, W. A., Maloney-Wilensky, E., Troxel, A. B., Levine, J. M., & Le Roux, P. D. (2010). Brain tissue oxygen-directed management and outcome in patients with severe traumatic brain injury, *J Neurosurg*, Vol.113, No. 3, (Sep 2010), pp. 571-580, ISSN 1933-0693

Stein, S. C., Georgoff, P., Meghan, S., Mizra, K., & Sonnad, S. S. (2010). 150 years of treating severe traumatic brain injury: a systematic review of progress in mortality, *J Neurotrauma*, Vol.27, No. 7, (Jul 2010), pp. 1343-1353, ISSN 1557-9042

Stewart, L., Bullock, R., Rafferty, C., Fitch, W., & Teasdale, G. M. (1994). Propofol sedation in severe head injury fails to control high ICP, but reduces brain metabolism, *Acta Neurochir Suppl (Wien)*, Vol.60, No., 1994), pp. 544-546, ISSN 0065-1419

Stiefel, M. F., Spiotta, A., Gracias, V. H., Garuffe, A. M., Guillamondegui, O., Maloney-Wilensky, E., Bloom, S., Grady, M. S., & LeRoux, P. D. (2005). Reduced mortality rate in patients with severe traumatic brain injury treated with brain tissue oxygen monitoring, *J Neurosurg*, Vol.103, No. 5, (Nov 2005), pp. 805-811, ISSN 0022-3085

Tagliaferri, F., Compagnone, C., Korsic, M., Servadei, F., & Kraus, J. (2006). A systematic review of brain injury epidemiology in Europe, *Acta Neurochir (Wien)*, Vol.148, No. 3, (Mar 2006), pp. 255-268; discussion 268, ISSN 0001-6268 (Print)

Taya, K., Gulsen, S., Okuno, K., Prieto, R., Marmarou, C. R., & Marmarou, A. (2008). Modulation of AQP4 expression by the selective V1a receptor antagonist, SR49059, decreases trauma-induced brain edema, *Acta Neurochir Suppl*, Vol.102, No., 2008), pp. 425-429, ISSN 0065-1419

Taylor, S. J., Fettes, S. B., Jewkes, C., & Nelson, R. J. (1999). Prospective, randomized, controlled trial to determine the effect of early enhanced enteral nutrition on clinical outcome in mechanically ventilated patients suffering head injury, *Crit Care Med*, Vol.27, No. 11, (Nov 1999), pp. 2525-2531, ISSN 0090-3493

Tisdall, M. M., Tachtsidis, I., Leung, T. S., Elwell, C. E., & Smith, M. (2008). Increase in cerebral aerobic metabolism by normobaric hyperoxia after traumatic brain injury, *J Neurosurg*, Vol.109, No. 3, (Sep 2008), pp. 424-432, ISSN 0022-3085

Valadka, A. B., Furuya, Y., Hlatky, R., & Robertson, C. S. (2000). Global and regional techniques for monitoring cerebral oxidative metabolism after severe traumatic brain injury, *Neurosurg Focus*, Vol.9, No. 5, 2000), p. e3, ISSN 1092-0684

Valadka, A. B., Goodman, J. C., Gopinath, S. P., Uzura, M., & Robertson, C. S. (1998). Comparison of brain tissue oxygen tension to microdialysis-based measures of cerebral ischemia in fatally head-injured humans, *J Neurotrauma*, Vol.15, No. 7, (Jul 1998), pp. 509-519, ISSN 0897-7151

Valadka, A. B., & Robertson, C. S. (2007). Surgery of cerebral trauma and associated critical care, *Neurosurgery*, Vol.61, No. 1 Suppl, (Jul 2007), pp. 203-220; discussion 220-201, ISSN 1524-4040

Ventilation with lower tidal volumes as compared with traditional tidal volumes for acute lung injury and the acute respiratory distress syndrome. The Acute Respiratory Distress Syndrome Network. (2000). *N Engl J Med*, Vol.342, No. 18, (May 4 2000), pp. 1301-1308, ISSN 0028-4793

Vespa, P., Boonyaputthikul, R., McArthur, D. L., Miller, C., Etchepare, M., Bergsneider, M., Glenn, T., Martin, N., & Hovda, D. (2006). Intensive insulin therapy reduces microdialysis glucose values without altering glucose utilization or improving the lactate/pyruvate ratio after traumatic brain injury, *Crit Care Med*, Vol.34, No. 3, (Mar 2006), pp. 850-856, ISSN 0090-3493

Vespa, P. M., McArthur, D., O'Phelan, K., Glenn, T., Etchepare, M., Kelly, D., Bergsneider, M., Martin, N. A., & Hovda, D. A. (2003). Persistently low extracellular glucose correlates with poor outcome 6 months after human traumatic brain injury despite a lack of increased lactate: a microdialysis study, *J Cereb Blood Flow Metab*, Vol.23, No. 7, (Jul 2003), pp. 865-877, ISSN 0271-678X

Vespa, P. M., Miller, C., McArthur, D., Eliseo, M., Etchepare, M., Hirt, D., Glenn, T. C., Martin, N., & Hovda, D. (2007). Nonconvulsive electrographic seizures after traumatic brain injury result in a delayed, prolonged increase in intracranial pressure and metabolic crisis, *Crit Care Med*, Vol.35, No. 12, (Dec 2007), pp. 2830-2836, ISSN 0090-3493

Vespa, P. M., Nuwer, M. R., Nenov, V., Ronne-Engstrom, E., Hovda, D. A., Bergsneider, M., Kelly, D. F., Martin, N. A., & Becker, D. P. (1999). Increased incidence and impact of nonconvulsive and convulsive seizures after traumatic brain injury as detected by continuous electroencephalographic monitoring, *J Neurosurg*, Vol.91, No. 5, (Nov 1999), pp. 750-760, ISSN 0022-3085

Vialet, R., Albanese, J., Thomachot, L., Antonini, F., Bourgouin, A., Alliez, B., & Martin, C. (2003). Isovolume hypertonic solutes (sodium chloride or mannitol) in the treatment of refractory posttraumatic intracranial hypertension: 2 mL/kg 7.5% saline is more effective than 2 mL/kg 20% mannitol, *Crit Care Med*, Vol.31, No. 6, (Jun 2003), pp. 1683-1687, ISSN 0090-3493

Vos, P. E., Lamers, K. J., Hendriks, J. C., van Haaren, M., Beems, T., Zimmerman, C., van Geel, W., de Reus, H., Biert, J., & Verbeek, M. M. (2004). Glial and neuronal proteins in serum predict outcome after severe traumatic brain injury, *Neurology*, Vol.62, No. 8, (Apr 27 2004), pp. 1303-1310, ISSN 1526-632X

Ward, J. D., Becker, D. P., Miller, J. D., Choi, S. C., Marmarou, A., Wood, C., Newlon, P. G., & Keenan, R. (1985). Failure of prophylactic barbiturate coma in the treatment of severe head injury, *J Neurosurg*, Vol.62, No. 3, (Mar 1985), pp. 383-388, ISSN 0022-3085

Waziri, A., Claassen, J., Stuart, R. M., Arif, H., Schmidt, J. M., Mayer, S. A., Badjatia, N., Kull, L. L., Connolly, E. S., Emerson, R. G., & Hirsch, L. J. (2009). Intracortical electroencephalography in acute brain injury, *Ann Neurol*, Vol.66, No. 3, (Sep 2009), pp. 366-377, ISSN 1531-8249

Weant, K. A., Martin, J. E., Humphries, R. L., & Cook, A. M. (2010). Pharmacologic options for reducing the shivering response to therapeutic hypothermia, *Pharmacotherapy*, Vol.30, No. 8, (Aug 2010), pp. 830-841, ISSN 1875-9114

Wintermark, M., van Melle, G., Schnyder, P., Revelly, J. P., Porchet, F., Regli, L., Meuli, R., Maeder, P., & Chiolero, R. (2004). Admission perfusion CT: prognostic value in patients with severe head trauma, *Radiology*, Vol.232, No. 1, (Jul 2004), pp. 211-220, ISSN 0033-8419

Woertgen, C., Rothoerl, R. D., & Brawanski, A. (2002). Early S-100B serum level correlates to quality of life in patients after severe head injury, *Brain Inj*, Vol.16, No. 9, (Sep 2002), pp. 807-816, ISSN 0269-9052

Young, N., Rhodes, J. K., Mascia, L., & Andrews, P. J. (2010). Ventilatory strategies for patients with acute brain injury, *Curr Opin Crit Care*, Vol.16, No. 1, (Feb 2010), pp. 45-52, ISSN 1531-7072

Zaloshnja, E., Miller, T., Langlois, J. A., & Selassie, A. W. (2008). Prevalence of long-term disability from traumatic brain injury in the civilian population of the United States, 2005, *J Head Trauma Rehabil*, Vol.23, No. 6, (Nov-Dec 2008), pp. 394-400, ISSN 1550-509X

Zemlan, F. P., Rosenberg, W. S., Luebbe, P. A., Campbell, T. A., Dean, G. E., Weiner, N. E., Cohen, J. A., Rudick, R. A., & Woo, D. (1999). Quantification of axonal damage in traumatic brain injury: affinity purification and characterization of cerebrospinal fluid tau proteins, *J Neurochem*, Vol.72, No. 2, (Feb 1999), pp. 741-750, ISSN 0022-3042

7

Growth Hormone and Kynesitherapy for Brain Injury Recovery

Jesús Devesa[1,2], Pablo Devesa[1,2], Pedro Reimunde[2] and Víctor Arce[1]
[1]Department of Physiology, School of Medicine, Santiago de Compostela
[2]Medical Center "Proyecto Foltra", Teo
Spain

1. Introduction

Acquired brain injury is a medical and social reality of growing magnitude and extraordinary severity requiring an increasingly specialised response to the extent permitted by technological advances and research. Although there are no accurate or reliable statistical data regarding the number of people affected by brain injury, scientific opinion maintains that brain injury represents one of the largest health problems in developed countries, both in terms of the number of deaths caused and the high number of people left suffering from some sort of functional and cognitive disability as a result of the sequelae caused by the damage occurred in the brain.

The most frequent causes of acquired brain injury are pre/perinatal hypoxia/ischemia or post-natal infections (for example, meningitis), cranial traumas, stroke. One of the first consequences of acquired brain injury is the loss of consciousness; the duration and degree of it are one of the most significant indicators of the severity of the injury. After the progressive recovery of the level of consciousness and the spatial orientation, most patients suffer a wide range of cognitive and motor sequelae; the nature and severity of them depend on the location and extent of brain damage, and the age of the patient as well.

The multiple functional and social impairments caused by the brain injury and the motor impairments affecting memory, speech or behaviour require a multi-disciplinary treatment approach from the critical-acute stage, calling for the highest level of specialisation until the patient can readjust back into the community. There is consensus among specialists regarding the damaged brain's ability to recover part of its functions spontaneously, a process that may take several months or even years. Experts also agree on the need for early neurorehabilitation to improve these natural mechanisms and achieve the best possible functional and social recovery, considering the complexity of the sequelae (motor, cognitive, emotional) caused in varying combinations by brain injury. However, access to rehabilitation facilities specialized in brain injury is marked by the shortage of public or private resources, with a huge difference in the availability of such facilities among the different countries. This shortage, scarcity or non-existence of public or private rehabilitation facilities in many countries, together with the enormous cost of these services offered by private centres, make access to rehabilitation and recovery difficult or even impossible for many people. Therefore, as a result of not seeing the benefit of potential recovery and social integration, this leads to a greater dependence and burden on the family. Therefore, acquired brain injury is a major public health, and yet medical science has little to offer for the persistent symptoms that prevent many of these individuals from fully re-entering society.

Until few years ago it was thought that recovery from a brain injury would occur through the reinforcement of the mechanisms of neural plasticity. Establishing new synaptic connections between surviving neurons would partially allow to recover lost functions. There are evidences that environmental enrichment induces epigenetic changes that facilitate synaptogenesis and memory in models of brain plasticity. On this basis special units for brain recovery should be the closest correpondence for an enriched environment for patients with brain injury. Anything that can be done to optimize the hospital and rehabilitation environment should be beneficial. No study was shown to what extent the beneficial effect is due to specific rehabilitation strategies, to the time spent in physiotherapy and occupational therapy, and a non-specific effect of a more stimulating environment with competent staff that can encourage and support the patients and family members, but all these factors are likely to be important. In all, it is likely that admission to an acute rehabilitation unit would benefit the recovery after a brain damage (Johansson, 2011).

Today we know that appart of brain plasticity, the development of any brain injury quickly leads to enhanced proliferation of neural stem cells. From the damaged cerebral areas a number of cytokines would be released for activating the migration and differentiation of newborn cells. It has been recently identified a P2Y-like receptor GPR17 that is a sensor of brain damage and a new target for brain repair (Lecca et al., 2008). Upon brain injury, the extracellular concentrations of nucleotides and cysteinyl-leukotrienes (cysLTs), two families of endogenous signaling molecules, are markedly increased at the site of damage, suggesting that they may act as "danger signals" to alert responses to tissue damage and start repair. In brain telencephalon, GPR17, a recently deorphanized receptor for both uracil nucleotides and cysLTs (e.g., UDP-glucose and LTD4), is normally present on neurons and on a subset of parenchymal quiescent oligodendrocyte precursor cells. Induction of brain injury using an established focal ischemia model in the rodent induces profound spatiotemporal-dependent changes of GPR17. In the lesioned area, an early and transient up-regulation of GPR17 in neurons expressing the cellular stress marker *Heat shock protein 70* (Hsp70, *Heat shock protein 70)* is observed. Magnetic resonance imaging in living mice showed that the *in vivo* pharmacological or biotechnological *knock down* of GPR17 markedly prevents brain infarct evolution, suggesting GPR17 as a mediator of neuronal death at this early ischemic stage. At later times after ischemia, GPR17 immuno-labeling appeared on microglia/macrophages infiltrating the lesioned area to indicate that GPR17 may also acts as a player in the remodeling of brain circuitries by microglia. At this later stage, parenchymal GPR17+ oligodendrocyte progenitors started proliferating in the periinjured area, suggesting initiation of remyelination. The *in vitro* exposure of cortical pre-oligodendrocytes to the GPR17 endogenous ligands UDP-glucose and LTD4 promoted the expression of myelin basic protein, confirming progression toward mature oligodendrocytes. Thus, GPR17 may act as a "sensor" that is activated upon brain injury on several embrionic distinct cell types, and may play a key role in both inducing neural death inside the ischemic core and in orchestrating the local/remodeling repair response (Lecca et al., 2008).

According to these concepts two different mechanisms are involved in trying to repair brain damage: 1) quick proliferation of neural precursors, and 2) development of neural plasticity. Both are independent but complementary of each other. Neural stem cells proliferation and brain plasticity require the intervention of neurotrophic factors. This concept is showed in Figure 1.

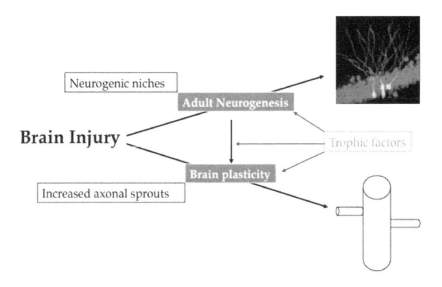

Fig. 1. Physiological responses to a brain injury. After a brain injury adult neurogenesis starts in neurogenic niches. Later, adequate rehabilitation and rich environment facilitate the development of brain plasticity. Both responses require the intervention of neurotrophic factors.

The knowledge of these and other events occurring after brain injury led to investigate how to enhance and improve mechanisms involved in brain repair.

In this chapter we will analyze current concepts about brain stem cells proliferation for brain repair and the effect of administering a neurotrophic and neuroprotective agent, growth hormone together with specific kynesitherapy, on the recovery of different kind of patients with acquired brain injury.

2. Adult neurogenesis

The complexity and specialization of neural functions increase as animal species ascend in the zoological scale. It is clear that the degree of specialization achieved, with so many and so complex interactions and functions, requires a long period of time for morphogenesis, in which not only cell proliferation and differentiation occurs, but also apoptosis must take place in a perfectly scheduled sequential expression of many different genes; later, after birth, the morphogenetic development of central nervous system is modulated by learning phenomena and the environment. However, this classical concept about neural development establishing that no new neurons are formed after birth has been changed when it was reported that new neurons are produced daily in several niches of the adult brain in many mammal species, including humans (Kuhn et al., 1996; Eriksson et al., 1998; Kempermann et al., 2004). This production is particularly important in the subventricular zone of the lateral ventricles and the subgranular zone of the dentate gyrus of the hippocampus, where neural progenitors reside primarily in the subgranular layers (Gould et al., 1999; Fukuda et al., 2003; Kronenberg et al., 2003).

The paradigm about a central nervous system unable to replace the daily loss of neurons began to be questioned in the mid-60's. However, the pioneer studies carried out in these years were not taken into account mainly due to technical and methodological issues (Altman & Gas, 1965; Kaplan & Hinds, 1977). Later, the notorious advance of the immunohistochemistry, cytology and molecular biology changed the dominant paradigm. Researchers, as Goldman (Goldman & Nottebohm, 1983) suggested that the generation of new neurons, neurogenesis, could be a normal phenomenon in the adult canary brain. The same group demonstrated later that the new formed neurons were incorporated into functional circuits (Paton et al., 1984). In the early 90's, cells with properties of neural precursors were isolated in the striatum of mice (Reynolds & Weiss, 1992). Soon the subventricular zone was identified as a niche were neural precursors were formed (Lois & Alvarez-Buylla, 1993). Lastly, at the end of 90's, it was described that adult neurogenesis is a phenomenon that also occurs in higher primates, including humans (Eriksson et al., 1998; Gould et al., 1999), a concept now widely accepted.

2.1 Where adult neurogenesis occurs and what is its functional significance?

Constitutive neurogenesis takes place in the rodent adult mammalian brain, and particularly in the subventricular zone. This zone harbors a population of stem cells that proliferate and give rise to neurons and glial cells. Neuroblasts formed here migrate long distances along the rostral migratory stream toward the olfactory bulb, where they differentiate into GABA and dopaminergic interneurons, involved in odor discrimination (Betarbet el al. 1996; Gheusi et al., 2000). Following cerebral injuries, such as ischemia, epileptogenesis, or focal neuronal degeneration, neurogenesis increases in the subventricular zone and the newly formed neurons are able to repopulate damaged areas (Parent, 2002; Romanko et al., 2004; Zhang et al., 2004). Appart of the subventricular zone and the subgranular zone of the dentate gyrus, recent data indicate that adult neurogenesis can also occur in other brain areas. It is thought that in the adult mammal brain physiological anti-neurogenic influences can be removed in pathological conditions or after any specific injury. This has been recently demonstrated in a model of unilateral vestibular neurectomy (UVN) that mimics human pathology in adult cats (Dutheil et al., 2011). UVN promoted an intense reactive cell proliferation in the deafferented vestibular nuclei located in the brainstem. The new cells survived up to one month, differentiated into glial cells - microglia or astrocytes - or GABAergic neurons, so highlighting a GABAergic neurogenesis. Surprisingly, post-UVN reactive cell proliferation contributed successfully to fine restoration of vestibular posturo-locomotor functions. Moreover, following brain injury, glia outside known neurogenic niches acquire or reactivate stem cell potential as part of reactive gliosis (Robel et al., 2011). A comparison of molecular pathways activated after injury with those involved in the normal neural stem cell niches highlights strategies that could overcome the inhibition of neurogenesis outside the stem cell niche and instruct parenchymal glia towards a neurogenic fate. This new view on reactive glia therefore suggests a widespread endogenous source of cells with stem cell potential, which might potentially be harnessed for local repair strategies (Robel et al., 2011).

Evenmore interesting is the fact that in the dentate gyrus of the adult hippocampus a continuous incorporation of new neurons exists. These new neurons slowly integrate into the existing dentate gyrus network: inmature adult-born neurons appear to function as pattern integrators of temporally adjacent events, thereby enhancing pattern separation for events separated in time; whereas maturing adult-born neurons it is likely that contribute to pattern separation by being more amenable to learning new information, leading to dedicated groups of granule cells, the principal projection neurons of the dentate gyrus, that respond to experienced environments (Aimone et al., 2010). This continuous neurogenesis is important for hippocampal function. At different stages in its maturation, each new neuron has different properties and, at any given time, the dentate gyrus population consists of excitatory granule cells of many different ages. The youngest, apparently more excitable in the network, could complement the pattern separation function of matures by adding a degree of similarity between events experienced close in time. Several models suggest that directing plasticity towards maturing neurons can preserve the representations of old memories in the dentate gyrus while maintaining its capacity to learn new information (Aimone et al. 2010).

Thus, although the role of this continuous adult neurogenesis remains to be fully established, a number of data suggest that it contributes to promote brain repair after injuries (Abdipranoto et al., 2008; Abdipranoto-Cowley et al., 2009). On the other side, it has been suggested that neurogenesis may be impaired in neurodegenerative disorders such as Parkinson's disease and Alzheimer's disease, and this might contribute to the pathogenesis of these chronic neurodegenerative disorders (Abdipranoto et al., 2008; Yu et al., 2008).

2.2 How adult neurogenesis is regulated?

The knowledge about how adult neurogenesis is regulated may provide adequate therapeutic tools for trying to repair the brain after an injury. However this is a difficult task, because many factors seem to be involved, directly or indirectly, in this process. We will analyze here the role of some of these putative neurogenic factors for trying later to establish then a relationship between them and the effects of growth hormone on neurogenesis.

Since some years ago we know that adult neurogenesis can be modulated by several physiological processes including learning, exercise, environmental enrichment, or stress (Kempermann et al., 1997; Nilsson et al., 1999; van Praag et al., 1999; Trejo et al., 2001; Lledo et al., 2006; Zhao et al., 2008). Many, if not all, of these effects are related to signals mediated by hormones or growth factors.

2.2.1 Gonadal steroids and adult neurogenesis

In adult songbirds, integration and survival of new neurons in the vocal control nucleus is modulated by the gonadal steroids testosterone and estradiol (Nordeen EJ & Nordeen KW, 1989; Rasika et al., 1994; Hidalgo et al., 1995; Johnson & Bottjer, 1995). In mammals, estrogen has been implicated in hippocampal function, with sex differences observed in long-term potentiation (Maren et al., 1994) and performance of hippocampal-dependent tasks (Roof & Havens, 1992; Roof et al., 1993; Galea et al., 1996). During proestrus, a time when estrogen levels are high, cell proliferation in the subgranular zone of the dentate gyrus increases, compared with estrus and diestrus, when estrogen levels are lower (Tanapat et al, 1999). Estradiol exerts extensive influence on brain development and is a powerful modulator of hippocampal structure and function. Surprisingly, the remarkable increase in ovarian hormones existing during the first and third trimester of pregnancy has no effect on cell proliferation in the subgranular zone of the dentate gyrus, suggesting that concomitants changes in oher factors, perhaps glucocorticoids, may counterbalance the positive regulation of cell proliferation by estradiol.

There is a sex difference in rates of cell genesis in the developping hippocampus of the laboratory rats, most likely occurrying because of the effects of estradiol on brain during critical periods of neural development (Bowers et al., 2010). Males generate more new cells than females. A recent study shows that exogenous estradiol treatment promotes cell proliferation and survival in the neonatal female but not the male hippocampus, whereas antagonizing endogenous estradiol synthesis or action reduces cell proliferation in the male but not in the female hippocampus (Bowers et al., 2010). Moreover, in the adult female hippocampus, estradiol stimulates cell proliferation and survival and increases dendritic synapse density, while the adult male hippocampus is insensitive to the spinogenesis or cell genesis inducing effects of estradiol treatment. However, inhibiting aromatase activity or blocking estrogen receptor binding reduces cell proliferation in the developing male but not in the female hippocampus (Bowers et al., 2010). Both the amount of endogenous estradiol and aromatase activity in the developing hippocampus are very low compared to the hypothalamus and do not appear to be sexually dimorphic (Konkle & McCarthy, 2010), suggesting that hippocampal sensitivity to estradiol is high and differs between sexes.

The possibility exists that the effects of estradiol are not mediated directly at the hippocampus but, instead, were secondary to changes in other brain areas projecting to the hippocampus (Bowers et al., 2010). Cholinergic neurons of the medial septum/diagonal band of Broca are essential for estradiol-induced spinogenesis in adult CA1 hippocampus (Lam & Leranth, 2003) and cholinergic input modulates maturation and integration of adult born dentate gyrus granule cells (Campbell et al., 2010). Gonadally intact males release more acetylcholine into the hippocampus than females during locomotor tasks and this sex difference is organized by estradiol during development (Mitsushima et al., 2009a; Mitsushima et al., 2009b). The cholinergic system matures relatively early and more new septal cholinergic neurons are born in males during a brief period of gestation but the sex difference does not persist into adulthood (Schaevitz & Berger-Sweeney, 2005). Nonetheless, it is possible that the effects observed in the study of Bowers et al. are the results of estradiol-induced acetylcholine release into the neonatal hippocampus during the early postnatal period. It is also possible that estradiol is acting outside the central nervous system (Bowers et al., 2010). At this time it is important to remark that acetylcholine is a powerful inducer of pituitary growth hormone release (Devesa et al., 1992).

With regard to progesterone, it seems that enhances the survival of newborn neurons, rather than its proliferation, via the Src-ERK and PI3K pathways (Zhang et al., 2010). In fact, progesterone attenuates the estradiol-induced enhancement of cell proliferation (Galea et al., 2006).

2.2.2 Adrenal steroids and adult neurogenesis

Antidepressants increase adult hippocampal neurogenesis in animal models, an effect already described by Elizabeth Gould soon after discovering that adult neurogenesis occurs in non human primates (Gould et al. 1999); however, the underlying molecular mechanisms responsible for this effect of antidepressants were not known. Recent sudies have suggested that glucocorticoids are involved in the neurogenic action of antidepresssants (David et al., 2009; Huang & Herbert 2006). Glucocorticoids release is the main response of the organism to acute and chronic stress. Chronic exposure to stress results in a reduction of hippocampal neurogenesis and of hippocampal volume.

The antidepressant-induced changes in neurogenesis are dependent on the glucocorticoid receptor. Specifically, the selective serotonin reuptake inhibitor antidepressant, sertraline, increases neuronal differentiation and promotes neuronal maturation of human hippocampal progenitor cells via a glucocorticoid receptor-dependent mechanism that is associated with glucorticoid receptor phosphorylation via protein kinase A signaling, therefore increasing cytosolic cAMP levels. Interestingly, this effect is only observed when sertraline is present during the proliferation phase, and it is accompanied by exit of cells from the cell cycle, as shown by reduced proliferation and increased glucocorticoid receptor-dependent expression of the cyclin-dependent kinase 2 inhibitors, p27[Kip1] and p57[Kip2] (Anacker et al., 2011). These effects of antidepressants are only seen in the presence of glucocorticoids; however, the molecular processes that lead to increased neuronal differentiation are activated directly by antidepressants alone and do not require glucocorticoids (Anacker at al., 2011). That is, regulation of neurogenesis by antidepressants is complex; it involves different glucocorticoid receptor-dependent mechanisms that lead to enhanced cell proliferation without changes in neuronal differentiation, or enhanced neuronal differentiation in the presence of decreased cell proliferation.

The fact that antidepressants induce adult neurogenesis via glucocorticoid receptor-dependent mechanism is not in contradiction with previous studies demonstrating that adrenal steroids inhibit adult neurogenesis by supressing cell proliferation in the hippocampal subgranular zone (Lennington et al., 2003). Aged rats and monkeys exhibit diminished cell proliferation in the subgranular zone as well as elevated levels of circulating glucocorticoids (Kuhn et al, 1996; Sapolsky, 1992). Removal of adrenal steroids by adrenalectomy increases cell proliferation in the subgranular zone in both aged and young adult (Cameron & McKay, 1999). Moreover, the number of new subgranular zone cells in adrenalectomized aged rats was threefold higher than the number in young control rats, indicating that adrenalectomized aged rats have rates of proliferation that surpass those normally found in young adults (Cameron & McKay, 1999). Moreover, a study on human post-mortem brain tissue has found that antidepressants increase the number of neural progenitor cells in patients with major depression to levels above those present in controls, and depressed patients are generally characterized by elevated endogenous levels of glucocorticoids (Boldrini et al., 2009). In the study of Anacker et al. (Anacker et al., 2011) the cell cycle-promoting genes, CCND1 and HDM2, were upregulated only by sertraline and dexamethasone co-treatment, the only condition which increases cell proliferation. In contrast, dexamethasone increased expression of the cell cycle-inhibiting genes, FOXO1 and GADD45B, which may explain the reduced cell proliferation and reduced neuronal differentiation with this treatment.

Experience has shown that therapy using music for therapeutic purposes has certain effects on neuropsychiatric disorders (both functional and organic disorders). However, the mechanisms of action underlying music therapy remain unknown, and scientific clarification has not advanced. The results of past studies have clarified that music influences and affects cranial nerves in humans from fetus to adult. The effects of music at a cellular level have not been clarified, and the mechanisms of action for the effects of music on the brain have not been elucidated. It has been proposed that listening to music facilitates the neurogenesis, the regeneration and repair of cerebral nerves by adjusting the secretion of steroid hormones, ultimately leading to cerebral plasticity. Music affects levels of such steroids as cortisol, testosterone and oestradiol, and it is likely that music also affects the receptor genes related to these substances, and related proteins (Fukul & Toyoshima, 2008).

2.2.3 Pituitary hormones and adult neurogenesis

Prolactin is a hormone that increases durig the pregnancy and also at postpartum, signaling lactation. The study of Shingo et al. (Shingo et al., 2003) showed that neurogenesis rates increase in the subventricular zone during pregnancy by 65% and again after delivery. In addition to observing cell proliferation, this study tracked integration of new neurons in the olfactory bulb, indicating that olfactory discrimination is critical for recognition and rearing of offspring. A doubling of olfactory interneurons may thereby enhance olfactory function following pregnancy, providing the mother with enhanced olfactory capability (Shingo et al., 2003). A similar mechanism has been recently described in male mice. Paternal-adult offspring recognition behavior in mice is dependent on postnatal offspring interaction and is associated with increased neurogenesis in the paternal olfactory bulb and hippocampus. Newly generated paternal olfactory interneurons are preferentially activated by adult offspring odors, but disrupting prolactin signaling aboslishes increased paternal neurogenesis and adult offspring recognition (Mak & Weiss, 2010).

Prolactin is a regulator of the stress response and stimulator of neurogenesis in the subventricular zone, but also protects neurogenesis in the dentate gyrus of chronically stressed mice and promotes neuronal fate (Torner et al. 2009). Neural stem and progenitors cells express the prolactin receptor and prolactin signals in these cells via ERK 1/2, however *in vitro* studies did not observe any effect of prolactin on these neural precursors proliferation, differentiation or survival, suggesting that prolactin action on *in vivo* neurogenesis occurs via an indirect mechanism (Wagner et al. 2009).

The effects of growth hormone on adult neurogenesis will be widely analyzed later in this chapter.

Recently it has been described that Oxytocin, but not Vasopressin, stimulates adult neurogenesis in the hippocampus of rats, even in animals subjected to glucocorticoid administration or cold water swim stress, indicating that the hormone stimulates neuronal growth and may protect against the suppressive effects of stress hormones on hippocampal plasticity (Leuner et al., 2011).

2.2.4 Growth factors and adult neurogenesis

When dissociated from the adult subventricular zone, neural stem cells require either epidermal growth factor (EGF) or basic fibroblast growth factor (FGF2) for self-renewal and long-term survival in culture (Reynolds & Weiss, 1992; Kuhn et al., 1997). Analysis of EGF and FGF2 responsiveness in the developing telencephalon indicates that early growth factor choice is temporally regulated (Tropepe et al., 1999; Maric et al., 2003). In the adult, the vast majority of subventricular zone cells expressing EGFR also express FGFR1 supporting the finding that most EGF-responsive cells can also be stimulated by FGF2 (Gritti et al., 1999). However, EGF and FGF2 appear to differ in their mechanisms of support, with EGF promoting faster expansion of the stem cell-like pool (symmetric division) compared to FGF2 (Gritti et al., 1999). This may be the result of differential control of cell cycle length by each growth factor, with SVZ stem-like cells cycling faster in the presence of EGF (Gritti et al., 1999). Alternatively, since the subventricular zone has two subsets of mitotically active cells, the neural stem cells (a relatively quiescent population with a cell cycle length up to 28 days) (Morshead & van der Kooy, 1992; Morshead et al., 1994), and the transitory amplifying progenitor (TAP) cells (cell cycle length approximately 12 h), these two growth factors may preferentially target one cell type. The latter appears to be supported by the work of Kuhn et al. (Kuhn et al., 1997) and Doetsch et al. (Doetsch et al., 2002). Kuhn et al.

(Kuhn et al., 1997) found that intracerebroventricular infusion of FGF2 into the lateral ventricle resulted in increased numbers of new neurons in the olfactory bulbe, while EGF infusion reduced the number of neurons reaching the olfactory bulbe, but substantially increased generation of astrocytes in the olfactory bulbe and the neighboring striatum. Extension of this study by Doetsch et al. (Doetsch et al., 2002) suggests that TAP cells are EGF receptive and these cells become invasive and glia-like, diverting neurogenesis to gliogenesis.

Recent studies using long-term ventricular infusion of EGF demonstrate intense cell proliferation around the ventricular wall, implicating the presence of EGF-reactive cells also outside the classical neurogenic lateral niche. Intraventricular injection of EGF induces within minutes CREB and ERK phosphorylation in astrocyte-like progenitor cells (type B cells) and EGF receptor-expressing transit-amplifying progenitor cells-both in the striatal and septal ventricular walls (Gampe et al., 2011). EGF infusion for 6 days induced continued CREB and ERK activation in nestin+ cells paralleled by intense periventricular cell proliferation. In addition, the ependyma became EGF receptor-immunoreactive, revealed intense CREB phosphorylation and underwent partial de-differentiation. These results demonstrate that intraventricular application of EGF induces CREB and ERK phosphorylation along the entire ventricular walls and thus permits a direct identification of EGF-responsive cell types. They further support the notion that not only the striatal ventricular wall where the subependimal zone is located but also the septal ventricular wall carries latent potential for the formation of neurons and glial cells (Gampe et al., 2011). Basal activity of CREB is required for the mitogenic signaling of EGF in neural stem cells at a level between ERK activation and SRE-mediated transcriptional activation (SRE: serum response element, a promoter sequence regulating c-fos gene expression) (Iguchi et al., 2011).

Interestingly, recent findings have shown that cells derived from subventricular zone Type-B cells (neural stem cells in the subventricular zone) actively respond to EGF stimulation becoming highly migratory and proliferative. A subpopulation of these EGF-activated cells expresses markers of oligodendrocyte precursor cells (OPCs). When EGF administration is removed, subventricular zone-derived OPCs differentiate into myelinating and pre-myelinating oligodendrocytes in the white matter tracts of corpus callosum, fimbria fornix and striatum. In the presence of a demyelinating lesion, OPCs derived from EGF-stimulated subventricular zone progenitors contribute to myelin repair. Given their high migratory potential and their ability to differentiate into myelin-forming cells, subventricular zone neural stem cells represent an important endogenous source of OPCs for preserving the oligodendrocyte population in the white matter and for the repair of demyelinating injuries (Gonzalez-Perez & Alvarez-Buylla, 2011). Of interest here is the fact that growth hormone induces EGF and EGFR expression in many territories (Pan et al., 2011) and activates EGFR by tyrosine phosphorilation as an essential element leading to MAP kinase activation and gene expression (Yamauchi et al., 1998).

Another growth factor involved in neurogenesis is the hematopoietic growth factor erythropoietin (EPO). mRNA and protein of EPO and its receptor (EPOR) are detected in a number of brain areas during brain development as well as *in vitro* in neurons, astrocytes, oligodendrocytes, microglia and cerebral endothelial cells. Expression of EPO and EPOR in the adult brain is stress-reponsive and is regulated by oxygen supply; both are upregulated after hypoxia or ischemia. Other stimuli such as hypoglycemia and IGF-I activate hypoxia-inducible factor and lead to increased expression of EPO (Byts & Sirén, 2009). The tissue protective functions EPO are independent of its action on erythropoiesis. Peripherally administered EPO crosses the blood-brain barrier and activates in the brain anti-apoptotic, anti-oxidant and anti-inflammatory signaling in neurons, glial and cerebrovascular endothelial cells and stimulates angiogenesis and neurogenesis. These mechanisms underlie its potent tissue protective effects in experimental models of stroke, cerebral hemorrhage, traumatic brain injury, neuroinflammatory and neurodegenerative disease (Byts & Sirén, 2009). Brain specific blockade of EPOR leads to deficits in neural cell proliferation and neuronal survival in the embryonic brain and in post-stroke neurogenesis in the adult brain (Chen et al., 2007; Tsai et al., 2006). Moreover, *in vivo* and *in vitro* data indicate hat EPO amplifies stroke-induced oligodendrogenesis that could facilitate axonal remyelination and lead to functional recovery after stroke (L. Zhang et al., 2010). Of interest here is that growth hormone induces EPO release from kidneys.

Brain injuries such as ischemia affect adult neurogenesis in adult rodents as both global and focal ischemic insults enhance the proliferation of progenitor cells residing in neurogenic niches. The ischemic insult increases the number of progenitor cells in monkey subgranular and subventricular zones, and causes gliogenesis in the ischemia prone hippocampal CA1 sector (Tonchev, 2011). The analysis of the expression at protein level of a panel of potential regulatory molecules, including neurotrophic factors and their receptors revealed that a fraction of mitotic progenitors were positive for the neurotrophin receptor Tyrosine kinase B (TrkB), while immature neurons expressed the neurotrophin receptor Tyrosine kinase A (TrkA). Astroglia, ependymal cells and blood vessels in subventricular zone were positive for distinctive sets of ligands/receptors indicating that a network of neurotrophic signals operating in an autocrine or paracrine manner may regulate neurogenesis in adult primate subventricular zone (Tonchev, 2011). The analysis of microglial and astroglial proliferation in postischemic hippocampal CA1 sector showed that proliferating postischemic microglia in adult monkey CA1 sector express the neurotrophin receptor TrkA, while activated astrocytes were labeled for nerve growth factor (NGF), ligand for TrkA, and TrkB, a receptor for brain derived neurotrophic factor (BDNF). These results implicate NGF and BDNF as regulators of postischemic glial proliferation in adult primate hippocampus (Tonchev, 2011). Figure 2 summarizes how these hormones and growth factors act on adult neurogenesis.

2.2.5 Growth hormone/IGF-I system and adult neurogenesis

GH is a pleiotropic hormone expressed not only in the pituitary but in almost any tissue (Devesa et al., 2010b). Thus, far beyond of its classical actions on body growth and intermediate metabolism, GH exerts an important role in the regulation of cell proliferation and survival in several tissues, including the CNS (Costoya et al., 1999; Sanders et al., 2009; McLenachan et al., 2009; Aberg et al., 2009).

The hypothesis that Growth Hormone (GH) and IGF-I play a role on brain repair after an injury has been postulated years ago. The existence of GH expression within the CNS has been reported by several authors, however its physiological role and, in particular, its possible contribution in the reparation of neurologic injuries remain poorly understood despite of that the positive effects of GH treatment on adult neurogenesis have been demonstrated in laboratory animals (McLenachan et al., 2009; Christophidis et al., 2009; Svensson et al., 2008; P. Devesa et al., 2011), and recent data from our group and others (Devesa et al., 2009; High et al., 2010; Reimunde et al., 2010; Reimunde et al., 2011; Devesa et al., 2011) suggest that the hormone may play a similar role in humans. GH-driven neurogenesis may also depend on the local production of GH (P. Devesa et al., 2011), the so called perypheral GH system that may be activated under both physiological and pathologic conditions (Devesa et al., 2010b).

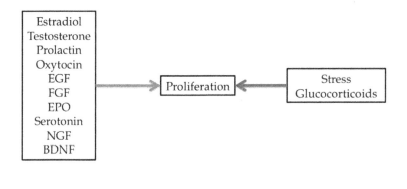

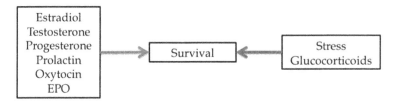

Blue lines indicate stimulation of neural precursors cells proliferation and/or survival, while red lines indicate inhibition.

Fig. 2. Factors involved in adult neurogenesis control.

In keeping with previous reports, we have found that hippocampal cells express GH under basal conditions and, more interestingly, the number of GH-expressing cells seems to increase after brain injury induced by kainate acid administration in rats (P. Devesa et al., 2011). Furthermore, using a double-labeling immunofluorescence we were able to notice that almost all GH-positive cells also showed BrdU immunoreactivity, thus suggesting the existence of a strong correlation between GH expression and cell proliferation (P. Devesa, 2011) (Figure 3).

Interestingly, data from Katakowski et al. (Katakowski et al., 2003) demonstrate that the activation of PI3K/Akt signal transduction pathway mediates the migration of neuroblasts to damaged brain areas after stroke, most likely for inducing regeneration. PI3K/Akt is a key signaling pathway for the intracellular effects of GH (Costoya et al., 1999). Moreover, the group of Scheepens demonstrated that the expression of GH and its receptor is strongly upregulated after brain injury and specifically associated with stressed neurons and glia (Scheepens et al., 2000). More recently, the same group demonstrated that during recovery from an ischemic brain injury, a cerebral growth hormone axis is activated; the level of GHR immunoreactivity in the ipsilateral SVZ was significantly increased 5 days after injury vs. the contralateral SVZ, coinciding both spatially and temporally with injury-induced neurogenesis. The population of GHR immunopositive cells in the ipsilateral SVZ at this time was found to include proliferating cells, neural progenitor cells and post-proliferative migratory neuroblasts (Christophidis et al., 2009).

As indicated before, several lines of evidence support a role for GH in neurogenesis. The GH receptor is expressed in regions of the brain in which neurogenesis occurs during embryonic brain development (García-Aragón et al., 1992; Turnley et al., 2002) and in neurogenic regions of the postnatal rat brain (Lobie et al., 1993). Growth hormone itself is also found in cells of the ventricular zone during embryonic neurogenesis (Turnley et al., 2002), and is produced endogenously within the postnatal hippocampus (Donahue et al., 2002; Donahue et al., 2006; Sun et al., 2005a; Sun et al., 2005b). Interestingly, GH gene expression within the hippocampus is increased by some factors known to increase neurogenesis (Parent, 2003), including learning (Donahue et al., 2002) and estrogen (Donahue et al., 2006).

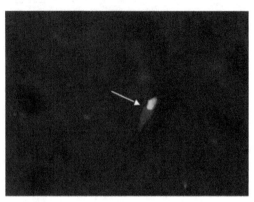

The detection of irBrDU in the nucleus of the cell (green) indicated by the arrow demonstrates that it is a newly born cell in rat hippocampal CA3 area showing irGH (brown), after brain injury induced by kainate acid administration and GH treatment, in its cytoplasm. Newly born neurons formed in the subgranular layer of the dentate gyrus migrate to the CA3 zone after commencing to mature in the granular area. Thus, it is feasible that the detection of irGH in CA3 cells may be related to a trophic and survival role of the hormone. Taken from Pablo Devesa, Doctoral thesis, 2011. University of Santiago de Compostela, Spain.

Fig. 3. Immunofluorescence (60x). Colocalization of GH and BrdU in a newly born hippocampal cell.

However, the role of GH in the hippocampal dentate gyrus has been related to neuronal survival rather than generation, as altered hippocampal GH levels have no effect on cell proliferation but do affect the survival of immature neurons (Sun et al., 2005b; Sun et al., 2007; Lichtenwalner et al., 2006). Studies of the effects of GH on embryonic rat cerebral cortical (Ajo et al., 2003) and hippocampal (Byts et al., 2008) neuronal cultures found that it induces the proliferation and differentiation of these cells. Overall, these findings indicate that GH may facilitate the proliferation, differentiation and survival of new neurons in response to brain injury. Further studies will reveal whether or not GH is "called" for brain repair after GPR17 activation.

On these bases, we explored a potential role for GH and its receptor on the proliferation, differentiation and survival of neural stem cells (NSCs) *in vitro*. NSCs were isolated from the SGZ of the DG from 9 days old C57/BL6 mice and cultured as neurospheres.

Western blot and immunofluorescence studies showed that neurospheres derived from these NSCs were demonstrated to express both GH and its receptor either in conditions of proliferation and differentiation showing colocalization with nestin (Figure 4) and SOX2 (Figure 5), markers of undifferentiated cells or cells in development. Migrating cells from neurospheres also showed irGHR (Figure 6). In all, these results indicate that GH and its receptor seem to be needed for the physiological neurogenesis.

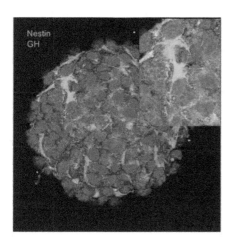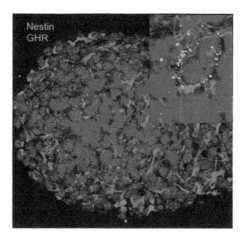

Neurospheres derived from NSCs obtained from the dentate gyrus of 9days old mice in proliferation medium showing irGH (left, green) and irGHR (right, green dots). The detection of ir for Nestin (red) indicates that cells in neurospheres are undifferentiated or in development. Taken from Pablo Devesa, Doctoral thesis, 2011. University of Santiago de Compostela, Spain.

Fig. 4. Confocal microscopy. Colocalization of GH and GHR with Nestin in mice neurospheres.

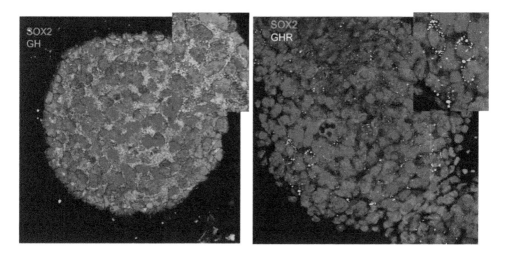

Neurospheres derived from NSCs obtained from the dentate gyrus of 9days old mice in proliferation medium showing irGH (left, green) and irGHR (right, green dots). The detection of ir for SOX2 (red) indicates that cells in neurospheres are undifferentiated or in development. Taken from Pablo Devesa, Doctoral thesis, 2011. University of Santiago de Compostela, Spain.

Fig. 5. Confocal microscopy. Colocalization of GH and GHR with SOX2 in mice neurospheres.

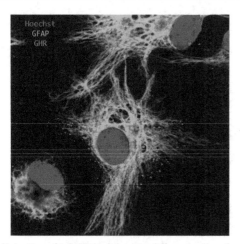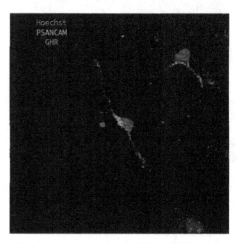

Detection of irGHR (red dots) in different cells migrating from neurospheres formed from NSCs
obtained from the dentate gyrus of 9days old mice. The detection of irGFAP (left, green) indicates that
these cells are astrocytes, while the detection of irPSANCAM (right, green) indicates that this cell is a
migrating neuron. Cells nuclei are stained in blue. Taken from Pablo Devesa, Doctoral thesis, 2011.
University of Santiago de Compostela, Spain.

Fig. 6. Confocal microscopy. Detection of GHR in cells migrating from mice neurospheres.

However, from these studies we could not be able for establishing the exact role that the
GH–GHR system plays on this mechanism. This is why we explored what would happen
when adding the hormone to the culture media either in conditions of proliferation and
differentiation.

As reported in other studies (Christophidis et al., 2009) treating NSCs with GH in the
presence of BrdU significantly increased the proportion of cells incorporating BrdU almost
doubling it (Figure 7). That is, despite of the fact that NSCs express the hormone, the
addition of exogenous GH increased stem cells proliferation. This effect is similar to that we
observed in animals with kainate acid-induced brain injury (P. Devesa et al., 2011).

It has been suggested that the GHR may actually play a greater role in the survival,
migration or differentiation of neurons generated in response to hypoxia/ischemia than in
proliferation (Christophidis et al., 2009). Consistent with a role for GHR in survival, GH
protects both mature neurons (Möderscheim et al., 2007; Byts et al., 2008; Silva et al., 2003)
and primary neurospheres derived from embryonic mouse NSCs (van Marle et al., 2005)
from death *in vitro*. Also, the survival of newborn neurons in the subgranular zone of adult
rat dentate gyrus is impaired as a result of GH deficiency (Lichtenwalner et al., 2006), and
elevated GH levels within the hippocampus reduce apoptosis (Sun et al., 2007). A role for
GH in neuronal differentiation is supported by a recent study that found that physiological
concentrations of human GH stimulate neurite initiation and arborization of embryonic
hippocampal neurons by activating the PI3K/Akt signalling pathway (Byts et al., 2008).
Other studies have found that high concentrations of human GH reduce neuronal
proliferation but enhance differentiation of these cells instead (Ajo et al., 2003; Lyuh et al.,
2007). Indeed, it appears that GH promotes proliferation of neural cells at the expense of
their differentiation, as neurosphere cultures derived from GHR *knockout* mice proliferate
less than those of *wt* mice due to their inability to respond to autocrine GH, yet they exhibit

accelerated neuronal differentiation (McLenachan et al., 2008). Interestingly, treatment of neurospheres derived from newborn or adult mouse neural stem cells with 100 ng/mL rat GH, which stimulates proliferation (Christophidis et al., 2009), significantly reduced neuronal differentiation (Turnley et al., 2002; Scott et al., 2006).

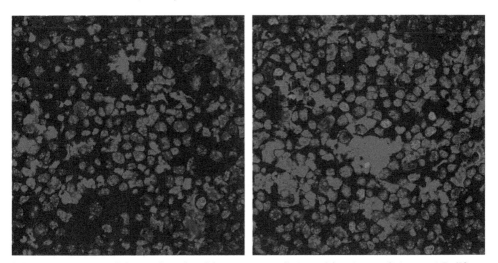

GH treatment increased the number of proliferating stem cells in proliferation conditions, as irBrdU (red) shows. Left: control, saline treated cells. Right: GH treated cells. Taken from Pablo Devesa, Doctoral thesis, 2011. University of Santiago de Compostela, Spain.

Fig. 7. *In vitro* effects of GH treatment on proliferating neural stem cells.

Overall, it appears that the effect of GH on neuronal differentiation depends upon the concentration of GH and proliferative potential of the cells used.

We also analyzed the role of GH on NSCs survival. In basal conditions there is a physiological rate of apoptosis that is significantly reduced by adding GH to the culture media in differentiation conditions. The antiapoptotic role of the hormone was clearly demonstrated by treating the cells with the GH agonist pegvisomant. This drug binds to the GHR but is unable to induce any kind of intracellular response because inhibits the dimerization of the GHR needed for intracellular signalling. In these conditions, basal apoptosis was significantly increased indicating that the autocrine interplay GH−GHR is key for NSCs survival. Moreover, treating the cells with GH did not modify the increased apoptosis elicited by pegvisomant (Figure 8).

GH effects are mediated via the GHR, which is a member of the cytokine receptor superfamily. The critical step in initiating GH signaling is the activation of receptor-associated Janus kinase 2 (JAK2), which induces cross-phosphorylation of tyrosine residues in the kinase domain of JAK2 and GHR. Phosphorylated residues on JAK2 and GHR form docking sites for the members of the STAT family of transcription factors (Perrini et al., 2008). Phosphorylation of the STATs by JAK2 results in their dissociation from the receptor and translocation to the nucleus, with subsequent binding to DNA and regulation of gene expression. Among the target genes, GH regulates the expression of suppressor of cytokine signaling (SOCS), a family of negative regulators that terminate the GH signaling cascade (Hansen et al., 1999). SOCS proteins bind to phosphotyrosine residues on the GHR or JAK2 and suppress GH signaling by inhibiting JAK2 activity, competing with STATs for binding to the GHR, or inducing degradation of the GHR complex.

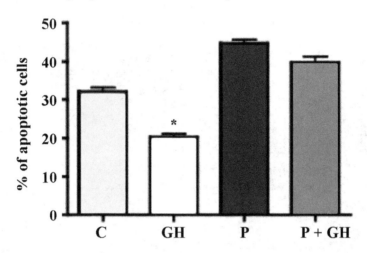

GH administration significantly reduced basal apoptosis in cultured NSCs cells (*p < 0.01 vs. control). Treatment with pegvisomant abolished the antiapoptotic effect of GH. C: control; P: pegvisomant. Taken from Pablo Devesa, Doctoral thesis, 2011. University of Santiago de Compostela, Spain.

Fig. 8. *In vitro* effects of GH treatment on the survival of mice neural stem cells.

The RAS/mitogen-activated protein kinase (MAPK) pathway has also been shown to be activated by GH. The GHR–JAK2 complex has been shown to recruit the adapter protein SHC, resulting in SHC tyrosine phosphorylation and binding to GRB2, and activation of RAS, RAF, MAPK/extracellular-regulated protein kinase (MEK), and ERK-1/2 (Vanderkuur et al., 1997). Alternatively, it has been suggested that GH might also regulate the activation of ERK by a SRC-dependent, JAK2-independent mechanism which involves phopholipase D (Zhu et al., 2002). This JAK2- independent mechanism has been recently demonstrated *in vivo* (Barclay et al., 2010). Tyrosine phosphorylation of a GRB2-binding site in the epidermal growth factor receptor could also be involved in GH-mediated MAPK activation (Yamauchi et al., 1997).

GH signaling via SHC and ERK can be interrupted after blocking insulin receptor substrate-1 (IRS-1) (Wang et al., 2009). IRS-1 is a docking protein tyrosine phosphorylated in response to insulin, IGF-I, GH, and other cytokines. IRS-1 greatly enhances GH-induced ERK.

GH has also been shown to stimulate the PI3K pathway through JAK2-mediated tyrosine phosphorylation of the insulin receptor substrates (IRS-1 to IRS-3), leading to their association with PI3K regulatory subunits (Zhu et al., 2001). In addition, direct binding of the p85 and p85β subunits to phosphotyrosine residues in the carboxyl terminus domain of the GHR has also been demonstrated (Moutoussamy et al., 1998).

As stated before, GH stimulation of PI3K is linked to the stimulation of the antiapoptotic serine protein kinase B or Akt (Costoya et al., 1999). Akt activation has been shown to be dependent on the presence of the JAK2-binding region of GHR, and to promote cell survival through the inhibition of the proapoptotic protein caspase 3 (Sanders et al., 2006). The role of PI3K/Akt on cell survival is well known after the pioneer study of our group (Costoya et al.,

1999). Inhibiting PI3K/Akt with a potent inibitor of phosphoinositide 3-kinases led to a significant increase in apoptosis in NSCs, however GH treatment was able to clearly decrease the rate of apoptosis observed by blocking PI3K/Akt signaling. This indicates that the hormone is able for signaling through other different pathways acting on cell survival (P. Devesa, 2011). We then studied the effects of inhibiting another cell survival pathway such as ERK. Inhibiting ERK phosphorylation significantly increased NSCs apoptosis in differentiation conditions, but again the treatment with GH was able to revert the proapoptotic effect of blocking ERK signaling.

Since GH was able to revert the propapoptotic effects of the inhibition of both PI3K/Akt and ERK, we decided to study signalling pathways located upstream, specifically mTOR. This is a master regulator of cell mass and metabolism, which is in part regulated by growth factor signalling through the canonical RTK (receptor tyrosine kinase)-PI3K/Akt axis and by nutrient (through class III PI3Ks), hypoxia or AMP.

Rapamycin is an allosteric mTOR inhibitor. As expected, treating NSCs with rapamycin led to a significant increase in apoptosis, but once more this effect on cellular death was reverted when GH was added together with rapamycin. This seems to be surprising given the importance of mTOR in signalling cell survival, and again indicated that the hormone uses different pathways for promoting cell survival. However, evidence exists showing that mTOR inhibition can lead to pathway reactivation: abrogation of the negative-feedback loop which is normally initiated by the direct substrate p70S6K (p70 S6 kinase) on insulin receptor substrate proteins can lead to strong PI3K/Akt pathway reactivation, most likely producing ERK pathway reactivation in a PI3K/Akt dependent manner (Carracedo et al., 2008). For a better understanding of such a concept see the scheme shown in Figure 9.

Thus, while PI3K/Akt inhibition would allow GH to act through ERK pathway, ERK inhibition would not impede PI3K/Akt to be the survival-signalling pathway. Of interest here is the fact that both kind of inhibitions only were reverted when exogenous GH was added. This means that the autocrine production of the hormone by NSCs is not enough for blocking intense cell death signals.

We then blocked simultaneously ERK and mTOR activation. Once more the intense apoptosis observed after pharmachological blockade of these pathways was reverted when GH was added together with them. The only explanations for this result is that the hormone may act directly at a upper level in the stream of signaling pathways for cell survival or the effect is due to the overactivation of PI3K occurred as a result of blocking those two other signaling pathways. To test the first possibility we used SP600125, an anthrapyrazolone inhibitor of Jun N-terminal kinase (Bennett et al., 2001). That is we were acting at the terminal level in the stream. In this case the clear increase in apoptosis produced by the inhibitor could not be reverted by administering GH together with the drug. It suggests either a direct effect of the hormone on JNK activation for cell survival or a direct effect of overactivated PI3K on JNK (as postulated by Zhu et al., 1998).

In summary, our results (P. Devesa, 2011), together with other studies previously described, demonstrate that GH is able for promoting NSCs proliferation, and also plays a key role on the survival of these cells. With regard to the antiapoptotic role of GH, it seems to be exerted trough different signaling pathways: PI3K/Akt, ERK and pJNK (Figure 10). Since culture media contain insulin our results do not allow us to conclude whether the effect of GH on pJNK is a direct effect or it results from the known crosstalk between GH and insulin at the cellular level (Xu & Messina, 2009) or from the overactivation of PI3K directly enhancing JNK activity (Zhu et al., 1998). In any case GH effects a very strong effect on the survival of NSCs.

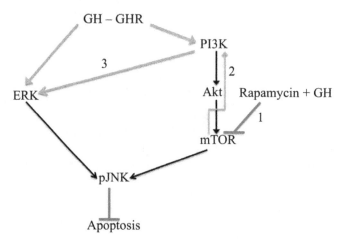

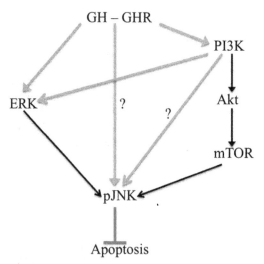

As showed in the scheme, rapamycin treatment inhibits mTOR, thus leading to a feedback activation of the PI3K/Akt pathway [2]. Physiologically this would lead to increased ERK activation [3], but this not occurs unless exogenous GH is given together with rapamycin [1]. Red lines indicate inhibition; blue lines indicate activation. Taken from Pablo Devesa, Doctoral thesis, 2011. University of Santiago de Compostela, Spain.

Fig. 9. Schematic representation of the cell survival signaling pathways studied.

The scheme shows how GH may act on cell survival in NSCs according to the results we obtained. The possibility of a direct effect of the hormone on JNK phosphorylation could not be demonstrated here; another possibility is that the activation of JNK occurs because of overactivation of PI3K after mTOR and ERK blockade. Red line indicates inhibition; blue lines indicate activation. Taken from Pablo Devesa, Doctoral thesis, 2011. University of Santiago de Compostela, Spain.

Fig. 10. Schematic representation about the putative role of GH in NSCs survival.

A number of studies indicate that the neurobiological consequences of the decline in GH/IGF-I, that occurs physiologically during aging, include decreased neurogenesis in the dentate gyrus of the hippocampus (Lichtenwalner et al., 2001; Lichtenwalner et al., 2006), where IGF-I appears to affect primarily the survival of newborn neurons, but also may influence the maturation and differentiation of newborn cells (Aberg et al., 2000; Darnaudery et al., 2006).

Despite that neurogenesis is dramatically reduced during senescence, newborn granule cells in the aged dentate gyrus retain the capacity for participation in functional hippocampal networks (Marrone et al., 2011); this is in agreement with the aforementioned hypothesis, suggesting that it is the age-associated lack of neurotrophic factors (GH/IGF-I?) the cause of decreased neurogenesis. In fact, growth hormone prevents neuronal loss in the aged rat hippocampus (Azcoitia et al., 2005).

GH induces IGF-I expression in liver and other tissues; however it is not the only factor responsible for it. In fact, there are a number of pathological situations in which a clear divergence exists between GH production and plasma levels of IGF-I. This is the case, for instance, of Anorexia Nervosa; in these patients, while large burst of pituitary GH are released into the blood, IGF-I plasma levels are consistently lower than normal. The opposite situation can be observed in obese children; GH secretion is deficient in these children, but plasma IGF-I levels are normal and growth velocity is above the mean for age (Devesa et al., 1992). The common link between these two situations seems to be plasma glucose levels, low in Anorexia Nervosa and showing a tendency to hyperglycemia in obesity. Thus, it has been postulated that glucose is needed for the hepatic production of IGF-I; more particularly a product of intracellular metabolism of glucose, since 2-deoxiglucose (who can not be metabolized) is unable to induce hepatic IGF-I expression. Therefore, although GH usually is the factor responsible for the hepatic production of IGF-I, in terms of neural effects both hormones may follow different paths. In fact, studies in rats submitted to moderate and severe hypoxia showed that the spatial distribution of the neuroprotection conveyed by growth hormone correlates with the spatial distribution of the constitutive neural growth hormone receptor, but not with the neuroprotection offered by IGF-I treatment in this model. These results suggest that some of the neuroprotective effects of growth hormone are mediated directly through the growth hormone receptor and do not involve IGF-I induction (Scheepens et al., 2001).

The effects of the GH/IGF-I axis on cell turnover in the adult brain probably are not limited to neuronal progenitors, since IGF-I can promote proliferation of oligodendrocyte progenitor cells (OPCs) and differentiation and survival of oligodendrocytes (McMorris & McKinnon, 1996; Mason et al., 2000; Aberg et al., 2007; Pang et al., 2007), an effect also induced by EGF (Gonzalez-Perez & Alvarez-Buylla, 2011) whose expression and that of its receptor may also be induced by GH (Pan et al., 2011). Thus, it is likely that the aging-related decline in GH/IGF-I and dependent changes in oligodendrocyte genesis and/or maturation may contribute to impaired remyelination in the central nervous system of aged individuals (Gilson & Blakemore, 1993; Shields et al., 1999; Franklin et al., 2002; Sim et al., 2002) and to a decline in normal cognitive function. In fact, GH has positive cognitive effects when given to GH-deficient patients.

In all, the system GH/IGF-I exerts both neuroprotective and regenerative effects at the CNS. In line with this a recent study in human patients describes that a high serum IGF-I during the rehabilitation phase of stroke correlates to better recovery of long-term function (Aberg et al., 2011).

It is likely that some of the positive effects of GH at central level are not directly exerted by the hormone but they are mediated trough the induction and release of a number of neurotrophic factors, as shown in Figure 11.

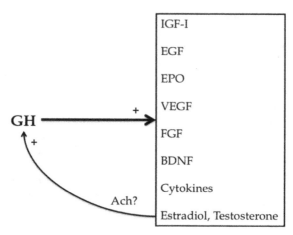

Some of the neurotrophic effects of GH *in vivo* could be mediated and/or enhanced through the induction of the expression and release of a number of neurotrophic factors. GH induces the expression of IGF-I, EGF, EPO; VEGF and FGF. The GH-effects on the induction of BDNF expression have not been tested yet but it is likely that they occur, directly or indirectly. GH induces an acute and strong release of neutrophiles from the bone marrow, then allowing the release of neurotrophic cytokines. GH has trophic effects on the gonads, thus facilitating estradiol and testosterone production. In turn, it is likely that the neurotrophic effects of these sexual steroids may be partially due to a positive effect on the pituitary GH release mediated by Ach and noradrenaline (Devesa et al., 1992).

Fig. 11. GH induction of the expression and/or release of a number of factors with known neurotrophic activity.

3. Effects of GH treatment combined with kynesitherapy on the recovery of patients with brain injuries

3.1 Cerebral palsy children

Cerebral palsy (CP) is a catastrophic acquired disease, occurring during development of the fetal or infant brain. It mainly affects the motor control centres of the developing brain, but can also affect cognitive functions, and is usually accompanied by a cohort of symptoms including lack of communication, epilepsy, and alterations in behavior.

Major causes for CP include abnormal intrauterine developments, due to fetal-maternal infections, asphyxia before birth, hypoxia during delivery, brain trauma during labor and delivery, and complications in the perinatal period. Apart from these, prematurity is responsible for 40%–50% of cases of CP. Periventricular leucomalacia (PVL) and parenchymal venous infarction complicating germinal matrix/intraventricular hemorrhage have long been recognized as the two significant white matter diseases responsible for the majority of cases of cerebral palsy in survivors of preterm birth.

However, in more recent studies using magnetic resonance imaging to assess the preterm brain, two new appearances have been documented, adding to the spectrum of white matter disease of prematurity: punctate white matter lesions, and diffuse excessive high signal intensity. These appear to be more common than PVL but less significant in terms of their impact on individual neurodevelopment. They may, however, be associated with later cognitive and behavioral disorders known to be common following preterm birth.

Most CP children often have poor linear growth during childhood, resulting in a diminished final adult height. However the number of studies in which it has been reported whether or not GH secretion is impaired in CP is quite limited. These studies reflect that GH provocative testing induced a GH deficient secretion. In a recent study it was indicated that diminished circulating IGF-1 and GH concentrations may explain why children with CP are smaller than normally growing children (Ali et al., 2007a). On the other hand, osteopenia is a common finding in children with CP, and seems to be associated with decreased IGF-1 and IGFBP3 plasma levels, usual markers of deficient GH secretion. The large percentage of CP children with GH deficiency (GHD) has been reported to be noteworthy. However, given the complexity of GH neurorregulation (Devesa et al., 1992) it seems to be logical that severe brain damage may affect a number of neurotransmitter pathways involved in GH control, thus affecting the normal secretion of the hormone.

Other possible causes of decreased growth in CP include psychosocial deprivation and suboptimal nutritional status, but these are also involved in subnormal GH secretion (Devesa et al., 1992).

We studied whether GH secretion was affected in 46 CP children (28 males, 18 females; aged 3 to 11 years old). Our results indicated that 70% of the patients seemed to have deficient GH secretion (Devesa et al, 2010a), therefore they were candidates to benefit from GH replacement therapy.

In few studies have the benefits of GH-replacement therapy in children with CP been reported, and most of these studies only reflect the increased growth observed during the treatment period with the hormone (Coniglio & Stevenson, 1995; Shim et al., 2004; Ali et al., 2007b).

Neuropsychological assessments have demonstrated that GHD is associated with reduced cognitive performance; specifically, in the majority of studies it has been found that GHD can lead to clinically relevant changes in memory, processing speed, attention, vocabulary, perceptual speed, spatial learning, and in reaction time tests. Cognitive dysfunction appears to be specifically related to GH deficiency; this hypothesis is supported by the positive correlations between serum IGF-I concentration and IQ, whereas poorer emotional well-being and reduced perceptual-motor performance are attributed to other pituitary hormone deficiencies.

In a recent study we described (Devesa et al., 2011) the positive effects of GH therapy together with psychomotor and cognitive stimulation in 11 children (7 males, 4 females; aged 3 to 7 years old) with CP and GHD. Cognitive performances in the children studied were assessed by using the Battelle Developmental Inventory Screening Test (BDIST) (Newborg et al., 1988). Tests were performed at admission, two months after commencing psychomotor and cognitive stimulation and two months after adding GH replacement therapy to psychomotor and cognitive stimulation. Before admission all these CP children had been intensively stimulated, most of them since they were 1 year old. Psychomotor and cognitive stimulation were adapted to the specific needs of each patient. Psychomotor stimulation involved tasks aimed at improving tonic–postural control, laterality, breathing and relaxation, static and dynamic balance, motor coordination and dissociation, body image, oculomotor coordination, spatial and temporal orientation, and gross and fine motor skills. Cognitive stimulation involved tasks directed at improving interaction with the environment, communication, attention, perception, memory, reasoning, and concept learning. These therapies were carried out for 45 minutes per day, 5 days per week during 4 months. Recombinant human GH was given subcutaneously, 30 µg/kg/day, 5 days/week, during 2 months (after 2 months of psychomotor and cognitive stimulation).

Patients did not improve their psychomotor and cognitive status during the pretreatment period, during which only psychomotor and cognitive stimulation were performed. However, significant improvements in all BDIST domains were observed when GH was administered together with psychomotor and cognitive stimulation; specifically, patients improved in personal and social skills, adaptive behavior, gross motor skills and total psychomotor abilities, receptive and total communication, cognitive skills, and in the total score of the scale ($p < 0.01$), and in fine motor skills and expressive communication ($p < 0.02$). As expected, plasma IGF-1 and IGFBP3 significantly increased after GH treatment.

These results led us to conclude that the combined therapy involving GH replacement and psychomotor and cognitive stimulation is useful for the appropriate neurodevelopment of children with CP and GHD (Devesa et al., 2011). Since these children had received an intensive neurostimulation without significant improvements before being treated with GH, it seems to be clear that the hormone, and/or IGF-1 was the main factor responsible for the results obtained. Moreover, since exogenous GH combines with locally produced GH for repairing brain injuries (P. Devesa et al., 2011) it is feasible to assume that GH treatment may be used too in CP children without GHD.

In another study (Reimunde et al., 2011), we assessed the effects of growth hormone treatment (30 µg/kg/day) combined with physical rehabilitation in the recovery of gross motor function in children with GHD and CP (four males and six females, mean age 5.63 ± 2.32 years) as compared with that observed in a similar population of CP children (five males, five females, mean age 5.9 ± 2.18 years) without growth hormone deficiency treated only with physical rehabilitation for two months. The Gross Motor Function Measure (GMFM-88) and Modified Ashworth Scale were performed before commencing the treatment and after completion thereof. The GMFM-88 is a scale constructed for evaluation of change in gross motor function in children with cerebral palsy and consists of 88 items grouped into five dimensions, ie, dimension A (lying and rolling, 17 items), dimension B (sitting, 20 items), dimension C (crawling and kneeling, 14 items), dimension D (standing, 13 items) and dimension E (walking, running, and jumping, 24 items).

Scores for each dimension are expressed as a percentage of the maximum score for that dimension, adding the scores for all dimensions, and dividing by 5 to obtain the total score. The reliability, validity, and responsiveness of the GMFM-88 scores are documented for children with cerebral palsy (Palisano et al., 2000). The Modified Ashworth Scale is used for measuring spasticity in spastic patients (Bohannon & Smith MB, 1987).

In children with CP and GHD, Dimension A ($p < 0.02$), dimension B ($p < 0.02$), and dimension C ($p < 0.02$) of the GMFM-88, and the total score of the test ($p < 0.01$) significantly improved after the treatment; dimension D and dimension E did not increase, and four of five spastic patients showed a reduction in spasticity. However, in children with cerebral palsy and without growth hormone deficiency, only the total score of the test improved significantly after the treatment period. Plasma IGF-I values (previously low in GHD CP children) were similar in both groups at the end of the treatment period, indicating that growth hormone replacement therapy was responsible for the large differences observed between both groups in response to physical rehabilitation.

According to these results it is likely that GH administration plays a key role in recovering from a brain injury, independently or not that a GH deficiency exists. In this regard, voluntary physical exercise is known to be a factor increasing neurogenesis and also enhancing learning and memory (Beckinstein et al., 2011). However few positive effects are obtained in CP chidren undergoing exhaustive daily physical work, as our data also reflect. Exercise is a powerful stimulus for endogenous growth hormone release, most likely through enhanced central NA tone (Devesa et al., 1992). It has been demonstrated that inhibiting PI3K/Akt signaling, one of the pathways by which GH acts (Costoya et al., 1999), blocks exercise-mediated enhancement of adult neurogenesis and synaptic plasticity in rats (Bruel-Jungerman et al., 2009). The possibility exists that the lack of significant improvements in CP children submitted to intensive physical work is due to an impaired GH secretion, as it seems to occur whenever a brain injury exists, independently that current provocative tests do not reflect the existence of a GH deficiency.

As described before, blindness is a common finding in CP children. We studied 20 children with CP occurring as a consequence of prematurity leading to Periventricular Leukomalacia (11 males, 9 females, aged 2,05 ± 1,43 years; mean ± SD of the mean) with critical impairment of vision and marked pallor of the optic nerve. They were treated with GH and visual stimulation performed with a tachistoscope (repetitive white light flashes, 100-150 ms, carried out in 10 phases lasting 1 min each one, 80 flashes/min; 5 days/week). Stimulation was performed in a dark isolated room. Visual evoked potentials (VEP) were recorded before commencing the treatment and after finishing it. Treatment lasted for 5 ± 2.65 months. The rationale for interrupting visual stimulation and GH treatment was based on clinical observations (for example, visual interaction with the environment, looking at objects or relatives, taking objects with the hands...).

Results from this study (unpublished data) show that the children we studied presented severe visual deficiencies, characterized by a delayed conduction from the retina to the occipital cortex, as VEP showed, but these were corrected at the end of treatment period, as Figure 12 shows. Latencies were significatly decreased, while no significant changes were observed in amplitudes.

Delayed conduction from the retina to the occipital cortex means a deficient myelination. This may be related to a delayed maturation of the CNS, but it is unlikely that this was the reason in these CP children since they suffered brain injuries produced by prematurity leading to Periventricular Leukomalacia in which cerebral white matter is consistently affected. Moreover, some of these children were older than 2 years old, a period of time from which it is considered that a brain damage is already established and significant improvements are unlikely to appear. Injuries involving the optic radiations, such as it happens in Periventricular Leukomalacia, have a bad prognosis (Hoyt, 2003) and most of these children are expected to remain visually handicapped.

We utilized a tachistoscope as a stimulation method of both visual hemifields, but it is unlikely that visual stimulation alone could be responsible for the clinical and VEP changes observed after the treatment. Despite the fact that there was not a control group in our study and this could lead to missinterpretating the results obtained, most of these children had been receiving intense stimulation previously without achieving significant results.

A recent study describe that plasma levels of GH/IGF-I influence glial turnover in the white matter (Hua et al., 2009). It is not clear whether the maintenance of Oligodendrocyte Precursor Cells (OPCs) and oligodendrocyte turnover in the adult brain serves normal function or only provides a rapidly recruitable population of cells for myelin repair following damage. Proliferation of oligodendrocyte precursors and recruitment of new, myelinating oligodendrocytes from immature precursors contribute to myelin repair following demyelinating lesions. Following demyelination, proliferation of OPCs and commitment, differentiation and survival of adult-born oligodendrocytes all appear to be targets of regulation by inflammatory cytokines and growth factors.

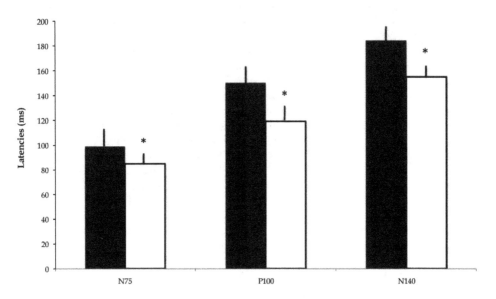

The figure shows changes observed in the latencies of Visual Evoked Potential waves registered in CP children before (black bars) and after (white bars) the treatment with GH and visual stimulation. * p < 0.005 vs. pretreatment.

Fig. 12. Latencies of Visual Evoked Potential waves in blind CP children.

The GH/IGF-I system appears to play a particularly critical role in myelin repair. IGF expression is induced in multiple models of demyelination and is increased during remyelination (Fushimi & Sharabe, 2004). Treatment with IGF-I or overexpression of IGF-I in transgenic mice inhibits oligodendrocyte death during demyelination and/or enhances remyelination following demyelinating lesions (McMorris & McKinnon, 1996; Mason et al., 2000; Kumar et al., 2007).

The possibility exists that remyelination observed in our study, as showed by the improvements in VEPs latencies, might be due to increased plasma IGF-I values. This does not exclude a direct effect of GH on myelination. As described before, GH induces EGF and EGF-R expression, factors recently involved on central nervous system remyelination (Gonzalez-Perez & Alvarez-Buylla, 2011).

Thus, it is feasible to assume that GH treatment played a significant role in the visual recovery elicited by specific visual stimulation.

Case report

At age 3 weeks a CP baby was admitted for rehabilitation in our Center. He suffered a massive bleeding *in utero* that produced a 20-minute cardiac arrest. A MRI carried out at age

2 weeks showed a severe encephalopathy with cystic cavities in both occipital lobes. VEP and auditory evoked potentials were isoelectric without any signs of conduction. Prognosis could not be worst: blind, deaf, dumb and spastic tetraparesia.

After obtaining signed informed consent from the parents we commenced an intensive rehabilitation with him. Visual stimulation, auditory stimulation, sensorial and physical stimulation and GH treatment (0.04 mg/kg/day). Three months later the child was showing signs of positive evolution. There was electrical conduction from the retina to the cortex, he responded to auditory stimuli and spasticity was decreased. GH treatment lasted for 4 months, but physical and sensorial stimulation continued for 12 months. At this time the child was absolutely normal as functional physical and cognitive tests revealed. Currently, at age 17 months, he walks, he speaks, he laughs, he plays, he is like any other child of his age. No sequelae have been observed and the treatment did not produce any kind of adverse effects.

A new MRI taken when he was 1 year old showed that the brain was completely regenerated. Cystic cavities disappeared and occipital lobes were fully functional. Voxels based morphometry comparing both MRI indicated that a number of brain areas experienced a significant regeneration; this was particularly significant in thalamus.

Figures 13 and 14 respectively show MRI and voxels based morphometry studies in this child.

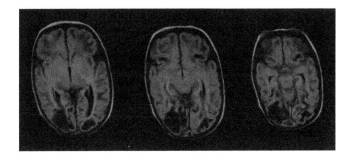

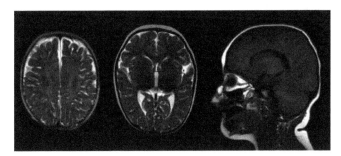

Upper images were taken at age 2-weeks. Notice the cavities affecting occipital lobes. Lower images were taken at age 1-year; no occipital cysts exist.

Fig. 13. Some images of MRI studies in the child described as a Case report.

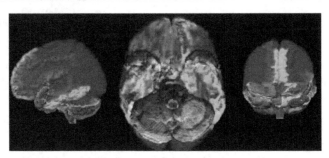

These images were obtained after comparing MRI studies carried out at 1-year interval in the child described as a Case report. The intensity of red colours is associated to greater regeneration.

Fig. 14. Voxels based morphometry.

To our knowledge this is the first description about complete human brain regeneration demonstrated with brain images. Brain plasticity may be responsible for achieving important functional recoveries in patients after a brain injury. In our case these recoveries were found not only by clinical and specific physical and cognitive tests, but they have been demonstrated with brain images. It is clear that the age at which we commenced the treatment of this child had a significant influence on the results obtained; brain development continues for 1 year after birth, approximately, but it also clear that physical and cognitive stimulation alone are not able for achieving a complete and functional recovery of the brain. Since the system GH/IGF-I has been involved in playing a very important role during embryonic brain development it seems that the treatment with the hormone was the main factor responsible for results achieved in this study. This supports our previous postulate about commencing GH treatments as soon as possible after a brain injury (Devesa et al., 2010a).

3.2 Traumatic brain injury

Traumatic brain injury (TBI) is an important health problem and a leading cause of death and disability worldwide, mainly in people under 40. Specifically, TBI is an important identified risk factor for cognitive deficits, such as attention, concentration, learning, memory, conceptual thinking, problem-solving or language (Vogenthaler, 1987). Recent studies have demonstrated that hypopituitarism, and particularly growth hormone deficiency (GHD), is common among survivors of TBI tested several months or years following head trauma (Popovic, 2005a; Popovic et al., 2005b). The subjects at risk are those who have suffered moderate-to-severe head trauma, although mild intensity trauma or even minor head injuries may precede hypopituitarism (Popovic et al., 2005b). Complex pituitary deficits are found in 35–40% of TBI patients; severe GHD occurs in 10–15% and partial GHD in 15% of TBI patients (Popovic et al., 2005b).

Neuropsychological assessments have demonstrated that GHD is associated with reduced cognitive performance; specifically, most of the studies indicate that GHD can lead to clinically relevant changes in memory, processing speed, attention, vocabulary, perceptual speed, spatial learning and in reaction time tests as well (van Dam, 2006; Falletti et al., 2006; Nieves-Martinez et al., 2010).

Cognitive dysfunction appears to be specifically related to GH deficiency; this hypothesis is supported by the positive correlations between serum IGF-I concentration and IQ. Thus, it has been shown that cognitive disorders secondary to GHD may be reversed by GH replacement (Maruff & Falletti, 2005).

We studied (Reimunde et al., 2010) 20 male adult patients with TBI suffered in the previous 10 years. Main brain injuries occurred because of frontal contusions affecting brain frontal lobes. Eleven of them presented GHD (mean age: 53.36 ± 17.35 years), while GH secretion seemed to be normal in the other nine patients (mean age: 47.12 ± 14.55 years).

All patients received daily cognitive rehabilitation, 1 hour per day, 5 days per week during 3 months. The contents of cognitive rehabilitation were aimed to improve the spatial, temporal and personal orientation, visual, auditory and tactile discrimination and perception, body recognition, planning and execution of motor acts, all memory types and processes, oral and writing language, calculation and executive function tasks. GHD patients were given human GH (0.5 mg/day during 20 days and then 1 mg/day, 5 days per week, for 3 months). Control patients were given placebo.

To assess different cognitive abilities we used a widely recognized neuropsychological test battery, the Wechsler Adults Intelligence Scale (WAIS) (Wechsler, 1990). This assessment battery involves several sections that specifically measure multiple cognitive functions. WAIS test was performed before commencing the treatment and after 3 months of treatment in all patients.

Results from our study demonstrate that individuals treated only with cognitive rehabilitation improved, specifically, their attentional functioning. However, the group treated with GH and cognitive rehabilitation improved their attentional functioning too, but moreover showed specific improvements in memory, understanding, associative thinking skills, information management and storing, learning, visual-motor dexterity and speed of execution.

In addition, the GHD group reached greater improvements in aspects related with memory, understanding, associative thinking skills and information management and storing information than the control patients.

These data correlated with previous results showing that GH-deficient subjects treated with GH experience significant improvements in concentration and attention, different memory modalities and learning.

It has been described that memory performance is weakly related to the mean daily GH dose, but there was a stronger positive correlation between the increase in mental performance and the GH-induced rise in serum IGF-I; this phenomenon can be explained by the large inter-individual differences in GH sensitivity (Deijen et al., 1998). However, in our study, no significant differences between plasma IGF-I levels in both groups of patients were observed at the end of the treatment period. Thus, it is unlikely that the IGF-I rise could be responsible for the results here obtained.

In conclusion, our study demonstrated, for the first time, the utility of a combination therapy involving GH replacement and cognitive rehabilitation in the recovery of cognitive impairments in patients who had suffered a TBI and a subsequent GHD. Our data show that the combination therapy has significantly greater effects than those achieved by carrying out only cognitive rehabilitation in patients with cognitive impairments secondary to a TBI without GHD. GH administration seems to be responsible for the results obtained. On these bases, we concluded that it woud be interesting to test whether GH administration to no GHD patients would improve cognitive functions in a number of neurological disorders (Reimunde et al., 2010).

4. Conclusions

Throughout this chapter we have reviewed the evidence showing that adult neurogenesis is a physiological mechanism to repair brain damage. We analyzed a number of factors directly involved in this process.

We demonstrated that both GH and its receptor are expressed in neural precursors in mice, and we showed that after a brain injury, in rats, the treatment with the hormone increases the number of newly born stem cells produced in response to the damage. We demonstrated that GH is present in the cytoplasm of these newly born cells, most likely for facilitating their migration from neurogenic niches. Our data in cell cultures obtained from mice stem cells demonstrate that the hormone plays a key role for neural cells survival.

In human patients with brain injury and GH-deficiency, we demonstrated that GH treatment together with physical and cognitive stimulation is responsible for the recovery of motor and cognitive abilities. GH treatment also appears to play a key role for remyelination of the visual pathways in children with cerebral palsy.

For the first time we showed here that an early treatment with the hormone can recover a brain injury in the first months of the life.

Although not presented here, GH treatment may repair central neurogenic dysphagias (Devesa et al., 2009; Reimunde et al., 2011, submitted for publication).

By analyzing the role of many factors positively involved on adult neurogenesis, we postulate that some of the positive effects of GH at the central level may be due to GH-induced expression of a number of neurotrophic factors and/or to enhanced release of some of them.

We conclude that GH treatment is a powerful tool for being used in a number of brain injuries, including neurodegenerative non-genetical diseases (for example, multiple sclerosis, Alzheimer, etc). It seems that there is no need that GH-deficiency exists for the hormone being useful.

GH treatments have to be well scheduled and short in time. The positive effects of the hormone remain in the time.

5. Acknowledgements

These studies were supported by Foundation Foltra (Teo, Spain). Studies in human patients were carried out in Medical Center Proyecto Foltra (Teo, Spain). Animal studies were carried out in the Department of Physiology, School of Medicine, Santiago de Compostela, Spain, under the direction of Professor Jesús Devesa and Professor Víctor Arce. Studies in NSCs were performed in the Institute of Neurosciences of the School of Medicine of Coimbra, Portugal, under the direction of Professor Joao Malva; his collaboration is greatly appreciated. Voxel based morphometries were performed by Brain Dynamics (Málaga, Spain).

6. References

Abdipranoto A, Wu A, Stayte S, et al. (2008). The role of neurogenesis in neurodegenerative diseases and its implications for therapeutic development. *CNS Neurol Disord Drug Targets.* 7:187-210.

Abdipranoto-Cowley A, Park JS, Croucher D, et al. (2009). Activin A Is Essential for Neurogenesis Following Neurodegeneration. *Stem Cells*. 27: 1330-46.

Aberg MA, Aberg ND, Hedbacker H, Oscarsson J & Eriksson PS. (2000). Peripheral infusion of IGF-I selectively induces neurogenesis in the adult rat hippocampus. *J Neurosci*. 20: 2896-2903.

Aberg ND, Johansson UE, Aberg MA, et al. (2007). Peripheral infusion of insulin-like growth factor-I increases the number of newborn oligodendrocytes in the cerebral cortex of adult hypophysectomized rats. *Endocrinology*. 148: 3765-3772.

Aberg ND, Johansson I, Aberg MA, et al. (2009). Peripheral administration of GH induces cell proliferation in the brain of adult hypophysectomized rats. *J Endocrinol*. 201:141-50.

Aberg D, Jood K, Blomstrand C, et al. (2011). Serum IGF-I levels correlate to improvement of functional outcome after ischemic stroke. *J Clin Endocrinol Metab*. 96:E1055-64.

Aimone JB, Deng W & Gage FH. (2010). Adult neurogenesis: integrating theories and separating functions. *Trends Cogn Sci*. 14: 325-37.

Ajo R, Cacicedo L, Navarro C & Sanchez-Franco F. (2003). Growth hormone action on proliferation and differentiation of cerebral cortical cells from fetal rat. *Endocrinology*. 144:1086-1097.

Ali O, Shim M, Fowler E, Cohen P & Oppenheim W. (2007a). Spinal bone mineral density, IGF-1 and IGFBP-3 in children with cerebral palsy. *Horm Res*. 68:316-320.

Ali O, Shim M, Fowler E, et al. (2007b). Growth hormone therapy improves bone mineral density in children with cerebral palsy: a preliminary pilot study. *J Clin Endocrinol Metab*. 92:932-937.

Altman J & Das GD. (1965). Autoradiographic and histological evidence of postnatal hippocampal neurogenesis in rats. *J Comp Neurol*. 124:319-35.

Anacker C, Zunszain PA, Cattaneo A., et al. (2011). Antidepressants increase human hippocampal neurogenesis by activating the glucocorticoid receptor. *Mol Psychiatry*. 16: 738-750.

Azcoitia I, Pérez Martín M, Salazar V., et al. (2005) Growth hormone prevents neuronal loss in the aged rat hippocampus. *Neurobiol Aging*. 5:697-703.

Barclay JL, Kerr LM, Arthur L, et al. (2010). In vivo targeting of the growth hormone receptor (GHR) Box1 sequence demonstrates that the GHR does not signal exclusively through JAK2. *Mol Endocrinol*. 24:204-17.

Beckinschtein P, Oomen CA, Saksida LM & Bussey TJ. (2011). Effects of environmental enrichment and voluntary exercise on neurogenesis, learning and memory, and pattern separation: BDNF as a critical variable? *Semin Cell Dev Biol*. Jul 7. [Epub ahead of print].

Bennett BL, Sasaki DT, Murray BW, et al. (2001). SP600125, an anthrapyrazolone inhibitor of Jun N-terminal kinase. *Proc Natl Acad Sci U S A*. 98:13681-6.

Betarbet R, Zigova T, Bakay RA & Luskin MB. Dopaminergic and GABAergic interneurons of the olfactory bulb are derived from the neonatal subventricular zone. *Int J Dev Neurosci*. 14: 921-30.

Bohannon RW & Smith MB. (1987) Interrater reliability of a modified Ashworth scale of muscle spasticity. *Phys Ther*. 67:206-207.

Boldrini M, Underwood MD, Hen R, et al. (2009). Antidepressants increase neural progenitor cells in the human hippocampus. *Neuropsychopharmacology.* 34:2376–2389.

Bowers JM, Waddell J & McCarthy MM. (2010). A developmental sex difference in hippocampal neurogenesis is mediated by endogenous oestradiol. *Biol Sex Differ.* 1:8-15.

Bruel-Jungerman E, Veyrac A, Dufour F, Horwood J, Laroche S & Davis S. (2009). Inhibition of PI3-Akt signaling blocks exercise-mediated enhancement of adult neurogenesis and synaptic plasticity in the dentate gyrus. *PloS One.* 4:e7901.

Byts N, Samoylenko A, Fasshauer T, et al. (2008). Essential role for Stat5 in the neurotrophic but not in the neuroprotective effect of erythropoietin. *Cell Death Differ.* 15:783–792.

Byts N & Sirén AL. (2009). Erythropoietin: a multimodal neuroprotective agent. *Exp Transl Stroke Med.* 1:4-11.

Cameron HA & McKay RD. (1999). Restoring production of hippocampal neurons in old age. *Nat Neurosci.* 2:894–897.

Campbell NR, Fernandes CC, Halff AW & Berg DK. (2010). Endogenous signaling through alpha7-containing nicotinic receptors promotes maturation and integration of adult-born neurons in the hippocampus. *J Neurosci.* 30: 8734– 8744.

Carracedo A, Ma L, Teruya-Feldstein J, et al. (2008). Inhibition of mTORC1 leads to MAPK pathway activation through a PI3K-dependent feedback loop in human cancer. *J. Clin. Invest.* 118:3065–3074.

Chen ZY, Asavaritikrai P, Prchal JT & Noguchi CT. (2007). Endogenous erythropoietin signaling is required for normal neural progenitor cell proliferation. *J Biol Chem.* 282:25875–25883.

Christophidis LJ, Gorba T, Gustavsson M, et al. (2009). Growth hormone receptor immunoreactivity is increased in the subventricular zone of juvenile rat brain after focal ischemia: a potential role for growth hormone in injury- induced neurogenesis. *Growth Horm IGF Res.* 19:497-506.

Coniglio SJ & Stevenson RD. (1995). Growth hormone deficiency in two children with cerebral palsy. *Dev Med Child Neurol.* 37:1013–1015.

Costoya JA, Finidori J, Moutoussamy S, Señaris R, Devesa J & Arce VM. (1999). Activation of growth hormone receptor delivers an antiapoptotic signal: evidence for a role of Akt in this pathway. *Endocrinology.* 140:5937-43.

Darnaudery M, Perez-Martin M, Belizaire G, Maccari S & Garcia-Segura LM. (2006). Insulin-like growth factor 1 reduces age-related disorders induced by prenatal stress in female rats. *Neurobiol Aging.* 27:119–127.

David DJ, Samuels BA, Rainer Q, et al. (2009). Neurogenesis-dependent and -independent effects of fluoxetine in an animal model of anxiety/depression. *Neuron.* 62:479–493.

Devesa J, Lima L & Tresguerres JA. (1992). Neuroendocrine control of growth hormone secretion in humans. *Trends Endocrinol Metab.* 3:175-83.

Devesa J, Reimunde P, Devesa A, et al. (2009). Recovery from neurological sequelae secondary to oncological brain surgery in an adult growth hormone-deficient patient after growth hormone treatment. *J Rehabil Med.* 41:775-7.

Devesa J, Casteleiro N, Rodicio C, López N & Reimunde P. (2010a). Growth hormone deficiency and cerebral palsy. *Ther Clin Risk Manag.* 6:413-8.

Devesa J, Devesa P & Reimunde P. (2010b). [Growth hormone revisited]. *Med Clin (Barc)* 6:413-18.

Devesa J, Alonso B, Casteleiro N, et al (2011). Effects of recombinant growth hormone (GH) replacement and psychomotor and cognitive stimulation in the neurodevelopment of GH-deficient (GHD) children with cerebral palsy: a pilot study. *Ther Clin Risk Manag.* 7:199-206.

Devesa P, Reimunde P, Gallego R, Devesa J & Arce VM. (2011). Growth hormone (GH) treatment may cooperate with locally-produced GH in increasing the proliferative response of hippocampal progenitors to kainate-induced injury. *Brain Inj.* 25: 503-10.

Devesa P. (2011). Effects of growth hormone on the central and peripheral neural repair. *Doctoral thesis.* University of Santiago de Compostela, Spain.

Deijen JB, de Boer H & van der Veen EA. Cognitive changes during growth hormone replacement in adult men. *Psychoneuroendocrinology.* 23:45–55.

Doetsch F, Petreanu L, Caille I, Garcia-Verdugo JM & Alvarez-Buylla A. (2002). EGF converts transit-amplifying neurogenic precursors in the adult brain into multipotent stem cells. *Neuron.* 36:1021–1034.

Donahue CP, Jensen RV, Ochiishi T, et al. (2002). Transcriptional profiling reveals regulated genes in the hippocampus during memory formation. *Hippocampus.* 12:821–833.

Donahue CP, Kosik KS, & Shors TJ. (2006). Growth hormone is produced within the hippocampus where it responds to age, sex, and stress. *Proc. Natl. Acad. Sci.* 103:6031–6036.

Dutheil S, Lacour M & Tighilry B. (2011). Discovering a new functional neurogenic zone-The vestibular nuclei of the brainstem. *Med Sci (Paris).* 27: 605-613.

Eriksson PS, Perfilieva E, Björk-Eriksson T, et al. (1998) Neurogenesis in the adult human hippocampus. *Nat Med.* 4:1313- 7.

Falleti MG, Maruff P, Burman P & Harris A. (1996). The effects of growth hormone (GH) deficiency and GH replacement on cognitive performance in adults: A meta-analysis of the current literature. *Psychoneuroendocrinology.* 31: 681– 691.

Franklin RJ, Zhao C & Sim FJ. (2002). Ageing and CNS remyelination. *Neuroreport.* 13: 923-928.

Fukuda S, Kato F, Tozuka Y, Yamaguchi M, Miyamoto Y & Hisatsune T. (2003). Two distinct subpopulations of nestin- positive cells in adult mouse dentate gyrus. *J Neurosci* .23:9357-66.

Fushimi S & Shirabe T. (2004). Expression of insulin-like growth factors in remyelination following ethidium bromide- induced demyelination in the mouse spinal cord. *Neuropathology.* 24:208–218.

Fukul H & Toyoshima K. (2008). Music facilitates the neurogenesis, regeneration and repair of neurons. *Med Hypotheses* 271 : 765-9.

Galea LA, Kavaliers M & Ossenkopp KP. (1996). Sexually dimorphic spatial learning in meadow voles Microtus pennsylvanicus and deer mice Peromyscus maniculatus. *J Exp Biol.* 199: 195–200

Galea LA, Spritzer MD, Barker JM & Pawluski JL. (2006). Gonadal hormone modulation of hippocampal neurogenesis in the adult. *Hippocampus.* 16: 225-32.

Gampe K, Brill MS, Momma S, Götz M & Zimmermann H. (2011). EGF induces CREB and ERK activation at the wall of the mouse lateral ventricles. *Brain Res.* 1376:31-41.

García-Aragón J, Lobie PE, Muscat GE, Gobius KS, Norstedt G & Waters MJ. (1992). Prenatal expression of the growth hormone (GH) receptor/binding protein in the rat: a role for GH in embryonic and fetal development?. *Development*. 114: 869–876.

Gheusi G, Cremer H, McLean H, Chazal G, Vincent JD & Lledo PM. (2000). Importance of newly generated neurons in the adult olfactory bulb for odor discrimination. *Proc Natl Acad Sci U S A*. 97: 1823-8.

Gilson J & Blakemore WF. (1993). Failure of remyelination in areas of demyelination produced in the spinal cord of old rats. *Neuropathol Appl Neurobiol*. 19:173–181.

Goldman SA & Nottebohm F. (1983). Neuronal production, migration, and differentiation in a vocal control nucleus of the adult female canary brain. *Proc Natl Acad Sci*. 80:2390-4.

Gonzalez-Perez O & Alvarez-Buylla A. (2011). Oligodendrogenesis in the subventricular zone and the role of epidermal growth factor. *Brain Res Rev*. 67: 147-56.

Gould E, Reeves AJ, Graziano MS & Gross CG. (1999). Neurogenesis in the neocortex of adult primates. *Science*. 286: 548- 52.

Gritti A, Frolichsthal-Schoeller P, Galli R, et al. (1999). Epidermal and fibroblast growth factors behave as mitogenic regulators for a single multipotent stem cell-like population from the subventricular region of the adult mouse forebrain. *J Neurosci*. 19: 3287–3297.

Hansen JA, Lindberg K, Hilton DJ, Nielsen JH & Billestrup N. (1999). Mechanism of inhibition of growth hormone receptor signaling by suppressor of cytokine signaling proteins. *Molecular Endocrinology*. 13:1832–1843.

Hidalgo A, Barami K, Iversen K & Goldman SA. (1995). Estrogens and non-estrogenic ovarian influences combine to promote the recruitment and decrease the turnover of new neurons in the adult female canary brain. *J Neurobiol*. 27:470–487.

High WM, Briones-Galang M, Clark JA, et al. (2010). Effect of Growth Hormone replacement therapy on cognition after traumatic brain injury. *J Neurotrauma*. 27:1565-75.

Hua K, Forbes EM, Lichtenwalner RJ, Sonntag WE & Riddle DR. (2009). Adult-onset deficiency in growth hormone and insulin-like growth factor-I alters oligodendrocyte turnover in the corpus callosum. *Glia*. 57:1062-71.

Hoyt, CS. (2003). Visual function in the brain-damaged child. *Eye*. 17:369–384.

Huang GJ & Herbert J. (2006). Stimulation of neurogenesis in the hippocampus of the adult rat by fluoxetine requires rhythmic change in corticosterone. *Biol Psychiatry*. 59:619-624.

Iguchi H, Mitsui T, Ishida M, Kaba S & Arita J. (2011). cAMP response element-binding protein (CREB) is required for epidermal growth factor (EGF)-induced cell proliferation and serum response element ativation in neural stem cells isolated from the forebrain subventricular zone of adult mice. *Endocr J*. Jun 24. [Epub ahead of print].

Johansson BB. (2011). Current trends in stroke rehabilitation. A review with focus on brain plasticity. *Acta Neurol Scand*. 123: 147-59

Johnson F & Bottjer SW. (1995). Differential estrogen accumulation among populations of projection neurons in the higher vocal center of male canaries. *J Neurobiol*. 26:87-108.

Kaplan MS & Hinds JW. (1977). Neurogenesis in the adult rat: electron microscopic analysis of light radioautographs. *Science*. 197:1092-4.

Katakowski M, Zhang ZG, Chen J., et al. (2003). Phosphoinositide 3-kinase promotes adult subventricular neuroblast migration after stroke. *J Neurosci Res.* 74:494-501.

Kempermann G, Kuhn HG & Gage FH. (1997). More hippocampal neurons in adult mice living in an enriched environment. *Nature.* 386: 493-5.

Kempermann G, Wiskott L & Gage FH. (2004). Functional significance of adult neurogenesis. *Curr Opin Neurobiol.* 14:186-91.

Konkle AT & McCarthy MM. (2010). Developmental time course of Estradiol, Testosterone, and Dihydrotestosterone levels in discrete regions of male and female rat brain. *Endocrinology.* 152: 223-35.

Kronenberg G, Reuter K, Steiner B, et al. (2003). Subpopulations of proliferating cells of the adult hippocampus respond differently to physiologic neurogenic stimuli. *J Comp Neurol.* 467:455- 63.

Kuhn HG, Dickinson-Anson H & Gage FH. (1996). Neurogenesis in the dentate gyrus of the adult rat: age-related decrease of neuronal progenitor proliferation. *J Neurosci.* 16:2027-2033.

Kuhn HG, Winkler J, Dempermann G, Thal LJ & Gage FH. (1997). Epidermal growth factor and fibroblast growth factor- 2 have different effects on neural progenitors in the adult rat brain. *J Neurosci.* 17:5820-5829.

Kumar S, Biancotti JC, Yamaguchi M & de Vellis J. (2007). Combination of growth factors enhances remyelination in a cuprizone-induced demyelination mouse model. *Neurochem Res.* 32:783-797.

Lam TT & Leranth C. (2003). Role of the medial septum diagonal band of Broca cholinergic neurons in oestrogen- induced spine synapse formation on hippocampal CA1 pyramidal cells of female rats. *Eur J Neurosci.* 17:1997- 2005.

Lecca D, Trincavelli ML, Gelosa P, et al. (2008). The recently identified P2Y-like receptor GPR17 is a sensor of brain damage and a new target for brain repair. *PLos One.* 3:e3579.

Lennington JB, Yang Z & Conover JC. (2003). Neural stem cells and the regulation of adult neurogenesis. *Reprod Biol Endocrinol.* 1:99-105.

Lichtenwalner RJ, Forbes ME, Bennett SA, Lynch CD, Sonntag WE & Riddle DR. (2001). Intracerebroventricular infusion of insulin-like growth factor-I ameliorates the age-related decline in hippocampal neurogenesis. *Neuroscience.* 107:603-613.

Lichtenwalner RJ, Forbes ME, Sonntag WE & Riddle DR. (2006). Adult-onset deficiency in growth hormone and insulin- like growth factor-I decreases survival of dentate granule neurons: insights into the regulation of adult hippocampal neurogenesis. *J Neurosci Res.* 83:199-210.

Leuner B, Caponiti JM & Gould E. (2011). Oxytocin stimulates adult neurogenesis even under conditions of stress and elevated glucocorticoids. *Hippocampus.* Jun 20. doi: 10.1002/hipo.20947. [Epub ahead of print].

Lledo PM, Alonso M & Grubb MS. (2006). Adult neurogenesis and functional plasticity in neuronal circuits. *Nat Rev Neurosci.* 7: 179-93.

Lobie PE, Garcia-Aragon J, Lincoln DT, Barnard R, Wilcox JN & Waters MJ. (1993). Localization and ontogeny of growth hormone receptor gene expression in the central nervous system. *Brain Res Dev Brain Res.* 74:225-33.

Lois C, & Alvarez-Buylla A. (1993). Proliferating subventricular zone cells in the adult mammalian forebrain can differentiate into neurons and glia. *Proc Natl Acad Sci.* 90:2074-7.

Lyuh E, Kim HJ, Kim M, et al. (2007). Dose-specific or dose-dependent effect of growth hormone treatment on the proliferation and differentiation of cultured neuronal cells. *Growth Horm. IGF Res.* 17: 315-322.

Mason JL, Ye P, Suzuki K, D'Ercole AJ & Matsushima GK. (2000). Insulin-like growth factor-1 inhibits mature oligodendrocyte apoptosis during primary demyelination. *J Neurosci.* 20: 5703-5708.

McLenachan S, Lum MG, Waters MJ & Turnley AM. (2009). Growth hormone promotes proliferation of adult neurosphere cultures. *Growth Horm IGF Res.* 19:212-8.

McMorris FA & McKinnon RD. (1996). Regulation of oligodendrocyte development and CNS myelination by growth factors: prospects for therapy of demyelinating disease. *Brain Pathol.* 6: 313-329.

Mak GK & Weiss S. (2010). Paternal recognition of adult offspring mediated by newly generated CNS neurons. *Nat Neurosci.* 13: 652-3.

Maren S, De Oca B & Fanselow MS. (1994). Sex differences in hippocampal long-term potentiation (LTP) and Pavlovian fear conditioning in rats: positive correlation between LTP and contextual learning. *Brain Res.* 661:25-34.

Maric D, Maric I, Chang YH & Barker JL. (2003). Prospective cell sorting of embryonic rat neural stem cells and neuronal and glial progenitors reveals selective effects of basic fibroblast growth factor and epidermal growth factor on self-renewal and differentiation. *J Neurosci.* 23:240-251.

Marrone DF, Ramirez-Amaya V & Barnes CA. (2011). Neurons generated in senescence maintain capacity for functional integration. *Hippocampus.* Jun 21. doi: 10.1002/hipo.20959. [Epub ahead of print].

Maruff P & Falleti M. (2005). Cognitive function in growth hormone deficiency and growth hormone replacement. *Hormone Research.* 64(Suppl 3):100-108.

Mason JL, Ye P, Suzuki K, D'Ercole AJ & Matsushima GK. (2000). Insulin-like growth factor-1 inhibits mature oligodendrocyte apoptosis during primary demyelination. *J Neurosci.* 20 :5703-5708.

McLenachan S, Lum MG, Waters MJ & Turnley AM. (2009). Growth hormone promotes proliferation of adult neurosphere cultures. *Growth Horm IGF Res.* 19:212-8.

Mitsushima D, Takase K, Takahashi T & Kimura F. (2009a). Activational and organisational effects of gonadal steroids on sex-specific acetylcholine release in the dorsal hippocampus. *J Neuroendocrinol.* 21:400-405.

Mitsushima D, Takase K, Funabashi T & Kimura F. (2009b). Gonadal steroids maintain 24 h acetylcholine release in the hippocampus: organizational and activational effects in behaving rats. *J Neurosci.* 29:3808-3815.

Möderscheim TA, Christophidis LJ, Williams CE & Scheepens A. (2007). Distinct neuronal growth hormone receptor ligand specificity in the rat brain. *Brain Res.* 1137:29-34.

Morshead CM & van der Kooy D. (1992). Postmitotic death is the fate of constitutively proliferating cells in the subependymal layer of the adult mouse brain. *J Neurosci.*12:249-256.

Morshead CM, Reynolds BA, Craig CG, et al. (1994). Neural stem cells in the adult mammalian forebrain: a relatively quiescent subpopulation of subependymal cells. *Neuron.* 13:1071–1082.

Moutoussamy S, Renaudie F, Lago F, Kelly PA & Finidori J. (1998). Grb10 identified as a potential regulator of growth hormone (GH) signaling by cloning of GH receptor target proteins. *Journal of Biological Chemistry.* 273:15906– 15912.

Newborg J, Stock JR, Wnek L, et al. (1988).*Battelle Developmental Inventory with Recalibrated Technical Data and Norms: Screening Test Examiner's Manual.* 2nd ed. Allen, TX: DLM, Inc.

Nieves-Martinez E, Sonntag WE, Wilson A, et al. (2010). Early-onset GH deficiency results in spatial memory impairment in midlife and is prevented by GH supplementation. *Journal of Endocrinology.* 204:31–36.

Nilsson M, Perfilieva E, Johansson U, Orwar O & Eriksson PS. (1999). Enriched environment increases neurogenesis in the adult rat dentate gyrus and improves spatial memory. *J Neurobiol.* 39:569-78.

Nordeen EJ & Nordeen KW. (1989). Estrogen stimulates the incorporation of new neurons into avian song nuclei during adolescence. *Brain Res Dev Brain Res.* 49:27–32.

Palisano RJ, Hanna SE, Rosenbaum PL, et al. (2000). Validation of a model of gross motor function for children with cerebral palsy. *Phys Ther.* 80:974–985.

Pan SN, Ma HM, Su Z, Zhang CX, Zhu SY & Du ML. (2011). Epidermal growth factor receptor signaling mediates growth hormone-induced growth of chondrocytes from sex hormone-inhibited adolescent rats. *Clin Exp Pharmacol Physiol.* Jun 1. doi: 10.1111/j.1440-1681.2011.05547.x. [Epub ahead of print].

Pang Y, Zheng B, Fan LW, Rhodes PG & Cai Z. (2007). IGF-1 protects oligodendrocyte progenitors against TNF alpha- induced damage by activation of PI3K/Akt and interruption of the mitochondrial apoptotic pathway. Glia. 55:1099–1107.

Parent JM. (2002). The role of seizure-induced neurogenesis in epileptogenesis and brain repair. *Epilepsy Res.* 50: 179-89.

Parent JM. (2003). Injury-induced neurogenesis in the adult mammalian brain. *Neuroscientist.* 9: 261–272.

Paton JA & Nottebohm FN. (1984). Neurons generated in the adult brain are recruited into functional circuits. *Science.* 225:1046-8.

Perrini S, Natalicchio A, Laviola L, et al. (2008). Abnormalities of insulin-like growth factor-I signaling and impaired cell proliferation in osteoblasts from subjects with osteoporosis. *Endocrinology.* 149:1302–1313.

Popovic V. (2005a). GH deficiency as the most common pituitary defect after TBI: Clinical implications. *Pituitary* 8: 239– 243.

Popovic V, Aimaretti G, Casanueva FF & Ghigo E. (2005b). Hypopituitarism following traumatic brain injury. *Growth Hormone & IGF Research.* 15:177–184.

Rasika S, Nottebohm F & Alvarez-Buylla A. (1994). Testosterone increases the recruitment and/or survival of new high vocal center neurons in adult female canaries. *Proc Natl Acad Sci U S A.* 91:7854–7858.

Reimunde P, Rodicio C, López N, Alonso A, Devesa P & Devesa J. (2010). Effects of recombinant growth hormone replacement and physical rehabilitation in recovery of gross motor function in children with cerebral palsy. *Ther Clin Risk Manag.* 6:585-92.

Reimunde P, Quintana A, Castañón B. et al. (2011). Effects of growth hormone (GH) replacement and cognitive rehabilitation in patients with cognitive disorders after traumatic brain injury. *Brain Inj.* 25:65-73.

Reynolds BA & Weiss S. (1992). Generation of neurons and astrocytes from isolated cells of the adult mammalian central nervous system. *Science.* 255:1707-1710.

Robel S, Berninger B & Götz M. (2011). The stem cell potential of glia: lessons from reactive gliosis. *Nat Rev Reurosci.* 12: 88-104.

Romanko MJ, Rola R, Fike JR, et al. (2004). Roles of the mammalian subventricular zone in cell replacement after brain injury. *Prog Neurobiol.* 74: 77-99.

Roof RL & Havens MD. (1992). Testosterone improves maze performance and induces development of a male hippocampus in females. *Brain Res.* 572:310-313.

Roof RL, Zhang Q, Glasier MM & Stein DG. (1993). Gender-specific impairment on Morris water maze task after entorhinal cortex lesion. *Behav Brain Res.* 57:47-51.

Sanders EJ, Parker E & Harvey S. (2006). Retinal ganglion cell survival in development: mechanisms of retinal growth hormone action. *Experimental Eye Research.* 83:1205-1214.

Sanders EJ, Baudet ML, Parker E, & Harvey S. (2009). Signaling mechanisms mediating local GH action in the neural retina of the chick embryo. *Gen Comp Endocrinol.* 163:63-9.

Sapolsky RM. (1992). Do glucocorticoid concentrations rise with age in the rat? *Neurobiol Aging.* 13:171-174.

Schaevitz LR & Berger-Sweeney J. (2005). Neurogenesis of the cholinergic medial septum in female and male C57BL/6J mice. *J Neurobiol.* 65:294-303.

Scheepens A, Williams CE, Breier BH, Guan J & Gluckman PD. (2000). A role for the somatotropic axis in neural development, injury and disease. *J Pediatr Endocrinol Metab.* 13 Suppl 6:1483-91.

Scheepens A, Sirimanne ES, Breier BH, Clark RG, Gluckman PD & Williams CE. (2001).Growth hormone as a neuronal rescue factor during recovery from CNS injury. *Neuroscience.* 104:677-87.

Scott HJ, Stebbing MJ, Walters CE. et al. (2006). Differential effects of SOCS2 on neuronal differentiation and morphology. *Brain Res.* 1067:138-145.

Shields SA, Gilson JM, Blakemore WF & Franklin RJ. (1999). Remyelination occurs as extensively but more slowly in old rats compared to young rats following gliotoxin-induced CNS demyelination. *Glia.* 28: 77-83.

Shim ML, Moshang T Jr, Oppenheim WL & Cohen P. (2004). Is treatment with growth hormone effective in children with cerebral palsy? *Dev Med Child Neurol.* 46:569-571.

Shingo T, Gregg C, Enwere E, et al. (2003). Pregnancy-stimulated neurogenesis in the adult female forebrain mediated by prolactin. *Science.* 299:117-120.

Silva C, Zhang K, Tsutsui S, Holden JK, Gill MJ & Power C. (2003). Growth hormone prevents human immunodeficiency virus-induced neuronal p53 expression. *Ann. Neurol.* 54:605-614.

Sim FJ, Zhao C, Penderis J & Franklin RJ. (2002). The age-related decrease in CNS remyelination efficiency is attributable to an impairment of both oligodendrocyte progenitor recruitment and differentiation. *J Neurosci.* 22: 2451-2459.

Sun LY, Al-Regaiey K, Masternak MM, Wang J & Bartke A. (2005a). Local expression of GH and IGF-1 in the hippocampus of GH-deficient long-lived mice. *Neurobiol. Aging.* 26:929–937.

Sun LY, Evans MS, Hsieh J, Panici J & Bartke A. (2005b). Increased neurogenesis in dentate gyrus of long-lived Ames dwarf mice. *Endocrinology.* 146:1138–1144.

Sun LY & Bartke A. (2007). Adult neurogenesis in the hippocampus of long-lived mice during aging. *J. Gerontol. A – Biol. Sci. Med. Sci.* 62:117–125.

Svensson AL, Bucht N, Hallberg M & Nyberg F. (2008). Reversal of opiate-induced apoptosis by human recombinant growth hormone in murine foetus primary hippocampal neuronal cell cultures. *Proc Natl Acad Sci U S A.* 105:7304-8.

Tanapat P, Hastings NB, Reeves AJ & Gould E. (1999). Estrogen stimulates a transient increase in the number of new neurons in the dentate gyrus of the adult female rat. *J Neurosci.* 19:5792–5801.

Tonchev AB. (2011). The nerve growth factor in health and unhealth neurons. *Arch Ital Biol.* 149: 225-31.

Torner L, Karg S, Blume A, et al. (2009). Prolactin prevents chronic stress-induced decrease of adult hippocampal neurogenesis and promotes neuronal fate. *J Neurosci.* 29:1826-33.

Trejo JL, Carro E & Torres-Aleman I. (2001). Circulating insulin-like growth factor I mediates exercise-induced increases in the number of new neurons in the adult hippocampus. *J Neurosci.* 21: 1628-34.

Tropepe V, Sibilia M, Ciruna BG, Rossant J, Wagner EF & van der Kooy D. (1999). Distinct neural stem cells proliferate in response to EGF and FGF in the developing mouse telencephalon. *Dev Biol.* 208:166–188.

Tsai PT, Ohab JJ, Kertesz N, et al. (2006). A critical role of erythropoietin receptor in neurogenesis and post-stroke recovery. *J Neurosci.* 26:1269–1274.

Turnley AM, Faux CH, Rietze RL, Coonan JR & Bartlett PF. (2002). Suppressor of cytokine signaling 2 regulates neuronal differentiation by inhibiting growth hormone signaling. *Nat. Neurosci.* 5: 1155–1162.

Vanderkuur JA, Butch ER, Waters SB, Pessin JE, Guan KL & Carter-Su C. (1997). Signaling molecules involved in coupling growth hormone receptor to mitogen-activated protein kinase activation. *Endocrinology.* 138:4301–4307.

van Dam PS. (2006). Somatotropin therapy and cognitive function in adults with growth hormone deficiency: A critical review. *Treatment in Endocrinology.* 5:159-170.

van Marle G, Antony JM, Silva C, Sullivan A & Power C. (2005). Aberrant cortical neurogenesis in a pediatric neuroAIDS model: neurotrophic effects of growth hormone. *Aids.*19:1781–1791.

van Praag H, Christie BR, Sejnowski TJ & Gage FH. (1999). Running enhances neurogenesis, learning, and long-term potentiation in mice. *Proc Natl Acad Sci USA.* 96: 13427-31.

Vogenthaler DR. (1987). An overview of head injury: Its consequences and rehabilitation. *Brain Injury.* 1:113–127.

Wagner K, Couillard-Despres S, Lehner B., et al. (2009). Prolactin induces MAPK signaling in neural progenitors without alleviating glucocorticoid-induced inhibition of *in vitro* neurogenesis. *Cell Physiol Biochem.* 24:397-406.

Wang X, Yang N, Deng L, Li X, Jiang J, Gan Y & Frank SJ. (2009). Interruption of growth hormone signaling via SHC and ERK in 3T3-F442A preadipocytes upon knockdown of insulin receptor substrate-1. *Mol Endocrinol*. 23:486-96.

Wechsler D. (1990). *Manual for the Wechsler adult intelligence scale. 8th ed. Madrid: TEA.*

Yamauchi T, Ueki K, Tobe K et al. (1997). Tyrosine phosphorylation of the EGF receptor by the kinase Jak2 is induced by growth hormone. *Nature*. 390:91–96.

Xu J & Messina JL. (2009). Crosstalk between growth hormone and insulin signaling. *Vitam Horm*. 80:125-53.

Yamauchi T, Ueki K, Tobe K, et al. (1998). Growth hormone-induced tyrosine phosphorylation of EGF receptor as an essential element leading to MAP kinase activation and gene expression. *Endocr J*. Apr; 45 Suppl: S27-31.

Yu T-S, Zhang G, Liebl DJ & Kernie SG. (2008). Traumatic brain injury-induced hippocampal neurogenesis requires activation of early nestin-expressing progenitors. *J Neurosci*. 28: 12901-12.

Zhang R, Zhang Z, Wang L, et al. (2004). Activated neural stem cells contribute to stroke-induced neurogenesis and neuroblast migration toward the infarct boundary in adult rats. *J Cereb Blood Flow Metab*. 24: 441-8.

Zhang L, Chopp M, Zhang RL, et al. (2010) Erythropoietin amplifies stroke-induced oligodendrogenesis in the rat. *PloS One*. 5:e106.

Zhang Z, Yang R, Zhou R, Li L, Sokabe M & Chen L. (2010). Progesterone promotes the survival of newborn neurons in the dentate gyrus of adult male mice. *Hippocampus*. 20: 402-12.

Zhao C, Deng W & Gage FH. (2008). Mechanisms and functional implications of adult neurogenesis. *Cell*. 132:645-60.

Zhu T, Goh EL, LeRoith D & Lobie PE. (1998). Growth hormone stimulates the formation of a multiprotein signaling complex involving p130(Cas) and CrkII. Resultant activation of c-Jun N-terminal kinase/stress-activated protein kinase (JNK/SAPK). *J Biol Chem*. 273:33864-75.

Zhu T, Goh EL, Graichen R, Ling & Lobie PE. (2001). Signal transduction via the growth hormone receptor. *Cellular Signalling*. 13:599–616.

Zhu T, Ling L & Lobie PE. (2002). Identification of a JAK2-independent pathway regulating growth hormone (GH)- stimulated p44/42 mitogen-activated protein kinase activity. GH activation of Ral and phospholipase D is Src- dependent. *Journal of Biological Chemistry*. 277:45592-45603.

8

Decompressive Craniectomy: Surgical Indications, Clinical Considerations and Rationale

Dare Adewumi and Austin Colohan
Loma Linda University Medical Center Department of Neurosurgery
Loma Linda
USA

"If there's no CSF pressure, but brain pressure exists, then pressure relief must be achieved by opening the skull" -Kocher 1901

1. Introduction

The management of increased intracranial pressure is a common clinical scenario encountered in a large portion of medicine. It is encountered more often in the practices of trauma, neurology and neurological surgery and as such is very common in intensive care settings. Treatment approaches remain one of the more controversial fields in medicine. In this chapter we will address the treatment approaches for elevated intracranial pressure. Indications for assessment, clinical considerations and approaches to proper management of elevated pressures focusing mainly on the decompressive craniectomy. We will address the role of the decompressive craniectomy in trauma stroke and address the option of lumbar drainage.

2. Intracranial pressure

Intracranial pressure is defined as the pressure within the cerebral vault that the systemic perfusion must overcome in order to adequately perfuse the brain. A mathematical expression of this relationship is that of CPP (Cerebral Perfusion Pressure) = MAP (Mean Arterial Pressure) - ICP (Intracranial Pressure). This relationship predicts that under settings where intracranial pressure approaches or surpasses mean arterial pressure the perfusion pressure declines resulting in hypoxic brain injury. The Monro-Kellie doctrine is often highlighted in illustrations of intracranial pressure. It holds that the adult cranial vault is a rigid structure composed of brain parenchyma, cerebrospinal fluid, and blood. The cranial vault being a rigid bony structure offers very little compliance and is not easily subject to shifts in space composition. As such, expansion in any of these compartments results in an increase in the amount of pressure contained within the rigid vault. There are inherent safeguards that allow for an element of expansion without excessive effects on the intracranial pressure. However once a certain a threshold is surpassed further expansion results in marked elevation in intracranial pressure. As intracranial pressure rises beyond adequate perfusion, the resultant effect is reduced perfusion and oxygen availability to the cerebrum resulting in hypoxic injury and cell death. The autolytic cascade leads to an increase in cell volume as the cell membrane is unable to maintain the electrochemical gradient due to a break down of the ATP dependent Na/K ATPase pump. Water and calcium influx leads to the expansion in the cell volume and a feed-forward positive cycle where cell death causes more edema and swelling, which causes increased intracranial pressure, which in turn causes less brain perfusion and results in further cell death. CSF flow through normal pathways can also be obstructed resulting in further elevation in intracranial pressure. The end result is often herniation as pressure becomes greater than the resistance of surrounding structures and brain structures actively transgress the boundaries established by dura mater and bone. There exist several ways to manage the complication of elevated intracranial pressure. Most of these are subdivided into a step wise systematic approach. One of such divides ICP management into two categories. Category 1 involves volume reduction. This utilizes the principles of the Monroe-Kellie doctrine. Removal of volume either in the form of CSF drainage or hyperosmotic diuresis will allow for more expansion of the edematous parenchyma. Category 2 describes the removal of mechanical constraints. This category primarily relies on the decompressive craniectomy. Removal of the rigid limitations preventing brain expansion would allow for more swelling thereby limiting and or preventing herniation (Scmidek H 2006). The AANS guidelines approach the management of elevated ICP similarly. The treatment paradigm is divided into 2 Tiers. Tier 1 involves the use of sedatives, paralytics, ventricular drainage, hyperosmolar therapy and mild hyperventilation. Tier 2 involves hypothermia, longer acting sedatives such as barbiturates, lumbar drainage via an intrathecal catheter and surgical decompression of the cranial vault. The decompressive craniectomy as we will discuss later allows for an outward herniation of brain structures as the limitations of the cranial vault are expanded theoretically minimizing any further injury the brain tissue would suffer by being forced into other compartments.

3. Management of elevated intracranial pressure

In this chapter we will focus primarily on the management of intracranial pressure in patients suffering from either stroke or traumatic brain injury. There remain other clinical scenarios where patients could suffer from elevated intracranial pressure. They include but are not limited to: infection, either meningeal or encephalitic, spontaneous intracerebral hemorrhage, and aneurysmal subarachnoid hemorrhage. Although decompressive craniectomy may play a role in these settings, it is beyond the scope of this chapter. The application of decompressive craniectomy in the posterior fossa will also not be addressed in this chapter.

Various cutoff values are used at different centers above which treatment of elevated intracranial pressure is indicated. Levels of 15, 20 and 25 are quoted but most centers use ICP > 20-25mmHg as the upper limit (Bullock 1995). There is a high mortality and even higher morbidity in patients with ICP persistently above 20mmHg. The physician's clinical discretion remains paramount in these settings. A 25 year-old trauma victim with an ICP of 30 but is awake, not intubated and following commands briskly is not as concerning as a 45 year-old with an ICP of 20 but has become acutely unresponsive. Several measurements can be employed in the management of elevated intracranial pressure. 1. Ensure adequate patient head positioning. The position of the patient's head can either optimize or hinder venous drainage. Venous congestion can lead to increased intracranial pressure. 2. Optimize the patient's vitals, specifically avoiding hypercarbia and hyperthermia. 3. Osmotic diuretics such as mannitol and hypertonic saline can also be utilized. In settings where adequate control of elevated ICP remains difficult, another option that can be employed is lumbar drainage. Lumbar drainage plays a role after ventriculostomy drainage has proven insufficient. At our institution we ensure patency of the ventriculostomy catheter with adequate drainage. If ICP remains elevated at this point a lumbar drain is placed. Initially the lumbar drain is left clamped and in most cases ICP control improves. However in situations where ICP elevation persists the lumbar drain is unclamped and placed at the same level as the ventriculostomy drain to minimize risk of brainstem herniation. The placement of lumbar drain plays a very valuable role in the reduction of elevated intracranial pressure (Munch E 2001; Murad A 2008).

4. Assessment of the trauma patient

The initial assessment of the trauma patient often begins in the emergency department. The basics must not be forgotten. Obtain a thorough history paying particular attention to mechanism of injury. Enough emphasis cannot be placed on obtaining a good overview of the situation. Even in the presence of an experienced trauma team the alert neurosurgeon can still play an additive role in helping to ensure that all bases are covered. A trauma team focused on placing a chest tube may not initially notice a lack of movement in a patient's lower extremities. The alert neurosurgeon would function well to inform the trauma team of this finding and help facilitate the appropriate imaging modality needed. Pay attention to the patient as a whole without focusing on the brain alone. In every trauma setting ensure that the ABC's of trauma (airway, breathing and circulation) are addressed before moving on to secondary surveys. A thorough physical and neurologic exam is always paramount. Initial head CT is indicated in settings where there are any moderate or high risk factors including but not limited to unresponsiveness, amnesia, altered mental status, deteriorating mental status (including intoxication), signs of calvarial fracture, focal neurologic deficits, penetrating skull injury, progressive headache, posttraumatic seizure, unreliable or inadequate history, multi-system trauma, severe facial injury, and significant subgaleal swelling (Stein S C 1992). Follow up Head CT remains at the clinical discretion of the physician and in the context of the nature of the presenting injury. A non-surgical epidural hematoma may require earlier follow up head CT than a small focal contusion. There exist practice guidelines and indications for ICP monitoring in the trauma setting. For salvageable patients with severe traumatic brain injury (GCS<8 after cardiopulmonary resuscitation), level II evidence dictates a need for ICP monitoring in patients with an abnormal Head CT. Level III evidence states a need for ICP monitoring in patients with a normal Head CT but with risk factors of elevated intracranial pressure, such as: age > 40 years, SBP < 90 mmHg, flexor or extensor posturing(Bullock 1995). However the final decision remains at the clinical discretion of the physician. Radiographic information can be used as an adjunct in determining a need for ICP monitoring but should not be used as a sole determinant. In one study 13% of patients with a normal CT scan will have elevated ICP, however patients with a normal CT and risk factors for elevated ICP have a 60% chance of elevated ICP (Narayan R

K 1082) . Decompressive craniectomy in trauma unlike in stroke remains controversial. In animal studies with artificially induced intracranial lesions, craniectomy has been linked to increased cerebral edema hemorrhagic infarcts and cortical necrosis (Moody R 1968; Cooper P 1979; Forsting M 1995). However decreased intracranial pressure, improved cerebral perfusion pressure and increased oxygen tension are also reported following craniectomy in trauma (Moody R 1968; Burkert W 1988). A review of more than 30 articles failed to demonstrate a clear benefit for craniectomy in the setting of trauma (Munch E 2000). A definitive answer to benefit of decompressive craniectomy still requires definitive randomized trials. At this point there does appear to be benefit especially in young patients with GCS >4.

Until the recently published DECRA trial (Cooper D 2011) no class I evidence supporting or disputing decompressive craniectomy in trauma existed. All previous evidence is class III at best. One of the more cited articles supporting decompressive craniectomy is a study designed at the University of Virginia (Polin 1997). In this study 35 bifrontal decompressive craniectomies were performed on patients with post-traumatic edema but no mass lesions between 1984 and 1993. The results were matched to control patients from the Traumatic Coma Data Bank. Their results showed good recovery and moderate disability in 37% of patients with mortality in 23% of patients as opposed to 16% moderate disability and 34% mortality in the Traumatic Coma Data Bank control. Post operative ICP control was better than the preoperative group and the control group. The study also found that patients with ICP>40 who underwent surgery >48hrs after time of injury did poorly.

A separate study published by the University of Maryland in Baltimore(Aarabi B 2006) discussed the findings of decompressive craniectomies performed between 2000-2004. 50 decompressive craniectomies were performed to control elevated ICP. 10 of these were performed before ICP elevation and 40 performed after ICP elevation. They found that decompressive craniectomies lowered the ICP to lower than 20 in 85% of patients. 14 of 50 patients died, 16 remained in a vegetative or severely disabled state, 20 had what was defined as a good outcome. Decompressive craniectomy was associated with a better than expected functional outcome in patients with medically uncontrollable ICP and or brain herniation compared with outcomes in other control cohorts reported in the literature.

A study out of Italy (Chibbaro S 2007) retrospectively reviewed 48 decompressive craniectomies and compared their outcomes to the Traumatic Coma Data Bank. They found that decompressive craniectomy reduced the midline shift and ameliorated basal cistern effacement. Younger patients (mean age of 31 years) had a better outcome. They also found that patients with early surgery, less than 16hrs of injury had, a better outcome than late intervention.

The DECRA trial as described earlier remains the only Class I evidence to date. The trial ran from December 2002 to April 2010. Eligibility criteria for inclusion in the study were patients between 15 and 59 years, patients with severe non-penetrating traumatic brain and patients with a GCS of 3 to 8. They excluded patients with dilated un-reactive pupils and those with mass lesions, including, but not limited to subdural and epidural hematomas. All patients had ICP monitoring and were treated medically if ICP was greater than 20. They defined early refractory ICP as a spontaneous elevation for more than 15 minutes continuously or intermittently within a 1 hour period despite first tier intervention. Patients were randomized within 72 hours to either surgery or standard care. The bifrontoparietal craniectomy technique used was based on the bifrontal craniectomy technique described by

Polin (Polin 1997). They randomly assigned 155 adults with severe traumatic brain injury and ICP refractory to first tier therapy to undergo either bifrontotemporoparietal decompressive craniectomy or standard medical care. 73 patients were enrolled in the surgical arm and 82 patients were enrolled in the medical arm. Patients in the the surgical group were found to have less time with elevated intracranial pressure, required fewer interventions for increased ICP post op and spent fewer days in the ICU. However patients undergoing craniectomy were found to have a worse outcome on the Glasgow outcome scale than those receiving standard care. The rates of death at 6 months were similar, 19% in the surgical arm and 18% in the medical arm.

The DECRA trial came under a large amount of criticism primarily related to the study design. The greatest word of caution arises in defining refractory ICP elevation has having reached levels greater than 20 for 15 minutes continuously or intermittently. Most neurosurgeons, neurologists and neurointensivists would address this as being too low a threshold for aggressive management of raised ICP. Some centers advocate the use of hyperosmotics such as Mannitol as a drip over 30 minutes instead of a bolus. Although "time is brain", operating on a patient based on an ICP elevation of 15 minutes can be seen as being very rapid and somewhat rash. Another criticism lies in the screening of 3,478 patients over a 7 year period to only enroll 155 patients. Finally the exclusion of patients with mass lesions is also a concern. Several of the patients involved in the DECRA trial with no mass lesion might fall into a category of diffuse axonal injury that did not require and would not be expected to benefit from a surgical decompression.

The RESCUEicp trial is a currently ongoing international prospective multi-center randomized controlled trial comparing the efficacy of decompressive craniectomy versus optimal medical management for the treatment of refractory intracranial hypertension following brain trauma. This study differs from the DECRA trial in terms of ICP threshold (25 vs 20 mmHg), timing of surgery (any time after injury vs within 72 hours post injury) and the acceptance of mass lesions. The RESCUEicp also holds a longer follow up period, 2 years as opposed to 6 months with the DECRA trial and a larger patient population with a goal of 400 (300 enrolled as of April 2011).

5. Assessment of the stroke patient

Decompressive craniectomy plays a vital role in patients diagnosed with malignant cerebral infarction. Malignant cerebral infarction refers to large territorial parenchymal strokes with ischemic edema and associated herniation. They typically involve occlusion of the MCA or ICA distribution causing infarction of the supplied territory. They account for approximately 15% of all strokes but mortality ranges from 50-80%. Patients typically present with rapid neurologic deterioration , gaze preference towards the infarcted hemisphere, contralateral hemiplegia and progressive decline in level of consciousness. Patients can rapidly progress from a state of being awake, alert, oriented and following commands to an obtunded state. The validity of decompressive craniectomy in stroke patients has been better studied and thereby better accepted in stroke patients than in trauma patients. Decompressive craniectomy in stroke patients as been show to reduce mortality from 50% to as as low as 32% in non-dominant hemisphere strokes with reduction of hemiplegia and in dominant hemisphere strokes only a mild-moderate aphasia. Better results occur with earlier surgery (Carter BS 1997). In 2007, three key landmark articles were published that proposed class I evidence supporting the use of decompressive craniectomy as valid treatment in the management of patients with malignant MCA infarction. The DECIMAL trial (Vahedi K 2007) was a study conducted in France after a poll of 47 neurology departments showed that only 2 departments were convinced of the efficacy of the decompressive craniectomy. The decompressive craniectomy in malignant MCA infarction trial was a multi center prospective randomized open but with blind evaluation of the primary end point study comparing early decompressive craniectomy versus standard medical therapy. It was conducted in 13 selected stroke centers including a stroke unit and a neurosurgery department from 2001 to 2005. Patients selected were between the ages of 18 and 55.

They included strokes as defined by an NIHSS > 16 within 24 hours of initial symptoms. The imaging criteria included head CTs that showed greater than a 50% MCA distribution involvement and MRI-DWI showing > 145 cm infarct volume. Exclusion criteria included patients with significant contralateral infarction, secondary hemorrhage of more than 50% of MCA territory pre-infarct significant disability, coagulopathy or use of tPA. For patients in the surgical arm of the study, decompressive craniectomy was performed less than 6hrs after randomization and up to 30hrs after initial onset of symptoms. 38 pts from 7 centers had been end enrolled when the study was prematurely ended (18 medical therapy, 20 surgical therapy). The study was ended due to slow recruitment of patients, a high difference in mortality between the 2 groups and to organize pooled data from the other ongoing trials, the DESTINY(Juttler E 2007) and HAMLET(Hotmeijer J 2009) trials. With the results gathered it was noted that the early decompression increased by more than half the number of patients with moderate disability and reduced by more than half the mortality rate at 1 year (mRS <3 of 50% in surgical group and 22% in medical group). The DECIMAL trial was able to conclude that in young patients (55yrs or younger) with malignant MCA infarction, early decompressive craniectomy had a great benefit on survival and led to a better functional outcome. No patients remained bedridden or had severe residual disability. Young patients had a significantly better outcome after surgery. However no patient had a complete recovery.

The DESTINY trial (Juttler E 2007)was a prospective, multi center, randomized, controlled clinical trial also based on a sequential design that used mortality after 30 days as the first end point. Although this trial was also ended prematurely it was able to show a statistically significant reduction in mortality after 32 patients had been enrolled. 15 of 17 patients randomized to the surgical group as opposed to 7 of 15 in the medical group survived after 30 days. DESTINY showed that hemicraniectomy reduces mortality in large hemispheric stroke patients. With only 32 patients enrolled the study was unable to demonstrate statistical superiority in functional outcome however the trial was terminated in light of the results of its joint analysis of the 3 European hemicraniectomy trials.

The HAMLET trial (Hotmeijer J 2009) was the third European trial and its aim was to assess the effect of decompressive surgery within 4 days of symptoms in patients with space-occupying hemispheric infarction. It showed that surgical decompression reduces fatality and poor outcome in patients with space occupying infarctions who are treated within 48hrs of stroke onset. The results however, showed no evidence that functional outcome is improved when decompression is delayed for up to 96hrs after stroke onset. They stress that the decision to operate should depend on the emphasis patients and relatives attribute to survival and dependency. Patient's lives can be saved but functional independence will either be severely impaired or completely lost.

A Meta-Analysis of the 3 randomized controlled trials found that hemicraniectomy within 48hrs after stroke onset resulted in reduced mortality and more favorable functional outcome. The trials were ongoing when the pooled analysis was planned. DESTINY and DECIMAL were stopped due to a clear reduction in mortality. HAMLET was still ongoing. The goal was to obtain results as soon as possible to avoid ongoing randomization in unnecessary and unethical situations. Indications include age <60 years. Stronger consideration in right hemisphere strokes and radiographic evidence of acute ICA or MCA infarcts with signs of impending severe brain swelling (Vahedi K 2007). 93 patients were included in the pooled analysis, (DESTINY 32pts, DECIMAL 38pts and HAMLET 23pts). More patients in the surgery group than in the medical group had mRS <4 (78% vs 24%). Also more patients in the surgical group survived than in the medical group (78% vs 29%). Interestingly certain rehab centers describe better improvement in patients with dominant hemisphere infarctions than in non-dominant hemisphere infarctions.

Perhaps this can be attributed to a retained capacity to learn activities of daily living. The most compelling argument for craniectomy in stroke patients regards the timing of surgery. This is supported by the 3 European trials as well as a retrospective study of 52 decompressions stratified by time of surgery into groups with intervention in under 6 hours from injury, intervention 6 hours after injury and no intervention. These showed mortality rates of 8%, 36% and 80% respectively. The average length of ICU stay was 12 days, 18 days and 7 days (shortened due to fatality)(Cho D 2003). A separate but similar study retrospectively stratified 63 interventions into decompression within 24 hours (early, 31 patients) and after 24 hours (late, 32 patients) of initial injury. Mortality was 16% for early decompression and 34% for late decompression. The average length of intensive care stay was 7 days for early decompression and 13 days for late decompression (Schwab S 1998). However early detection is only capable and confirmatory with adequate radiographic evidence.

MRI with DWI offers the best correlation to stroke severity and clinical outcome. The 90% sensitivity and 96% specificity of predictive value of malignant cerebral infarction with MRI-DWI are superior to the 60% and 70 to 90% specificity reported with Head CT (Arenillas J 2002; Manno E 2003). Given the limited availability of MRI either due to hospital constraints or patient co-morbidities, as well as the time restraints imposed by timely use of tPA in the setting of hyperacute stroke, the Head CT remains the most available and widely used radiographic reference tool.

At our institution we have developed a standard protocol applied to patients with malignant MCA stroke to assess their eligibility for decompressive craniectomy:

- LLUMC Protocol for Decompressive Craniectomy in Stroke
- Patients < 60 years old
- Large MCA stroke (greater than 145ml volume on DWI or greater than 50% MCA territory)
- Presentation within 48hrs of initial symptoms
- Exclude dilated un-reactive pupils
- Exclude bleeding diathesis
- Ventriculostomy placement ipsilateral to infarcted brain
- Lumbar drain if ICP remains elevated
- Cranioplasty between 6 weeks and 6 months

These parameters although not standardized nationally take into consideration the findings of other institutions and several published works. The ubiquity of factors such as age and timing of intervention are far reaching, as exhibited by the findings of Eghwrudjakpor and Allison (Eghwrudjakpor P 2010). They describe a glasgow coma core of 8 and above, age less than 50 years and early intervention as being the most significant determinants of prognosis.

6. Surgical considerations

A wide variety of surgical techniques have been reported for decompressive craniectomy. All approaches can be performed either unilaterally or bilaterally. The bone flap can be stored in various locations, the patients abdominal subcutaneous fat, cryopreservation and in situ using the hinge craniectomy method (Ko 2007). A standard trauma flap skin incision is made with the goal of exposing the following margins: anteriorly to the superior border of the orbital roof, avoiding entry into the frontal sinus, posteriorly to at least 2cm posterior to the external meatus, medially to a point 2cm lateral to the midline to avoid the sagittal sinus and inferiorly to the floor of the middle cranial fossa (Scmidek H 2006). The temporalis muscle is reflected anteriorly. Burrholes are placed at the keyhole, the root of the zygoma and as preferred along the planned craniotomy route. A high speed drill is used for the craniotomy. The lesser wing of the sphenoid is fractured and removed to the superior orbital fissure. The dural edges can be tacked up to the skull to minimize formation of epidural hematoma. Dura can be opened in several manners but typically is done in a stellate fashion. Dura closure is not mandatory at this point and can either be left open, with mild approximation of dural leaflets or replaced with dural substitute. The decompressive craniectomy alone without durotomy reduces the intracranial pressure by 15%. A duraplasty further reduces the intracranial pressure by an additional 55% (Scmidek H 2006). At our institution we rely more on the rapid closure technique as described by Guresir et al. This technique has been found to significantly shorten operation time without increased complication rates or additional complications (Guresir E 2011). There have been incidences of CSF leak attributed to open dural leaflets but this has not been our experience. In the setting of trauma, evacuation of hematoma or contusion can proceed as indicated by the nature of the injury.

The size of the craniectomy directly correlates with degree of expansion (Gaa M 1990; Yoo D 1999). Small craniectomies are associated with further infarction and hemorrhage at the sites of the craniectomy margin. Mortality rates have also been reported as elevated in small diameter craniectomies (Wagner S 2001). This is due to the venous congestion that occurs in the herniated brain tissue as it is restricted and compressed by the bony boundary of the skull defect. Brain parenchyma herniates through the bony defect which in essence is the desired effect but compression of parenchyma adjacent to the bony boundary in a small craniectomy leads to venous congestion, venous infarction and further damage to brain tissue. This is more common in craniectomies smaller than 8cm in diameter.

Doubling the diameter of a craniectomy from 6cm to 12cm increases the decompressed brain volume from 9ml to 86ml. A lower margin of craniectomy relative to the floor of the middle fossa has also been described with improved outcomes. This can be related to the state of decompression of the mesencephalic cisterns. Compression of the basal cisterns is known to impair clinical outcome, a larger craniectomy to the base of the brainstem could minimize brain stem compression (Toutant S 1984; Munch E 2000). The state of the mesencephalic cisterns correlates greatly with the distance of the craniectomy to the temporal cranial floor. As such decompression or out-fracturing of the temporal floor after removal of the bone flap remains exceedingly important. Compression of the cisterns impairs clinical outcome and a large craniectomy to the base of the cranium could minimize brain stem compression. A mortality rate of 77%, 39% and 22% as been described in those with absent, compressed and normal cisterns respectively. Patients presenting with a GCS of 7-8 who were expected to fair well did not recover as expected if the basal cisterns were compressed or absent in studies evaluated within the first 48hrs of admission(Toutant S 1984). As such recommendations for craniectomy size are typically in the range of 10x15cm with the lower margin extending to less than 1cm from the floor of the middle cranial fossa.

The frontal craniotomy is typically used in cases of frontal contusions or infarction. Bifrontal craniectomy is the most widely used. The surgical technique involves placing the patient supine. A bicoronal skin incision is planned posterior to the coronal suture. After incision the temporalis muscle is reflected inferiorly. Burr holes are made at the keyhole and at the root of the zygoma. Burr holes are also placed on either side of the sagittal sinus and along the planned craniectomy. Bilateral craniectomies are performed leaving a strip of bone covering the sagittal sinus.This strip of bone is then removed after freeing the sagittal sinus. A separate technique involves placing burrholes directly on the superior sagittal sinus and a burr hole at each key hole. The dura is then stripped from the bone, taking particular caution at the sinus. A bone flap is created connecting the keyhole burrholes with the most posterior burrhole at the sinus. Bilateral U shaped durotomies are created.

If the sinus is to be ligated and sacrificed, tributary veins are coagulated as they drain into the sinus. The sinus is then ligated at the most anterior margin as dictated by the craniotomy margin and posteriorly to a maximum of 1/3 of the length of the entire superior sagittal sinus. The ligated sinus can then be separated from the falx as it dives into the intercerebral hemisphere. Further consideration and care must be taken in settings of trauma with frontal skull fractures and frontal contusions. Bony structures may serve a tamponade effect on a lacerated sinus and may need to be left in place or anterior portions of the sinus may need to be sacrificed for adequate decompression. Bilateral dural openings are made into U-shaped flaps extending to the anterior portion of the sagittal sinus followed by ligation of the sinus. Some authors advocate preservation of the strip of bone overlying the sagittal sinus, others argue that sacrificing the anterior 1/3 of the sinus could lead to increased venous pressure and worsening cerebral edema (Polin 1997).

The removal of large areas of contused, infarcted or hemorrhagic theoretically further enhances the decompression. It also removes regions of disrupted blood brain barrier that could lead to further edema. Temporal lobectomy can be performed with removal of no more than 4-5cm of brain from the temporal tip on the dominant side and 6-7cm on the non-dominant side. Frontal lobectomy has also been described but neither has shown great therapeutic promise (Nussbaum E S 1991).

7. Recovery after hemicraniectomy

Decompressive hemicraniectomy, although life saving typically leaves survivors with severe disability. The alternative to this however being death. Most patients fail to ever re-attain functional independence. Patients typically have their bone flap replaced 6 weeks to 6 months after the initial injury to ensure resolution of the initial insult. Patients suffering from the post craniectomy syndrome may have their bone flap replaced sooner rather than latter.

Complications include but are not limited to intracerebral hematoma formation, extra-axial collections, cerebrospinal fluid leakage and cranioplasty failure. Post craniectomy hematoma formation primarily occurs due to inadequate surgical hemostasis or rupture of friable vessels as herniating brain tissue is compressed along the craniotomy margin. This is seen more often in small hemicraniectomies (Wagner S 2001).. The vast majority of these are clinically silent. Extra axial fluid accumulations occur as a result of CSF leakage through the dural leaflets or secondary to post traumatic extra axial hydrocephalus. Some patients may require a ventricular or sub-dural shunt.

CSF leak occurs in conjunction with open dura and inadequate closure of galea and skin. The incidence of this is in the range of 3% to 5% (Polin 1997; Wagner S 2001). Cranioplasty failure occurs as a result of bone flap resorption or infection. This occurs in 2% to 6% of cases. Poor graft fixation and approximation, excessive use of bone wax and a poorly vascularized or infected scalp can lead to this (Polin 1997). Patients with a compromised flap could subsequently require an acrylic bone flap. Postoperative seizure disorder are also reported in the range of 5% to 30%. The etiology of these remain unclear but can be attributed to the initial injury, resultant decompression, and a complicated hospital course.

8. Non-traumatic brain injury

In the setting of non-traumatic brain injury, the role of decompressive craniectomy remains unclear similar to traumatic brain injury. These include patients in categories including but not limited to subarachnoid hemorrhage secondary to ruptured aneurysm, intracerebral hemorrhage (ICH), and infectious processes. Kim et al (Ki-Tae Kim 2008) describe a series in which 75 patients underwent decompressive craniectomy and were analyzed retrospectively. In this group 28 patients were classified as traumatic brain injury, 24 as intracerebral hemorrhage and 23 with major infarction. Patients with a GCS score less than 8 and midline shift on head CT greater than 6mm were considered surgical candidates. Patients outcomes at 6 months revealed a mortality rate of 21.4% in TBI, 25% in ICH and 60.9% in major infarction.

Favorable outcomes defined by glasgow outcome score of 4-5 (moderate disability or better) were observed in 57.1% of patients with TBI, 50% with ICH and 30.4% with major infarction. They also describe changes in intracranial pressure that were further increased with dural opening regardless of the disease group. Although this study describes the decompressive craniectomy as being more effective in ICH and TBI patients, we would encourage the reader to bear in mind these findings relate to retrospective studies. As described earlier in the chapter there exists class I evidence supporting the use of decompressive craniectomy in major infarction or stroke patients provided certain parameters are met.

Hitchings and Delaney further describe a series of patients who underwent decompressive craniectomy for non trauma related conditions (Hitchings L 2010). They describe 54 patients who underwent 56 procedures. They noted that although intracranial pressure was reduced by the procedure. patients had long hospital stays and consumed a very significant amount of resources. Among survivors, two-thirds sustained a good outcome however most patients suffered residual deficits. They noted a mortality rate of 39%. These findings remain in concordance with the general concordance regarding decompressive craniectomies in that patients lives typically can be saved but functionality and quality of life suffer greatly.

9. Conclusion

Intracranial hypertension is a common sequelae of several illnesses and traumatic injury. Decompressive craniectomy provides an effective means of reducing and managing intracranial pressure. Lumbar drainage is also a useful adjunct in addition. Selection criteria remains in evolution primarily in the trauma setting but at the present time it appears the best outcomes are in young otherwise healthy patients. The decision to proceed with decompressive craniectomy should take into consideration several factors including family wishes and reasonable expectations of level of recovery.

10. References

Aarabi B, H. D., Ahn E, Aresco C, Scalea T, Eisenberg H (2006). "Outcome following decompressive craniectomy for malignant swelling due to severe head injury." *Journal of Neurosurgery* 104: 469-479.

Arenillas J, R. A., Molina C, et al (2002). "Prediction of early neurological deterioration using diffusion and perfusion weighted imaging in hyperacute middle cerebral artery stroke." *Stroke* 33: 2120-2197.

Bullock, R. C. R. M., Clifton G, et al (1995). Guidelines for the management of severe head injury. *The Brain Trauma Foundation*
The American Association of Neurological Surgeons
The Joint Section of Neurotrauma and Critical Care. New York,
Park Ridge, Illinois.

Burkert W, P. H. (1988). "Decompressive trephination in therapy refractory brain edema." *Zentralbl Neurochir* 50: 318-323.

Carter BS, O. C., Candia GJ, et al (1997). "One year outcome after decompressive surgery for massive nondominant hemisphere infarction." *Neurosurgery* 40: 1168-1176.

Chibbaro S, T. L. (2007). "Role of decompressive craniectomy in the management of severe head injury with refractory cerebral edema and intractable intracranial pressure, Our experience with 48 cases." *Surgical Neurology* 68: 632-638.

Cho D, C. T., Lee H (2003). "Ultra-early decompressive craniectomy for malignant middle cerebral artery infarction." *Surgical Neurology* 60: 227-232.

Cooper D, R. J., Murray L, Arabi Y, Davies A, D'Urso P, Kossman T, Ponsford J, Seppelt I, Reilly P, Wolfe R (2011). "Decompressive Craniectomy in Diffuse Traumatic Brain Injury." *The New England Journal of Medicine* 364: 1493-1502.

Cooper P, H. H., Clark W, et al (1979). "Enhancement of experimental cerebral edema after decompressive craniectomy: Implications for the management of severe head injuries." *Neurosurgery* 4: 296-300.

Eghwrudjakpor P, A. A. (2010). "Decompressive Craniectomy Following Brain Injury: Factors Important to Patient Outcome." *Libyan Journal of Medicine* 5(4620).

Forsting M, R. W., Schabitz W, et al (1995). "Decompressive Craniectomy for cerebral infarction: An experimental study in rats." *Stroke* 26: 259-264.

Gaa M, R. M., Lorenz M, et al (1990). "Traumatic brain swelling and operative decompression: A prospective investigation." *Acta Neurochirugica Supplementum* 51: 326-328.

Guresir E, V. H., Schuss P, Oszvald A, Raabe A, Seifert V, Beck J (2011). "Rapid closure technique in decompressive craniectomy." *Journal of Neurosurgery* 114: 954-960.

Hitchings L, D. A. (2010). "Decompressive Craniectomy for patients with severe non-traumatic brain injury: a retrospective cohort study." *Critical Care Resuscitation* 12: 16-23.

Hotmeijer J, K. L., Algra A, Amelink G, Van Gijn J, Van Der Worp H (2009). "Surgical decompression for space-occupying cerebral infarction (the Hemicraniectomy After Middle Cerebral Artery infarctin with Life-threatening Edema Trial [HAMLET]): a multicentre, open, randomised trial." *The Lancet* 8(4): 326-333.

Juttler E, S. S., Schiedek P, Unterberg A, Hennerici M, Woitzk J, Witte S, Ekkehart J, Hacke W (2007). "Decompressive Surgery for the Treatment of Malignant Infarction of the Middle Cerebral Artery (DESTINY)." *Stroke* 38: 2518-2525.

Ki-Tae Kim, J.-K. P., Seok-Gu Kang, Kyung-Suck Cho, Do-Sung Yoo, Dong-Kyu Jang, Pil-Woo Huh, Dal-Soo Kim (2008). "Comparison of the effect of decompressive craniecomty on different neurosurgical diseases." *Acta Neurochirurgica* 151(1): 21-30.

Ko, S. (2007). "In situ Hinge Craniectomy." *Neurosurgery* 60: 255-259.

Manno E, N. D., Fulgham J, et al (2003). "Computed tomographic determinants of neurologic deterioration in patients with large middle cerebral artery infarctions." *Mayo Clinic Proc* 78: 156-160.

Moody R, R. S., Mullan S (1968). "An evaluation of decompression in experimental head injury." *Journal of Neurosurgery* 29: 586-590.

Munch E, B. C., Horn P, Roth H, Schmiedek P, Vajkoczy P (2001). "Therapy of malignant intracranial hypertension by controlled lumbar cerebrospinal fluid drainage." *Critical Care Medicine* 29: 976-981.

Munch E, H. P., Schurer, L et al (2000). "Management of severe traumatic brain injry by decompressive craniectomy." *Neurosurgery* 47: 315-322.

Murad A, G. S., Colohan AR (2008). "Controlled lumbar drainage in medically refractory increased intracranial pressure. A safe and effective treatment " *Acta Neurochirurgica Supplementum* 102: 89-91.

Narayan R K, K. P. R. S., Becker D P, et al (1082). "Intracranial Pressure: To monitor or not to monitor?" *Journal of Neurosurgery* 56: 650-659.

Nussbaum E S, W. A. L., Sebring L, et al (1991). "Complete temporal lobectomy for surgical resucitation of patients with transtentorial herniation secondary to unilateral hemispheric swelling." *Neurosurgery* 29: 62-66.

Polin, R., Shaffrey M, Bogaev Ce, et al (1997). "Decompressive bifrontal craniectomy in the treatment of severe refractory posttraumatic cerebral edema." *Neurosurgery* 41: 84-92.

Schwab S, S. T., Aschoff A, et al (1998). "Early hemicraniectomy in patients with complete middle cerebral artery infarction." *Stroke* 29: 1888-1893.

Scmidek H, R. D., Ed. (2006). *Operative Neurosurgical Techniques Indications, Methods and Results*. Decompressive Craniectomy: Physiologic Rationale, Clinical Indications and Surgical Considerations. Philadelphia PA, Elsevier.

Stein S C, R. S. E. (1992). "Moderate head injury: A guide to initial management." *Journal of Neurosurgery* 77: 652-654.

Toutant S, K. M., Marshall L, et al (1984). "Absent of compressed basal cisterns on first CT scan: Ominous Predictors of outcome in severe head injury." *Journal of Neurosurgery* 61: 84-92.

Vahedi K, e. a. (2007). "Sequential-Design, Multicenter, Randomized, Controlled Trial of Early Decompressive Craniectomy in Malignant Middle Cerebral Artery Infarction (DECIMAL Trial)." *Stroke* 38: 2506-2517.

Vahedi K, H. J., Juettler E; et al (2007). "Early decompressive surgery in malignant infarction of the middle cerebral artery: A pooled analysis of three randomized controlled trials." *Lancet Neurology* 6: 215-222.

Wagner S, S. H., Aschoff A, et al (2001). "Suboptimum hemicraniectomy as a cause of additional cerebral lesions in patients with malignant infarction of the middle cerebral artery." *Journal of Neurosurgery* 94: 693-696.

Yoo D, K. D., Cho K et al (1999). "Ventricular pressure monitoring during bilateral decompression with dural expansion." *Journal of Neurosurgery* 91: 953-959.

9

The Role of Decompressive Craniectomy in the Management of Patients Suffering Severe Closed Head Injuries

Haralampos Gatos[1], Eftychia Z. Kapsalaki[2], Apostolos Komnos[3]
Konstantinos N. Paterakis[1] and Kostas N. Fountas[1]
[1]Departments of Neurosurgery, University Hospital of Larissa
School of Medicine, University of Thessaly, Larissa
[2]Diagnostic Radiology, University Hospital of Larissa
School of Medicine, University of Thessaly, Larissa
[3]Department of Intensive Care Unit, General Hospital of Larissa, Larissa
Greece

1. Introduction

Severe Traumatic Brain Injury (S-TBI) is the major cause of mortality, morbidity, and disability among people younger than 45 years old. It constitutes a major problem in developed countries, not only for the affected patients and their families but also for the society, with serious socio-economic ramifications. It cannot be overemphasized the society's burden from S-TBIs, which may exhaust even the most developed health care systems. During the last 30 years, advances in pre-hospital treatment, novel imaging modalities, intensive care monitoring improvements, rehabilitation advances, as well as better understanding of the S-TBI pathophysiology have decreased the overall mortality rate from 70-80% in 1970's to 30 % nowadays. Severe TBI is still associated with unfavorable outcome (death or severe disability) in up to 60%. Continuous efforts of the neurosurgical community focus not only on decreasing the S-TBI associated mortality, but also on improving the quality of life and the functional outcome of patients suffering S-TBIs [Danish, et al., 2009; Honeybul, et al., 2011].

It has been demonstrated by Marmarou and his colleagues [Marmarou et al., 1991] that increased intracranial pressure (ICP) is strongly associated with poor outcome in patients suffering S-TBIs, making thus intracranial hypertension the most frequent cause of death and disability. Moreover, it has been postulated that this association between increased ICP and poor outcome is linear. Frequently, the greatest challenge for a neurosurgeon treating a patient suffering a S-TBI is the management of increased ICP, which in a large number of cases overwhelms brain's ability to regulate cerebral blood flow (CBF), resulting thus to cerebral ischemia and consequently to severe disability and/or death. Elevated ICP is usually defined as an ICP above a threshold of 20 mmHg, measured within any intracranial space (subdural, intraventricular, extradural or intraparenchymal compartments). The cause of increased ICP in patients with S-TBIs is the result of an increase in brain parenchyma volume at the expense of one or more of the other two intracranial components (cerebral blood volume, cerebral spinal fluid). An increase in brain water content (edema), increased cerebral blood volume, and /or the presence of hematomas contribute significantly to increases of ICP in patients with S-TBI.

It has been proposed that the employment of DC may drastically lower the increased ICP by allowing expansion of the edematous cerebral hemispheres. Furthermore, it has been postulated that DC interrupts the vicious cycle of intracranial hypertension via the impairment of the cerebral perfusion pressure (CPP), which inevitably results into further ICP increasing and may eventually lead to cellular injury and death. In this chapter the historical evolution of the surgical technique of DC is presented along with a brief description of the various surgical types and techniques, which are currently utilized in clinical practice. Moreover, the current concepts and controversies, the ongoing clinical trials, and the procedure associated complications are presented and discussed.

2. Decompressive craniectomy: Historical landmarks

Decompressive craniectomy has been proposed for many years as a valid treatment option for severe medically refractory intracranial hypertension, caused by various pathological conditions such as, S-TBIs, extensive cerebral infraction, massive subarachnoid hemorrhage, large intraparenchymal hemorrhage, severe intracranial infections, and extensive venous sinus thrombosis.

Hippocrates was the first who clearly described the indications for trephination in severe head injuries. Indeed, trephination remained for centuries the major surgical intervention for managing patients with severe closed head injuries. The concept of decompression (removal of a variable amount of calvaria) was introduced in the late 1890 by Annandale. Kocher in 1901 proposed the opening of the skull for relieving increased intracranial pressure, while Harvey Cushing [Cushing, 1905] performed a subtemporal decompressive craniectomy for treating moribund edema caused by an intracranial neoplastic disorder.

The concept of large cranial and dural decompression along with the removal of any underlying masses was initially described by Miyazaki in 1966, while Kjellberr and Prieto refined this surgical technique in 1971. For decades, DC was known as an occasionally life saving procedure, associated however with numerous serious complications. Therefore, the vast majority of neurosurgeons were not very eager in incorporating DC in the trauma neurosurgical armamentarium. Characteristically, Clarke in 1968 stated that the only reason for reporting his experience from performing DCs in S-TBI patients was for warning other neurosurgeons to avoid performing similar surgery.

Decompressive craniectomy in its current form was recently re-introduced by Guerra and his coworkers [Guerra et al., 1999], who reported favorable outcome in more than 50% of their cases, undergoing DC after suffering S-TBIs. Since then, many non-randomized, usually retrospective, and small size clinical studies have suggested that DC may be a valuable treatment option, when maximal medical treatment has failed to control increased ICP. It has to be pointed out that the number of the published articles in the medical literature regarding the role of DC in the management of patients with S-TBI has been geometrically increased during the last decade (Fig. 1). However, the pertinent literature demonstrates a wide variation in clinical outcomes, and ill-defined indications for performing DC in patients with S-TBIs [Aarabi et al., 2006; Howard et al., 2008; Jagannathan, et al., 2007; Morgalla et al., 2008; Münch et al., 2000].

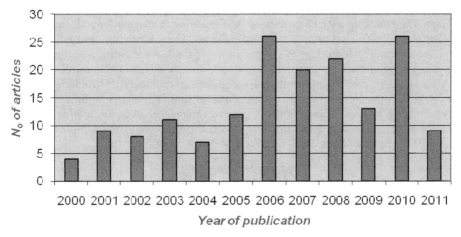

Fig. 1. Diagrammatic representation of the number of PubMed listed articles regarding the role of DC in S-TBI patients, during the decade 2000-2010.

2.1 Types of surgical decompression and surgical procedures

Historically, DC is defined as the removal of different parts and portions of the skull, with or without opening of the underlying dura, and augmentative duroplasty. A variety of operations have been proposed and different surgical techniques have been developed for brain decompression. These include: a) the classic and widely used fronto-temporo-parietal craniectomy (either unilateral or bilateral), b) the bifrontal (bicoronal) craniectomy, c) the subtemporal decompression or the recently modified temporal craniectomy, and d) the hinge (door-like) craniotomy.

The fronto-temporo-parietal craniectomy (hemicraniectomy), theoretically consists of extensive bone resection, exposing practically almost the whole underlying cerebral hemisphere. The patient is placed in supine position, with his/her head turned towards the opposite direction. An extended reverse questionmark skin incision is performed starting one cm in front of the tragus, extending above and behind the ipsilateral ear (approximately to the posterior mastoid line) and then curving forward one or two cm laterally from the midline, ending at or just behind the frontal hair line. Key points of the procedure are the extension of the decompression to the floor of the middle cranial fossa (all the way to the zygomatic arch with preservation of the superficial temporal artery and the branches of the facial nerve), (Fig. 2), and adequate size decompression with at least 12cm in its largest diameter (Fig. 3). Usually, the temporalis muscle is dissected in one plane (osteoplastic flap), by using monopolar cautery. According to another technique, the temporalis muscle may be mobilized separately, and its fascia may be dissected and harvested for the duraplasty. The pterion and the temporal bones have to be adequately exposed. Burr holes are placed to the pterion, temporal bone, posterior parietal and frontal regions, as close as possible to the scalp incision, taking advantage of the whole skin flap. Then, the underlying bulging dura is carefully stripped off the bone, in all the burr holes with the use of a fine dissector. The burr holes are connected by using a high-speed craniotome, and then the inferior rim of the temporal bone is carefully removed in pieces, by a large rongeur exposing thus the floor of the middle cranial fossa. At this point, the ipsilateral sphenoid wing can be drilled off, by using a diamond burr, if the patient's condition allows such a time-consuming maneuver. The bone flap may be preserved by implanting it in an abdominal subcutaneous pocket, or it can be freezed and appropriately stored. The underlying dura is incised and opened in a cruciate fashion (Fig. 4). Augmentative duraplasty is performed then by using either gallea aponeurotica, or temporal fascia, or commercially available dural substitutes. The importance of performing meticulous hemostasis cannot be overemphasized. The wound is closed in anatomical layers, avoiding any tension at the skin margins. The surgeon judges according to brain edema and ICP measurements, whether the temporal fascia is sutured back or just a few approximating sutures are placed to the temporalis muscle [Apuzzo, 1993; Huang & Wen, 2010; Valadka & Robertson, 2007].

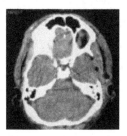

Fig. 2. Early postoperative CT scan showing adequate decompression of the middle cranial fossa in a patient undergoing decompressive craniectomy.

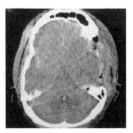

Fig. 3. Early postoperative CT scan demonstrating a large size decompressive craniectomy.

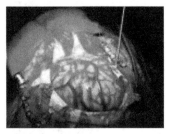

Fig. 4. Intraoperative picture showing cruciate opening of the dura. Please note the bulging, edematous brain, and the engorged cortical veins.

In bilateral hemicraniectomy, a bone ridge of approximately 3-4 cm in width is preserved over the superior sagittal sinus (SSS) (Fig 5). In bifrontal DC, a bicoronal skin flap is performed and bilateral frontal bones including the bone over the SSS are removed. A key point of this procedure is the careful elevation of the bone flap, which requires careful dissection of the underlying SSS.

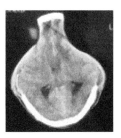

Fig. 5. Delayed CT scan of a patient undergoing bilateral hemicraniectomy. Please note the preservation of the bone over the superior sagittal sinus.

In the hinge craniotomy, the bone flap is repositioned in its place with the use of three titanium miniplates. A Y-shaped miniplate is placed just posterior to the coronal suture, a simple straight two-hole miniplate is placed at the sphenoid wing, and another miniplate at the posterior temporal region. It has to be emphasized, that only the Y-shaped miniplate is secured to the surrounding skull, while the other two miniplates are secured only at one side acting as buttress plates, preventing this way future bone flap settling, while allowing temporary expansion of the underlying edematous brain [Kenning, et al., 2009; Schmidt, et al., 2007].

In selected cases, DC can be combined with ipsilateral temporal lobectomy (anterior temporal lobectomy and uncusectomy), preventing thus the risk of transtentorial brain herniation. In this procedure the head of the patient should be turned 45⁰ towards the contralateral side, and a fronto-temporo-parietal craniectomy is performed. After the dural incision and under microscopic magnification, an anterior temporal lobectomy is performed, sparing the superior temporal gyrus. A sub-pial aspiration/resection technique is used for removing the anterior 4-5 cm of the inferior and middle temporal gyri, as well as the fusiform gyrus, the uncus, the parahippocampal gyrus, and potentially the mesial temporal structures [Chibbaro, et al., 2008].

A decompressive craniectomy may be performed either for preventing or for treating severe brain swelling. Prophylactic or primary DC is defined as the surgical decompression performed primarily for evacuation of an underlying mass of any type, whenever the surgeon decides that removal of the bone flap along with the overlying bone flap will benefit the patient. According to the Congress of Neurological Surgeons' guidelines, a prophylactic DC may be performed in: a) comatose patients with epidural hematoma, b) in patients with acute subdural hematoma with thickness greater than 10 mm, or midline shift greater than 5 mm, c) in patients with admitting GCS score <8 and traumatic parenchymal lesions greater than 50 cm^3 in volume, or greater than 20 cm^3 with midline shift of at least 5 mm and/or cisternal compression, and d) in patients with open (compound) depressed cranial fractures, greater in thickness than that of the adjacent cranium, or with underlying hematoma, dural penetration, pneumocephalus, infection, or frontal sinus involvement [Bullock, et al., 2006; Sahuquillo & Arikan, 2006]. Secondary DC or therapeutic decompression is defined as the surgical decompression performed in patients with massive unilateral or bilateral brain edema in order to control high ICP refractory to maximal medical therapy.

2.2 Current concepts and controversies

Decompressive craniectomy has recently become a valid, widely-performed treatment option for managing patients with medically refractory intracranial hypertension. The Brain Trauma Foundation (BTF) and the Brain Injury Consortium (BIC) consider DC as a second-tier therapy for medically intractable intracranial hypertension. The algorithm of treating increased ICP of traumatic origin is based on a set of therapeutic maneuvers and first-line measures as head elevation, maintenance of adequate oxygen tension, maintenance of normovolemia and normal osmosis, normothermia, appropriate sedation and analgesia, avoiding pyrexia and seizures, adequate CSF draining via an external ventriculostomy, mild to moderate hypocapnia, administration of mannitol and hypertonic solutions, and neuromuscular blockade. When these first-level measures fail, only a few therapeutic options are available. These second-tier therapies are the administration of high dose barbiturates, induction of hypothermia, and DC. The BIC state that DC may be considered in exceptional situations, while Bullock et al suggest that DC may be the procedure of choice in patients with post-traumatic edema, hemispheric swelling, or diffuse injury given the appropriate clinical context. This context however, remains to be defined [Brain Trauma Foundation [BTF], 2007; Bullock, et al., 2006; Maas, et al., 1997].

Numerous experimental models have demonstrated that DC reduces secondary brain injury. These effects are thought to be the result of an increase in collateral cerebral circulation, reduction in tissue edema, and improvement in oxygenation and energy metabolism [Stiver, 2009; Weiner et al., 2010]. Furthermore, postoperative radiological evaluation in cases of DC shows amelioration of midline shift, and improvement of the preoperative compression of the basal cisterns [Laalo, et al., 2009].

Despite the constantly increasing clinical employment of DC in the management of patients with S-TBIs, there are still several points of controversy, regarding its exact role in the treatment of these patients. The most important controversial points may be summarized to the following:

- Lack of clear indications and guidelines, regarding the selection of candidates for DC. Cochrane data base analysis in 2007 [Sahuquillo & Arikan, 2006] concluded that there was no evidence to support the routine use of secondary DC to reduce unfavorable outcome in adults suffering S-TBIs and refractory intracranial hypertension. Contrariwise, it seems that there is more solid evidence in pediatric trauma patients, in whom DC seems to reduce the risk of death and unfavorable outcome [Sahuquillo & Arikan, 2006].
- The exact role of ICP measurements and the ICP waveform type in selecting patients for DC. Many investigators suggest that a single episode of ICP> 20 mmHg lasting at least for 5 minutes is an indication for performing DC, while others suggest a higher ICP threshold of 25 to 30 mmHg.
- Patient's age. Most neurosurgeons are very reluctant to perform DC in patients over 60 years old. Indeed, outcome seems to be worse in elderly patients. However, this issue remains to be addressed.
- The presence of commorbitity. It appears that multi systemic trauma patients have worse outcome. The presence of cardiological and other systemic underlying pathology, as well as the preoperative use of anti-platelet or anticoagulant medication should be seriously assessed before deciding to perform a DC.
- Ideal timing for performing DC. The question of early versus late intervention remains still unanswered. It is apparent that surgical decompression needs to be performed

before irreversible brain stem compression and/or herniation occur [Ruf, et al., 2003; Timofeev, et al., 2008].

- Ideal size of decompression. It was previously mentioned that adequate decompression of the floor of the middle cranial fossa is essential for achieving optimal relaxation of the perimesencephalic cisterns. It has been also proven that small DCs and small dural openings may cause swollen brain tissue to herniate through the bony defect, causing strangulation, infarction and worsening of the brain swelling. The current trend is to perform large size DCs with a diameter larger than 12 cm. However, the issue of the appropriate size DC has to be addressed in a prospective, randomized study.
- The exact role of other parameters of neuromonitoring, such as brain tissue oxygen, markers of anaerobic metabolism (microdialysis), transcranial Doppler ultrasonography measurements, and electroencephalographic monitoring may provide further information, making the selection of ideal surgical candidate for DC more accurate [Bor-Seng-Shu, et al., 2006; Weiner, et al., 2010].
- The effect of DC in the functional outcome of patients with S-TBIs remains to be proven. Does the performance of DC provide better functional outcome? Several clinical studies have suggested that DC reduces ICP but the overall functional outcome remains essentially unchanged [Danish, et al., 2009; Howard, et al., 2008; Morgalla, et al., 2008].

During the last decade a systematic attempt was made to prospectively assess the role of DC in the management of patients suffering S-TBIs and/or presenting medically refractory intracranial hypertension [Ban, et al., 2010; Morgalla et al., 2008; Valadka & Robertson, 2007].Two independent, parallel, multi-centric, prospective clinical studies (the DECRA and the Rescue ICP trials) were designed and are underway for evaluating the exact role of DC in the management of patients with S-TBIs. These studies are supposed to address the issue of the efficacy of DC but also may clarify other DC-associated controversial points.

2.3 The DECRA clinical trial

The early DEcompressive CRAniectomy (DECRA) in patients with severe traumatic brain injury is a multi-centric, prospective, randomized trial, coordinated by The National Trauma Research Institute, the National Health and Medical Research Council of Australia, the Victorian Trauma Foundation, the ANZICS Foundation, and the Western Australian Institute for Medical Research. The primary objective of the trial is to determine whether early decompressive craniectomy compared to conventional management strategies in patients with severe diffuse traumatic brain injury and early refractory intracranial hypertension improves neurological outcomes, at six months post injury. The inclusion criteria are: severe diffuse traumatic brain injury defined as GCS<9 and CT-scan with evidence of brain swelling (Marshall score grade D2-4), or GCS score > 8 before intubation and Marshall score D3 or D4 on the obtained brain CT scan, age 15-60 years, ICP monitor insertion, decompression within 72 hours from the injury, and medically refractory ICP (defined as ICP> 20mmHg for more than 15 minutes continuously or cumulative during one hour) [Cooper, et al., 2008].

The exclusion criteria are: intracranial hemorrhage>3cm in diameter, intracranial mixed hemorrhagic contusion>5cm in long axis, previous craniectomy, presence of epi-dural and/or sub-dural hematoma > 0.5 cm in thickness, co-existent spinal cord injury, penetrating brain injury, arrest at the scene, unreactive pupils >4mm in diameter, GCS score =3, general contraindications for neurosurgical intervention, or no change of survival after careful consideration of the obtained brain CT and the patient's clinical examination.

The surgical technique used is the bifrontal decompressive craniectomy (as described by Polin and his coworkers) with a single fronto-temporal bone flap extending across the midline. The underlying dura could be opened either by making a bilateral cruciate incision or by employing a large L-shaped incision, with the lower corner of the L facing laterally. The dural openings are covered with dural or fascial patches [Polin, et al., 1997].

DECRA trial investigators presented their initial results in April 2011. They reported on 155 randomly assigned cases (73 patients underwent DC while 82 had standard care). According to their results the investigators concluded that in adults with severe diffuse traumatic brain injury and refractory intracranial hypertension, early bifronto-temporo-parietal decompressive craniectomy decreased intracranial pressure and the length of stay in the ICU. However, they found that patients undergoing craniectomy had worse scores on the Extended Glasgow Outcome Scale than those receiving standard care (odds ratio for a worse score in the craniectomy group: 1.84). Similarly, patients undergoing DC demonstrated a greater risk of an unfavorable outcome (odds ratio: 2.21). The observed death rates at six months were similar in the craniectomy group (19%) and the standard-care group (18%) [Cooper, et al., 2011].

It has to be emphasized however, that the DECRA study carries significant weaknesses and biases. It is of great interest that out of 3700 patients, who were potential candidates for participating in this study, only 155 were finally recruited. This may be a significant selection bias. In addition, the small number of study participants significantly decreases the statistical strength of the DECRA study. Furthermore, the utilized ICP threshold of 20 mmHg for assigning patients for DC may be considered too low for patients with S-TBIs.

2.4 The rescue ICP trial
The Randomized Evaluation of Surgery with Craniectomy for Uncontrollable Elevation of Intra-Cranial Pressure, is a multi-centric 48 (centers from 19 different countries) clinical study, organized as a collaborative research project between the university of Cambridge (Departments of Neurosurgery and Neurointensive Care), and the European Brain Injury Consortium. It is a randomized controlled trial comparing the efficacy of DC versus optimal medical management for the treatment of refractory intracranial hypertension following brain trauma. The inclusion criteria are: patients with S-TBI, age 10-65 y.o, with an abnormal CT-scan requiring ICP monitoring, and raised ICP > 25 mmHg for > 1 hour to 12 hours. Patients may have immediate operation for a mass lesion but not a decompressive craniectomy. Patients with immunological, hepatic, or renal compromise may be included in this study as long as there is a description of the type and the extent of their impairment. Contrariwise, patients with bilateral fixed and dilated pupils, bleeding diathesis, a devastating injury, inability to follow them, inability to monitor ICP, primary decompression, brainstem injury, or patients that were treated according to the Lund protocol, or have received barbiturates before their randomization, should be excluded from the study. The surgical treatment comprises of a large unilateral fronto-temporo-parietal craniectomy for unilateral brain edema or of large bilateral fronto-temporo-parietal craniectomies for diffuse bilateral hemisphere swelling. The craniectomy extends from the frontal sinus anteriorly to the coronal suture posteriorly, and to the pterion laterally. It is accompanied by a large dural opening (dural flap pedicles are based on the superior sagittal sinus medially, and also a division of the falx anteriorly is required).

The primary endpoint of the Rescue-ICP study will be the outcome assessment at discharge (GOS score), and then at six months after injury (Extended GOS score), while secondary endpoints will be: a) the assessment of outcome using the SF-36 and the SF-10 questionnaires, b) assessment of ICP control, c) length of stay in the ICU, d) hospital length of stay, and e) a detailed health-economic analysis of the collected data [Hutchinson, et al., 2006]. The results of the Rescue-ICP study are expected with great interest, and may greatly influence the future of DC and the overall management of patients suffering S-TBIs.

3. Decompressive craniectomy complications

Decompressive craniectomy has been associated with high mortality rates, mainly due to the severity of the underlying trauma, and also with numerous, and occasionally severe complications. Several factors have been identified as predisposing to the development of DC-associated complications. These include low GCS score upon admission, patient's old age, the presence of commorbidity, and the systematic preoperative anti-coagulant administration. Yang et al [Yang, et al., 2008] reported that the frequency of DC associated complications was 62% for admitting GCS scores 3-5, 39% for GCS scores 6-9, and 36 % for GCS scores >9. In addition, older patients (> 60 y.o) tend to have higher complications rates and prolonged ICU stay. Likewise, preoperative administration of anti-coagulant or antiplatelet medication increases the risk of intraoperative and/or postoperative bleeding.

The alterations in cerebral compliance, CBF autoregulation, and altered CSF dynamics associated with S-TBIs, are the main reason for developing DC-associated complications. Several theories suggesting that the sudden change from prolonged severe compression to a state of maximal vasolidation and hyperemia following DC may cause loss of autoregulation, and may be responsible for the occurrence of DC associated complications [Aarabi, et al., 2009; Yang, et al., 2008]. The most commonly occurred complications may be divided to:

1. Perioperative complications

a. Blossoming of pre-existing cerebral contusions. Expansion of pre-existing hemorrhagic contusions, as demonstrated on serial CT scans, has been reported as frequently as 40% of the cases, and may be considered inherent to the injury evolving process.
b. Evolution and expansion of contralateral masses. The decompression provided by DC allows the expansion of contralateral masses (hematomas), which that were preoperatively tamponated by the swollen brain.
c. External cerebral herniation. Expansion of the edematous brain through the bony defect may occur, especially during the first two postoperative weeks. The compression of the cortical veins of the herniated cerebral tissue leads to infarction, and unfortunately to further swelling. In small size decompressions, a mushroom-like herniation of the swollen parenchyma may occur. Therefore, most surgeons propose large craniectomies and wide dural openings for protecting the underlying cortical veins and for minimizing the risk of external cerebral herniation.

2. Early postoperative complications.

a. Subdural effusions and hygromas are very often developed in cases of DC (Fig 6). Aarabi and his coworkers [Aarabi, et al., 2009] have reported subdural effusions and hygromas in 50% of their cases. Alteration of CSF circulation after a DC may incite the development of hygromas, which may progressively expand in volume. However, the hygromas very rarely demand surgical evacuation, and they usually resolve spontaneously.

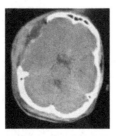

Fig. 6. Postoperative CT scan demonstrating the development of a subdural hygroma.

b. Impaired wound healing and infection may complicate a DC, and prolong patient's hospitalization. The performance of an extensive DC may compromise the skin flap blood supply (especially in the occipital area), and thus may increase the possibility of postoperative wound healing problems. Therefore, it is of paramount importance to maintain adequate skin flap blood supply by preserving the superficial temporal artery, and by avoiding tight skin suturing during closure. The observed high infection rate in patients undergoing DC may also be partially explained by the fact that the vast majority of these patients require prolonged ICU treatment and multiple interventions.

c. Post-DC hydrocephalus incidence has been reported to be as high as 15 %, and is associated with poorer clinical outcome (Fig 7). The treatment of hydrocephalus with CSF shunting remains controversial, and the timing of intervention before or after cranioplasty is still disputable.

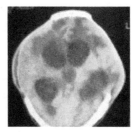

Fig. 7. Delayed postoperative CT scan demonstrating severe ventriculomegaly in a patient undergoing bilateral hemicraniectomy.

d. The syndrome of the trephined is a frequent delayed complication and its diagnosis is often overlooked. Occasionally it may be presented with delayed onset of focal neurological deficits.

e. Paradoxical herniation with brain stem compression and neurological deterioration is a very rare complication and may be precipitated by a lumbar puncture in a craniectomized patient.

3.1 Cranioplasty

One of the drawbacks of DC is the fact that a second surgical intervention is required to repair the bone defect. Autologous bone grafts may be used, which are preserved subcutaneously, or stored freezed under specific conditions in storage bone-banks. Tailor-made heterologous or synthetic bone grafts may also be used. The previous belief ofdelayed cranioplasty for minimizing the risk of infection, is seriously questioned nowadays, and an increasing number of surgeons prefer early surgical skull reconstruction. Several surgeons support the idea of immediate cranioplasty even during the initial hospitalisation, as early as 2-4 weeks after trauma, when there is no suspicion of infection. The possibility of a new head injury with the exposed brain unprotected must be taken into consideration. Moreover, the observation of better functional outcome after cranioplasty, may further increase the number of early cranioplasty cases [Beauchamp, et al., 2010; Morina, et al., 2011].

4. Conclusions

The management of refractory post-traumatic intracranial hypertension remains a challenge for neurosurgeons, anesthesiologists, and neuro-intensivists. Cerebral ischemia leading to severe disability or death is unfortunately the only result expected. In order to deal with this dramatic situation only few treatment options exist. The ultimate measure to relieve uncontrollable ICP is an extensive decompressive craniectomy. It is proven that DC increases the volumetric compensatory capacity and reduces ICP. However, the well-documented risks and drastically complications of DC have to be seriously considered before performing a DC. In carefully selected cases these risks may be outweighted by the expected benefit. The results of the two ongoing prospective, randomized, controlled trials are expected to enlighten us on the exact role of DC in the management of patients with S-TBIs, and its effect on their long-term functional outcome.

5. References

Aarabi, B., Hesdorffer, DC., Ahn, ES., Aresco, C., Scalea, TM., & Eisenberg, HM. (2006). Outcome following decompressive craniectomy for malignant swelling due to severe head injury. *J Neurosurg* Vol.104, No.4, (April 2006), pp. 469-79, ISSN 0022-3085

Aarabi, B., Chesler, D., Maulucci, C., Blacklock, T., & Alexander, M. (2009). Dynamics of subdural hygroma following decompressive craniectomy: a comparative study. *Neurosurg Focus* Vol.26, No.6, (June 2009), pp.E8, ISSN 1092-0684

Apuzzo, MLJ. (1993). Complication Avoidance and Management, In: *Brain Surgery,* Volume 2, part 4, pp.1283-1296, Churchill Livingstone Inc., ISBN 0-443-08709-1, New York

Ban, SP., Son, YJ., Yang, HJ., Chung, YS., Lee, SH., & Han, DH. (2010). Analysis of complications following decompressive craniectomy for traumatic brain injury. *J Korean Neurosurg Soc* Vol.48, No.3, (September 2010), pp.244-50, ISSN 1225-8245

Beauchamp, KM., Kashuk, J., Moore, EE., Bolles, G., Rabb, C., Seinfeld, J., Szentirmai, O., & Sauaia, A. (2010). Cranioplasty after post injury decompressive craniectomy: is timing of the essence? *J Trauma* Vol. 69, No.2, (August 2010), pp.270-4, ISSN 0022-5282

Bor-Seng-Shu, E., Hirsch, R., Teixeira, MJ., De Andrade, AF., & Marino, R Jr. (2006). Cerebral hemodynamic changes gauged by transcranial Doppler ultrasonography in patients with posttraumatic brain swelling treated by surgical decompression. *J Neurosurg* Vol.104, No.1, (January 2006), pp.93-100, ISSN 0022-3085

Brain Trauma Foundation BTF. (2007). Guidelines for the management of severe traumatic brain injury, 3rd edition. *J Neurotrauma* Vol. 24, No. 1, (2007), ISSN 0897-7151

Bullock, MR., Chesnut, R., Ghajar, J., Gordon, D., Hartl, R., Newell, DW., Servadei, F., Walters, BC., & Wilberger, JE. (2006). Guidelines for the Surgical Management of

Traumatic Brain Injury. *Neurosurgery* Vol. 58, No. 3, (March 2006), pp. S2-vi, ISSN 0148-396X

Chibbaro, S., Marsella, M., Romano, A., Ippolito, S., & Benericetti, E. (2008). Combined internal uncusectomy and decompressive craniectomy for the treatment of severe closed head injury: experience with 80 cases. *J Neurosurg* Vol.108, No.1, (January 2008), pp. 74-9, ISSN 0022-3085

Cooper, DJ., Rosenfeld, JV., Murray, L., Wolfe, R., Ponsford, J., Davies, A., D'Urso, P., Pellegrino, V., Malham, G., & Kossmann, T. (2008). Early decompressive craniectomy for patients with severe traumatic brain injury and refractory intracranial hypertension--a pilot randomized trial. *J Crit Care* Vol.23, No.3, (September 2008), pp. 387-93, ISSN 1541-6933

Cooper, DJ., Rosenfeld, JV., Murray, L., Arabi, YM., Davies, AR., D'Urso, P., Kossmann, T., Ponsford, J., Seppelt, I., Reilly, P., & Wolfe, R.; DECRA Trial Investigators; Australian and New Zealand Intensive Care Society Clinical Trials Group. (2011). Decompressive craniectomy in diffuse traumatic brain injury. *N Engl J Med* Vol.364, No.16, (2011 April 21), pp.1493-502, ISSN 0028-4793

Guerra, WK., Gaab, MR., Dietz, H., Mueller, JU., Piek, J., & Fritsch, MJ. (1999). Surgical decompression for traumatic brain swelling: indications and results. *J Neurosurg* Vol.90, No.2, (February 1999), pp.187-96, ISSN 0022-3085

Cushing H. (1905). The establishment of cerebral hernia as a decompressive measure for inaccessible brain tumors; with the description of intramuscular methods of making the bone defect in temporal and occipital regions. *Surg Gynecol Obstet* Vol.1, pp.297–314, ISSN 0039-6087

Danish, SF., Barone, D., Lega, BC., & Stein, SC. (2009). Quality of life after hemicraniectomy for traumatic brain injury in adults. A review of the literature. *Neurosurg Focus* Vol.26, No.6, (June 2009), pp.E2, ISSN 1092-0684

Honeybul, S., Ho, KM., Lind, CR., & Gillett, GR. (2011). Surgical intervention for severe head injury: ethical considerations when performing life-saving but non-restorative surgery. *Acta Neurochir (Wien)* Vol. 153, No.5, (May 2011), pp. 1105-10, ISSN 0001-6268

Howard, JL., Cipolle, MD., Anderson, M., Sabella, V., Shollenberger, D., Li, PM., & Pasquale, MD. (2008). Outcome after decompressive craniectomy for the treatment of severe traumatic brain injury. J *Trauma* Vol.65, No.2, (August 2008), pp.380-6, ISSN 0022-5282

Huang, X., & Wen, L. (2010). Technical considerations in decompressive craniectomy in the treatment of traumatic brain injury. *Int J Med Sci* Vol.7, No.6, (November 8), pp. 385-90, ISSN 1449-1907

Hutchinson, PJ., Menon, DK., & Kirkpatrick, PJ. (2005). Decompressive craniectomy in traumatic brain injury--time for randomised trials? *Acta Neurochir (Wien)* Vol.147, No.1, (January 2005), pp. 1-3, ISSN 0001-6268

Hutchinson, PJ., Corteen, E., Czosnyka, M., Mendelow, AD., Menon, DK., Mitchell, P., Murray, G., Pickard, JD., Rickels, E., Sahuquillo, J., Servadei, F., Teasdale, GM., Timofeev, I., Unterberg, A., & Kirkpatrick, PJ. (2006). Decompressive craniectomy in traumatic brain injury: the randomized multicenter RESCUE icp study (www.RESCUEicp.com). *Acta Neurochir Suppl* Vol.96, pp.17-20, ISSN 0001-6268

Jagannathan, J., Okonkwo, DO., Dumont, AS., Ahmed, H., Bahari, A., Prevedello, DM., Jane, JA Sr., & Jane, JA Jr. (2007). Outcome following decompressive craniectomy in children with severe traumatic brain injury: a 10-year single-center experience with long-term follow up. *J Neurosurg* Vol.106, No.4, (April 2007), pp.268-75, ISSN 0022-3085

Kenning, TJ., Gandhi, RH., & German, JW. (2009). A comparison of hinge craniotomy and decompressive craniectomy for the treatment of malignant intracranial hypertension: early clinical and radiographic analysis. *Neurosurg Focus* Vol.26, No.6, (June 2009),pp. E6, ISSN 1092-0684

Laalo, JP., Kurki, TJ., Sonninen, PH., & Tenovuo, OS. (2009). Reliability of diagnosis of traumatic brain injury by computed tomography in the acute phase. *J Neurotrauma* Vol. 26, No.12, (December 2009), pp. 2169-78, ISSN 1557-9042

Maas, AI., Dearden, M., Teasdale, GM., Braakman, R., Cohadon, F., Iannotti, F., Karimi, A., Lapierre, F., Murray, G., Ohman, J., Persson, L., Servadei, F., Stocchetti, N., & Unterberg, A. (1997). EBIC-guidelines for management of severe head injury in adults. European Brain Injury Consortium. *Acta Neurochir (Wien)* Vol.139, No.4, pp. 286-94, ISSN 0001-6268

Marmarou, A., Anderson, RL., Ward, JD., Choi, SC., Young, HF., Eisenberg, HM., Foulkes, MA., Marshall, LF., & Jane, JA. (1991). Impact of ICP instability and hypotension on outcome in patients with severe head trauma. *J Neurosurg Vol.* 75, (November 1991),pp. S59-66, ISSN 0022-3085

Morgalla, MH., Will, BE., Roser, F., & Tatagiba, M. (2008). Do long-term results justify decompressive craniectomy after severe traumatic brain injury? *J Neurosurg* Vol.109, No.4, (October 2008), pp.685-90, ISSN 0022-3085

Morina, A., Kelmendi, F., Morina, Q., Dragusha, S., Ahmeti, F., Morina, D., & Gashi, K. (2011). Cranioplasty with subcutaneously preserved autologous bone grafts in abdominal wall-Experience with 75 cases in a post-war country Kosova. *Surg Neurol Int* Vol.2, (May 28), pp. 72. ISSN 2152-7806

Münch, E. Horn, P., Schürer, L., Piepgras, A., Paul, T.,& Schmiedek, P. (2000). Management of Severe Traumatic Brain Injury by Decompressive Craniectomy. *Neurosurgery Vol.* 47, No. 2, (August 2000), pp. 315-323, ISSN 0148-396X

Polin, RS., Shaffrey, ME., Bogaev, CA., Tisdale, N., Germanson, T,. Bocchicchio, B, & Jane, JA. Decompressive bifrontal craniectomy in the treatment of severe refractory posttraumatic cerebral edema. (1997). *Neurosurgery* Vol.41, No.1, (July 1997), pp.84-92, ISSN 0148-396X

Ruf, B., Heckmann, M., Schroth, I., Hügens-Penzel, M., Reiss, I., Borkhardt, A., Gortner, L., & Jödicke, A. (2003). Early decompressive craniectomy and duraplasty for refractory intracranial hypertension in children: results of a pilot study. *Crit Care* Vol. 7, No.6, (December 2003), pp. R133-8, ISSN 1364-8535

Sahuquillo, J., & Arikan, F. (2006). Decompressive craniectomy for the treatment of refractory high intracranial pressure in traumatic brain injury. *Cochrane Database Syst Rev* Vol, 25, No.1, pp.CD003983

Schmidt JH, 3rd., Reyes, BJ., Fischer, R., & Flaherty, SK. (2007). Use of hinge craniotomy for cerebral decompression. Technical note. *J Neurosurg* Vol.107, No.3, (September 2007), pp.678-82, ISSN0022-3085

Stiver, SI. (2009). Complications of decompressive craniectomy for traumatic brain injury. *Neurosurg Focus* Vol.26, No.6, (June 2009), pp. E7, ISSN 1092-0684

Timofeev, I., Czosnyka, M., Nortje, J., Smielewski, P., Kirkpatrick, P., Gupta, A., & Hutchinson, P. (2008). Effect of decompressive craniectomy on intracranial pressure and cerebrospinal compensation following traumatic brain injury. *J Neurosurg* Vol.108, No.1, (January 2008), pp.66-73, ISSN 0022-3085

Valadka, AB., & Robertson, CS. (2007). Surgery of cerebral trauma and associated critical care. *Neurosurgery* Vol.61, No.1, (July 2007), pp.203-20, ISSN 1220-8841

Weiner, GM., Lacey, MR., Mackenzie, L., Shah, DP., Frangos, SG., Grady, MS., Kofke, A., Levine, J., Schuster, J., & Le Roux, PD. (2010). Decompressive craniectomy for elevated intracranial pressure and its effect on the cumulative ischemic burden and therapeutic intensity levels after severe traumatic brain injury. *Neurosurgery* Vol. 66,No.6, (June 2010), pp. 1111-8, ISSN 0148-396X

Yang, XF., Wen, L., Shen, F., Li, G., Lou, R., Liu, WG., & Zhan, RY. (2008). Surgical complications secondary to decompressive craniectomy in patients with a head injury: a series of 108 consecutive cases. *Acta Neurochir (Wien)* Vol.150, No.12, (December 2008), pp, 1241-7, ISSN 0001-6268

10

Novel Strategies for Discovery, Validation and FDA Approval of Biomarkers for Acute and Chronic Brain Injury

S. Mondello, F. H. Kobeissy, A. Jeromin, J. D. Guingab-Cagmat,
Z. Zhiqun, J. Streeter, R. L. Hayes and K. K. Wang
University of Florida and Banyan Biomarkers, Inc.
USA

1. Introduction

The proposed chapter outlines novel approaches that provide an infrastructure for discovery and validation of new biomarkers of acute brain injury. Approaches to validation can be also applied to existing biomarkers of brain injury in order to provide more rigorous assessment of their clinical utility. Importantly, there are currently no biomarkers of brain injury approved by Food and Drug Administration (FDA). The chapter reviews approaches critical for securing FDA approval of biomarkers of brain injury and disease, focusing on traumatic brain injury (TBI).

The chapter reviews proteomics techniques applied for the first time to discovery of biomarkers of central nervous system (CNS). These techniques include refined mass spectrometry technology and high throughput immunoblot techniques. Output from these approaches can identify potential candidate biomarkers employing systems biology and data mining methods that will also be described.

Once potential biomarkers have been identified, it is important to provide information on their clinical utility for diagnosis, management and prognosis of patients exposed to brain injuries. This section of the chapter will review both preclinical and clinical methods for biomarker validation. Preclinical models discussed include rodent models of closed head injury such as the controlled cortical impact (CCI) device. Consideration will also be given to the design and results from human clinical trials validating biomarkers of mild, moderate and severe traumatic brain injury (TBI). Human studies will include detailed analyses of the biokinetics of different biomarkers in order to understand their utility in acute, subacute and chronic phases of TBI. Consideration will also be given to relationships between levels of biomarkers and magnitude of acute injury, CT imaging profiles, occurrence of secondary insults and long term outcome.

To achieve practical clinical utility, it is important to develop highly sensitive and specific assays for individual biomarkers. Enzyme-linked immunosorbent assays (ELISAs) are the current choice for clinical use, since this assay technology provides reliable, quantitative and accurate data. ELISA technologies relevant to biomarker measurement will be discussed. Once ELISA assays for individual biomarkers have been developed, these assays need to be transferred to devices that are appropriate for the clinical application and medical environment in which biomarker analyses will be conducted. We will review devices for use in clinical laboratories, emergency rooms (ERs), intensive care units (ICUs) and austere medical environment. In addition, this section will include review developing technologies allowing concurrent assessment of multiple biomarkers (multiplex).

To date, studies of biomarkers for brain injury have been restricted to research applications only. Although there is broad recognition of clinical utility of biomarkers, the FDA has yet to approve any biomarkers of CNS injury of disease. This section of the chapter provides a detailed outline of the regulatory consideration necessary for a biomarker to file for approval by FDA. Importantly, many of these considerations need to be integrated into relatively early stages of biomarker validation, assay development and device selection.

2. Biomarker discovery: Methods and results

2.1 Proteomics/systems biology in the area of neurotrauma

The application of neuroproteomics/neurogenomics has revolutionized the characterization of protein/gene dynamics, leading to a greater understanding of post-injury biochemistry. Neuroproteomics and neurogenomics fields have undertaken major advances in the area of neurotrauma research focusing on biomarker identification. Several candidate markers have been identified and are being evaluated for their efficacy as biological biomarkers utilizing these "omics approaches". The identification of these differentially expressed candidate markers using these techniques is proving to be only the first step in the biomarker development process. However, to translate these findings into the clinic, data-driven development cycle incorporating data-mining steps for discovery, qualification, verification, and clinical validation is needed. Data mining steps extend beyond the collected data level into an integrated scheme of animal modeling, instrumentation, and functional data analysis.

Proteomics is the identification and quantification of all expressed proteins of a cell type, tissue or organism. The advancement in the field of proteomics has coincided with the completion of the human genome sequencing project (Fenn et al. 1989, Tanaka 1988, Karas & Hillenkamp 1988). In recent years, the term proteomics is often mentioned together with biomarker discovery, as proteomic studies have the capability of identifying sensitive and unique signature protein biomarkers from tissues or biofluids derived from animal models or human clinical samples inflicted with various diseases. Neuroproteomics and neurogenomics, the application of proteomics and genomics in the field of neuronal injury, have been identified as a potential means for biomarker discovery, with the ability to identify proteome dynamics in response to brain injury (Guingab-Cagmat 2009, Haskins et al. 2005, Davidsson & Sjogren 2005, Shin et al. 2002, Celis et al. 2004).

In the area of brain injury, several studies have demonstrated the role of proteomics (Denslow et al. 2003, Katano et al. 2006) and genomics (Redell et al. 2009, Ding et al. 2006) in providing significant insight into understanding changes, modifications and functions in certain proteins post TBI. In addition, genomics and proteomics are powerful, complementary tools that play an important role in the area of biomarker identification. Over the past few years, advances in the fields of neuroproteomics and neurogenomics have led to the discovery of many candidate biomarkers and are becoming the primary methods for initial candidate marker selection (Kobeissy et al. 2008, Wang et al. 2006, Ottens et al. 2007, Nogoy 2007, Ottens et al. 2006). The identification of differentially expressed candidate markers using these techniques is proving to be only the first step in the biomarker development process. However, to translate these into the clinic, these novel assays require a data-driven development cycle that incorporates data-mining steps for discovery, qualification, verification, and clinical validation (Rifai et al. 2006).

TBI neuroproteomics studies have utilized biofluids such as blood/serum in addition to injured tissue to identify clinical markers that may correlate with injury severity. One of the studies by Burgess et al, evaluated altered differential proteins in normal human post mortem cerebrospinal fluid (CSF) (Burgess et al. 2006). The rationale of using post-mortem CSF is that it resembles a model of massive brain injury and cell death which post-mortem, thus comparing protein profile of post-mortem CSF with brain injury CSF would be ideal for identifying protein markers of injury. Of the 229 proteins identified, a total of 172 were novel and not previously described. The findings showed that the use of post mortem CSF (non-TBI samples) to evaluate altered protein levels mimicked the changes occurring in the brain following a traumatic insult. Furthermore, the identification of differential proteins of intracellular origin in the CSF corroborates the suggestion that there is protein leakage into the CSF following brain injury (Dumont et al. 2004, Hammack et al. 2004). This is a key step in identifying protein markers since, neuronal specific proteins leak from injured brain directly to the CSF.

In one of the TBI studies conducted in our laboratory, 1D-differential gel electrophoresis (DIGE) protein separation in series with mass spectrometry analysis was used to discover putative TBI biomarkers in brain tissues from a rat model (Haskins et al. 2005). These included 57 downregulated and 74 upregulated proteins; however data were not so informative due to limited separation capability. In an advanced study, we utilized a multidimensional separation platform called (CAX-PAGE/RPLC-MSMS) which consisted of different levels of separation including ion chromatography, 1-D gel electrophoresis and mass spectrometry as a novel approach for identifying biomarkers and protein breakdown products (degradomes); for detailed reviews, refer to (Svetlov et al. 2006, Kobeissy et al. 2006). As an application, the CAX/neuroproteomic analysis was employed on cortical samples of rat subjected to controlled cortical impact (CCI) model of experimental TBI (48 hrs post injury). Of interest, our neuroproteomic analysis identified 59 differential protein components of which 21 decreased and 38 increased in levels after TBI. One main advantage of this technique is its ability to elucidate degradomic substrates of different protease systems; thus our data identified the elevated levels of the breakdown products of several proteins (Kobeissy et al. 2006). Several of these are now being investigated as potential biomarkers specific for TBI to assess severity and recovery by evaluating their levels at different time points post TBI.

2.1.1 Data mining coupled neurosystems biology analysis in brain Injury

Coupled to data-mining steps, systems biology (SB) represents a mathematical model capable of predicting the altered processes or functions of a complex system under normal and perturbed conditions. It combines experimental, basic science data sets, proteomic and genetic data sets, literature and text mining, integration with computational modeling, bioinformatics and pathway/interaction mapping methods. When constructed properly, SB databases can provided a context or framework for understanding biological responses within physiological networks at the organism level, rather than in isolation (Chen et al. 2007).

In this regard, "omics" output constitutes one key component of neurosystems biology. It discusses the global changes involved in neurological perturbations integrating the final outcomes into a global functional network map which incorporates potential biomarkers identified (Grant 2003, Grant & Blackstock 2001). In the area of brain injury, neurosystems biology platform harnesses data sets that, by themselves, would be overwhelming, into an organized, interlinked database that can be queried to identify non-redundant brain injury pathways or convert hot spots. These can be exploited to determine their utilities as diagnostic biomarkers and/or therapeutic targets. The ultimate goals of system biology are: first by exploring the systems component (gene, protein, small molecule, metabolite etc.), help biologist, pharmaceutical companies and doctors to better understand the mechanisms underlying the disease components. Thus, it allows for suitable targets for treatment. Secondly, the systems biology approach enables one to be able to predict the functions and behavior of various components of the system upon varying any on the interconnected component since the whole system will be viewed globally rather than on micro, individual component level (Beltrao et al. 2007).

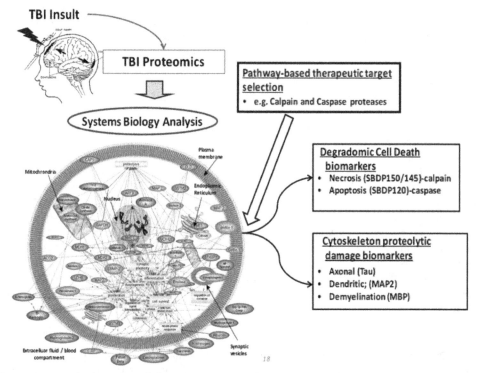

Fig. 1. Systems biology–based therapeutic target identification and target-specific biomarker selection.

In the field of neurotrauma, identifying and analyzing brain injury-related networks plays important and practical clues relating to biological pathways relevant to disease processes. However, the more important underlying goal in this analysis is to provide important clues that may suggest radically new approaches to therapeutics. Systems modeling and simulation is now considered fundamental to the future development of effective therapies. In the brain injury for example, it has been shown that calpain and caspase proteases are major components in cell death pathways taking part in two destructive proteolytic pathways that not only contribute to key forms of cell death (necrosis and apoptosis), but also in the destruction of important structural components of the axons (alphaII-spectrin breakdown products (SBDPs) and tau), dendrites (MAP2) and myelin (MBP) (Figure. 1). Interestingly, two different forms of SBDPs reflect either neuronal necrosis (SBDP150 and SBDP145 cleaved by calpain) or neuronal apoptosis (SBDP120 cleaved by caspase-3) (Wang et al. 2005). These SBDPs and other similar neural protein breakdown products can serve as target pathway specific biomarkers as illustrated in Figure 1.

Calpain and caspase proteases are used here as examples of therapeutic targets with proteolytic brain biomarkers representing non-redundant pathways relevant to the pathobiology of these therapeutic targets and the disease itself. TBI (traumatic brain injury); MAP2 (microtubule-associated protein 2); MBP (myelin basic protein); SBDP (spectrin breakdown product).

3. Biomarker validation: Methods and results

Traumatic injury to the brain results in a cellular activation and disintegration, leading to release of cell-type–specific proteins. Measurable amounts of these damage markers are present in cerebrospinal fluid (CSF) and blood. These markers not only indicate the pathoanatomic injury type and the severity of injury but also might provide specific

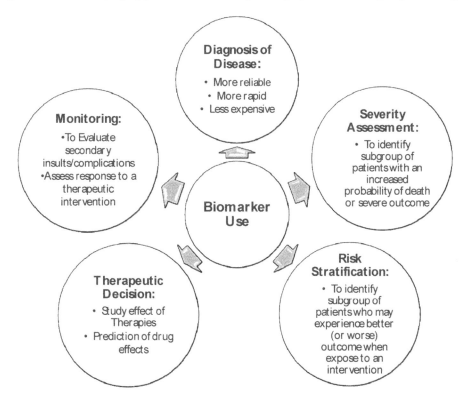

Fig. 2. Potential use of biomarkers in TBI

information about the pathophysiologic mechanisms which can be targeted by therapeutic interventions. Therefore, during the last decade, neurobiochemical markers for TBI have attracted increased attention, they can be used to screen for, diagnose or monitor the patients and to guide targeted therapy or assess therapeutic response (Etzioni et al. 2003, Vitzthum et al. 2005). (Figure. 2) Furthermore, biomarkers might be valuable tool in drug development (Blennow 2010).

3.1 Clinical evaluation

However, several studies have measured a variety of neurochemical substances in the CSF or blood, and a number of proteins synthesized in astroglial cells or neurons have been proposed as markers of cell damage in the CNS and after TBI, to date, none has been approved for clinical use. Critical criteria of the diagnostic performance of a clinically valid biomarker for TBI include its diagnostic accuracy and predictability.

The diagnostic accuracy of a test is the proportion of correctly classified patients (the sum of true positive and true negative tests) and is determined by calculating the test's sensitivity, specificity, likelihood ratio and receiver operating characteristic (ROC) curve (Bossuyt et al. 2003). Sensitivity is the ability to detect a disease in subjects in whom the disease is truly present (i.e., a true positive), and specificity is the ability to rule out the disease in subjects in whom the disease is truly absent (i.e., a true negative). Likelihood ratio (LHR), used to assess diagnostic value of a test, is the likelihood that a given test result would be expected in a patient with the specific disease compared to the likelihood that that same result would be expected in a patient without the target disorder. Two dimensions of accuracy might be considered, the LHR for a positive test (positive LHR) and the LHR for a negative test (negative LHR) (Albert 1982, Altman 1991). ROC curve is the graphical way of presenting the sensitivity (true positive rate) versus false positive rate (1 − specificity). A ROC curve enables the determination of appropriate cut-points, depending on the intended clinical utility of the test (Zweig& Campbell 1993). The area under the curve (AUC) is a measure of predictive discrimination: 50% is equivalent to random guessing and 100% is perfect prediction.

Although sensitivity and specificity are the most commonly provided variables in diagnostic studies, they do not directly apply to many clinical situations because the physician would rather know the probability that the disease is truly present or absent if the diagnostic test is positive or negative rather than probability of a positive test given the presence of the disease (sensitivity). This information is provided by the diagnostic predictability. Diagnostic predictability establishes the ability of the test to predict the presence or absence of disease for a given test result and is determined by calculating the positive and negative predictive values. The positive predictive value denotes the proportion of patients with positive test results who have the disease, and the negative predictive value defines the proportion of patients with a negative test who do not have the disease. The predictive values of a test vary with the prevalence of the disease in the population examined. Bayes' theorem allows calculation of the predictive values for any prevalence of disease using the prevalence and the sensitivity and specificity measures derived from previous studies (Altman 1991).

To demonstrate its clinical utility, a novel biomarker needs to be evaluated in a series of human studies (phase 1-4 trials) in order to establish the performance characteristics. The phase 1 examines whether the biomarker is significantly different for diseased patients as compared to those known not to have the disease. If a satisfactory discrimination between patients and controls is proven, the following step is to determine diagnostic accuracy (phase 2). Phase 3 evaluates the performance of the test in the target population (Sackett & Haynes 2002). Phase 3 assesses whether the measurement of the biomarkers modifies outcome and influence therapeutic interventions and the subsequent effect on health outcome (intervention studies) (Sackett & Haynes 2002). Phase 4 trial is also known as post-marketing surveillance trial because this phase can be done after the marker has been made commercially available.

3.2 Novel candidate biomarkers

Many publications can be found for candidate biomarkers, although the initially promising results have often not been confirmed. Here, we review novel biomarkers that have shown high sensitivity and specificity in at least two independent studies. Biomarkers reflect damage and release from each of the major cell types/structures in brain parenchyma, therefore they can be divided into neuronal/synaptic and glial biomarkers (Table 1). We also discuss selected candidate biomarkers related to cellular and subcellular origins.

Biomarker	Location	Function/ Pathogenic process	Comment
Neuronal and Axonal Markers			
NSE	Prominently in the cytoplasm of neurons	Upregulated NSE is released from damaged axons to maintain cellular homeostasis.	Also present in erythrocytes and platelets
UCH-L1	Cell Body (perikarya)	Protein de-ubiquitinization	Implicated in familial Parkinsonism
SBPDs	Axons	Cortical cytoskeleton matrix support	Pathology--dependent generation of αII-spectrin breakdown products (SBDPs): Calpain generates SBDP145 as a signature event in acute neuronal necrosis Caspase-3 generates SBDP120 as a signature event in delayed neuronal apoptosis.
Phosphorylated neurofilament	Predominantly in axons	Main component of the axonal cytoskeleton	Increased serum concentrations of this protein are expected to provide a specific measure of axonal injury
Glial Markers			
S100b			
GFAP	Major protein constituent of glial filaments in astrocytes	Cytoskeleton support	Induced during " reactive astrogliosis " after TBI

Table 1. Biomarkers for TBI

3.2.2 Neuronal and axonal markers

Neuronal and axonal proteins could prove to be valuable biomarkers as these molecules might correlate with cognitive function and long term outcome.

3.2.2.1 Neuron-specific enolase

Neuron-specific enolase (NSE) is a glycolytic pathway enzyme, localized predominantly in neuronal cytoplasm. Several studies demonstrated that NSE is a sensitive and specific indicator of neuronal cell death (Selakovic et al. 2005, Oertel et al. 2006). In addition, studies have been conducted examining CSF and serum NSE levels from adults with severe TBI, and their relationship with severity of injury and clinical outcome. Increased CSF and serum levels of NSE have been reported after TBI. NSE concentrations were also associated with severity of injury, CT scan findings and outcome (Selakovic et al. 2005, Herrmann et al. 2000, Ross et al. 1996). Although, NSE was originally identified in neurons, further studies have shown the protein in erythrocytes and platelets. False positive values have been reported in the setting of combined CNS injury plus shock and in the setting of hemolysis (Piazza et al. 2005).

3.2.2.2 Ubiquitin C-terminal hydrolase

Ubiquitin C-terminal hydrolase (UCH-L1), a neuron-specific cytoplasmic enzyme, is highly enriched in neurons representing between 1 and 5% of total soluble brain protein (Lincoln et al. 1999). This protein is involved in either the addition or removal of ubiquitin from proteins that are destined for metabolism (via the ATP-dependent proteosome pathway) (Laser et al. 2003), thus playing an important role in the removal of excessive, oxidized or misfolded proteins during both normal and neuropathological conditions, such as neurodegenerative disorders (Kobeissy et al. 2006). Because of the important function and its high brain specificity, UCH-L1 has been proposed as a novel biomarker for TBI. CSF levels of UCH-L1 in CSF have been found significantly increased in severe TBI patients compared with uninjured patients, with significant associations observed between levels of UCH-L1 in CSF, injury severity and clinical outcome (Papa et al. 2010). A study has been conducted investigating the exposure and kinetic metrics of UCH-L1 in adults with severe TBI, and their relationship with severity of injury and clinical outcome (Brophy et al. 2010). A strong correlation between CSF and serum median concentrations and biokinetics, especially during the acute period, and relationships with clinical outcome were observed (Brophy et al. 2011). Furthermore, a recent study reported that serum concentrations of UCHL1 were associated with abnormal blood brain barrier (BBB) permeability, suggesting that UCH-L1 might be used to monitor BBB disruption in patients with TBI (Blyth et al. 2011).

3.2.2.3 Spectrin Breakdown Products (SBDPs)

Alpha II-spectrin is primarily found in neurons and is abundant in axons and presynaptic terminals (Riederer et al. 1986). The protein is processed to breakdown products (SBDPs) of molecular weights 150 kDa (SBDP150) and 145 kDa (SBDP145) by calpain and is also cleaved to a 120-kDa product (SBDP120) by caspase-3. Calpain and caspase-3 are major executioners of necrotic and apoptotic cell death, respectively, during ischemia or TBI (Ringger et al. 2004, Pineda et al. 2007, Mondello et al. 2010). Thus, a unique feature of this technique is the ability to concurrently detect calpain and caspase-3 proteolysis of aII-spectrin, providing crucial information on the underlying cell death mechanisms. In addition, distinct temporal release patterns of CSF SBDP145 and SBDP120 were reported to reflect different temporal characteristics of protease activation (Mondello et al. 2010). Pineda et al., employing Western blot analyses, reported elevated levels of SBDPs in CSF from adults with severe TBI and their significant relationships with severity of injury and outcome (Pineda et al. 2007). Increased CSF SBDP levels were found to be significantly associated with mortality in patients with severe TBI. In addition, the temporal profile of SBDPs in nonsurvivors also differed from survivors (Mondello et al. 2010).These data suggest that SBDPs may provide crucial information not only on severity of brain injury, but also on underlying pathophysiological mechanisms associated with necrotic and apoptotic cell death.

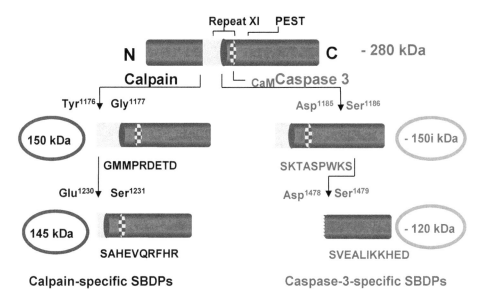

Fig. 3. Brain Injury-Dependent Generation of SBDPs

3.2.2.4 Phosphorylated neurofilament

A recent addition to the growing number of markers of brain injury is the heavily phosphorylated form of the major neurofilament subunit NF-H (pNF-H). Because pNF-H is specific for axons, increased serum concentrations of this protein are expected to provide a specific measure of ongoing axonal damage or degeneration. Increased pNF-H concentrations in serum and CSF have been observed following a variety of CNS damage and disease states, both in animal models and in human patients (Anderson et al. 2008, Boylan et al. 2009, Ganesalingam et al. 2011, Douglas-Escobar et al. 2010).

3.2.3 Glial markers
Several candidate glial markers have been proposed. In the section below, we focus on s100 and GFAP, which are the most extensively examined glial markers in TBI.

3.2.3.1 S100B
S-100b is a low-affinity calcium-binding protein that is primarily expressed and secreted astrocytes (Xiong et al., 2000). The biological function of S100B is still somewhat unclear.

Intracellularly, this protein is involved in in the regulation of a large variety of cell activities and in the regulation of cell morphology (Goncalves et al., 2008, Kleindienst & Bullock 2006). S100B is also released into the extracellular space where seems to have both toxic/degenerative and trophic/reparative roles depending on the concentration (Goncalves et al., 2008). S100B found in low levels in healthy individuals, rises rapidly after head injury. The serum half-life of s100 is about 30 to 90 minutes and can be detected soon after injury (Jonsson et al., 2000). Several studies have demonstrated effectiveness of S100B as a diagnostic marker in the setting of TBI (Romner et al. 2000, Raabe et al. 1999). Increased levels of this protein marker have been shown to correlate with injury severity, mortality, and poor neurologic outcome following severe TBI (Vos et al. 2004). In addition, since 1995 several studies have investigated the clinical utility of this biomarker to predict normal CT findings after minor head injury in adults (Ingebrigtsen et al. 1995, Biberthaler et al. 2006). However, several observations concerning S100B have tempered the original enthusiasm regarding the usefulness of this protein as brain damage biomarker. One of the limitations to the use of S100B as a potential screening agent for brain injury is the lack of specificity. Indeed, S-100b, originally considered specific to astroglia in the central nervous system, is present in other extracerebral tissues such as adipocytes, chondrocytes and bone marrow cells (Donato 2001). High serum S-100b levels have been observed after extracranial trauma and burns (Anderson et al. 2001, Romner &Ingebritsen 2001). In addition, increased S100B may reflect either glial damage or astrocytic reactions to neural injury, referred to as reactive astrogliosis, which might have beneficial or detrimental physiological purposes (Herrmann et al. 2003, Kleindienst et al. 2007). This has raised concerns as to whether the serum levels of this protein actually correlate with the degree of brain damage or are more reflective of other processes. Finally, because of the high normative values in the pediatric population, S100B is not a useful marker in children (Piazza et al. 2007, Berger et al. 2006).

3.2.3.2 Glial fibrillary acidic protein

Glial fibrillary acidic protein (GFAP), a monomeric intermediate filament protein found in the astroglial skeleton, is not found outside the central nervous system and is thus considered a marker worth focusing upon in the search for brain specificity (Vos et al. 2004, Missler et al. 1999). In addition GFAP can be measured in peripheral blood (van Geel et al. 2002, Missler et al. 1999).

Recent evidence indicates elevates serum GFAP levels in various types of brain damage, ranging from neurodegerative disorders (Baydas et al. 2003) and stroke (Herrmann et al. 2000) to traumatic brain injury (TBI) (Vos et al. 2004, Nylen et al. 2006, Pelinka et al. 2004). Clinical studies have proposed that the serum GFAP level is a reliable marker of primary brain damage after TBI with the further advantage that it is not released in situations of multiple traumas without brain injury (Vos et al. 2004, Pelinka et al. 2004). GFAP has also been demonstrated to be a potential useful biomarker to predict clinical outcome. Recently, Vos and colleagues showed a high specificity of GFAP in predicting death or unfavorable outcome at 6 months (0.93– 0.95), with a falsepositive rate for unfavorable outcome below 5% (Vos et al. 2010).

4. Assay development and hand-held devices

A variety of different analytical assay formats have been developed to measure biomarkers in biofluids such as cerebrospinal fluid (CSF) and plasma and serum (Mondello et al. 2011).

The most commonly used format is a two-sided enzyme-linked sandwich immunoassay (ELISA). This format is based on the coating of a solid surface in a plate to capture the biomarker/analyte of interest, followed by incubation with a directly or indirectly-labeled labeled detection antibody. In the ELISA, this label is of enzyme-based, but there are a variety of different surface structures, labels and detection methods available. These include fluorescence, chemiluminescence, optical (absorbance) and electro-chemiluminescence.

Key elements in the consideration of the assay format are the analytical performance of the assay in terms of sensitivity and specificity, which assessed as specific assay parameters. The importance of these assay parameters and their assessment can be found in a recent paper by Mondello et al. (Mondello et al. 2011). Over the past few years, a practical iterative approach "fit-for-purpose" approach to biomarker assay development and validation has evolved, which centers around the "intended use" of the assay and the regulatory requirements associated with it (Lee et al. 2006). Assays "evolve" through different stages from the original assay development phase through an analytical qualification and validation phase. The underlying concept here is to fully understand the analytical performance of these assays for their intended use, before testing on clinical samples. Laboratories performing testing on human specimen for diagnosis, prevention or treatment of any disease are certified under the Clinical Laboratory Improvement Amendments (CLIA) of 1988 or have similar accreditation outside the US. These standard practices frequently required for CLIA certification were published by the Clinical and Laboratory Standard Institute (CLSI). In May 2001, the Food and Drug Administration (FDA) issued guidance for industry for bioanalytical method validation of assay to support pharmacokinetic (PK) assessment of small molecule drugs (Guidance for Industry on Bioanalytical Method Validation: availability. Fed. Regist. 66, 28526-28527, 2001).

In view of the diverse of biomarker assays for either PK , drug development or diagnostic purposes, neither the FDA bioanalytical validation nor the CLSI guidelines fully meet the needs of drug development and diagnostic applications of biomarker assays, which has resulted in additional recommendations for example by the American Association of Pharmaceutical Scientists (AAPS). A more comprehensive overview can be found in Lee et al, 2006. While it is important to develop "fit-for purpose" biomarker assays and analytically define and understand their performance, this procedure should be mirrored in the standardized collection of biofluids to be analyzed. For example, the Alzheimer Disease Neuroimaging initiative (ADNI) has identified the crucial parameters in the collection and storage primarily of CSF, which has resulted in the formulation of standard operating procedures (SOPs) and the quality-control assessment of collected samples. This has also led to the formation of a global CSF consortium, which based on the availability of biofluids such as CSF collected under standardized conditions allowed the identification of the variability when performing biomarker assessment at multiple sites (Mattson et al. 2011).

The translation of a "fit-for-purpose assay into a clinically useful and commercially viable diagnostic product requires the transfer of such an assay onto an appropriate platform, suitable for its intended use. While the laboratory assays described above are typically performed in a clinical reference laboratory setting over a course of hours, it is desirable to perform the measurement of acute biomarkers of brain injury in point-of-care (POC) type setting, outside the clinical laboratory. This includes the accident site, emergency room, sidelines of a sports field and military field. Rather than performing the biomarker assay in a benchtop multiwell plate format, in these setting a smaller and portable POC system is desirable, which requires little to no sample preparation and can performed as a rapid diagnostic test in 30 min or less. In the battle field, these requirements are even more stringent in that the assay system should be carried around as handheld device, simple and lightweight and withstand extreme environments.

Over the last couple of years a variety of different POC platforms have been developed (Price & Kricka 2007). These POC assay platform comprise different design concepts and detection technologies based on their intended use. Glucose testing in diabetic patients is one of successful examples of POC test. The first blood glucose measurements were carried out with small paper strips invented and introduced by Ames in 1965. A measurement if performed by adding a drop of blood to a strip wherein the reaction of glucose in the blood results in the development of blue color and is compared to a color chart for analysis.

For tests, which do not require quantification, but simply detect the presence of a biomarker such as pregnancy test, a lateral flow-strip design might be sufficient. These are membrane strips, through which a small volume of sample liquid is transported by capillary action. These lateral flow strips are based on the binding of labels in the presence of biomarker through an immunochemical reaction, typically, small gold particles.

The assessment of biomarkers in the POC or handheld device format might require a more semi-quantitative assessment and here solutions have been developed, which mimic several of the assay steps a central laboratory test in a miniaturized format. One of the earliest examples is the i-STATR system (Abbott Laboratories, Abbott Park, IL) for measuring electrolyte, coagulation, glucose, cardiac markers such as troponin, and other tests. Wet assay reagents are stored in a cartridge and are actively pumped by the device through mechanical displacement to perform the various steps of the assays. Other examples such as AtolyzerR, originally developed by Atonomics, and the Roche cobas h232R exist and many more new technologies are being developed. A modification is the Philips MagnotechR system, which replace the liquid manipulation steps by magnetically controlled movement. The implementation of molecular-diagnostic-based POCs also shows promise for the future. These assays typically include a polymerase-chain reaction-based amplification step.

All these implementations of the POC tests in a miniaturized cartridge-type format are designed to allow a high level of assay control. The overall assay performance is influenced by minor variation for example in timing of the individual assay steps and can results in large overall assay performance variability. The successful adaptation of any biomarker assay to a POC/handheld device is dependent on the requirement for sensitivity and precision in its intended use. The development of new POC technologies and solutions shows great promise for the adaptation of CNS biomarker assays in unmet medical needs.

5. Strategy for regulatory approval by FDA

Biomarkers, whether proteomic based or based on more traditional technologies, can be used for a variety of purposes. Generally speaking, the term 'biomarker' describes any measurable diagnostic indicator used to assess the presence or risk of disease. For the US Food and Drug Administration (FDA), the term 'diagnostic' includes the diagnosis, screening and prediction of disease. But it also encompass other uses such as staging or the prognosis of disease, monitoring patients and the effectiveness of a treatment and/or optimizing treatment outcomes by aiding health-care providers in medical and therapeutic decision making.

The FDA has been involved in the regulation of medical devices, including in vitro diagnostic devices (IVDs) since 1976 when the US Congress established laws for the regulation of medical devices under the Medical Device Amendments act (REF. 8). According to the Medical Device Amendments act, for an in vitro diagnostic (IVD) device to enter the US market it must comply with a set of rules and regulations in order to prove safety and effectiveness for its intended use. In 21 CFR 860.7(d)(1) device safety requires "the probable benefit to health from use of device for its intended use and conditions of use ... outweigh any probable risk." In 21 CFR 860.7(e)(1) device effectiveness requires "that in a significant portion of the target population, the use of the device for its intended use and conditions for use ... will provide clinically significant results." In addition, a new assay is required to demonstrate an adequate analytical performance (appropriate accuracy and precision) and clinical performance (sensitivity, specificity and some indication of clinical utility) (21 CFR 807; 21 CFR 814).

In order to be commercialized in a kit, newly discovered biomarkers device must follow specific pathways. Investigational studies of diagnostic devices can be performed with various design configurations, but they must conform to FDA requirements. The researchers are required to apply for an investigational device exemption (IDE) before initiating the study, as described in Title 21 of the Code of Federal Regulations 812 (21 CFR 812)(US Food and Drugs Administration [FDA], 2006). The IDE submission should describe the nature of the proposed study, include details of informed consent and ensure patient protection and that the risks associated with participation in the study will be clearly communicated to individuals.

After the appropriate investigational studies have been completed, the FDA requires premarket submissions before a test can be approved for clinical use in the United States. Depending on the nature of the test and its classification, the product could be reviewed as a 510(k) premarketing clearance with a 90-day timeline or Premarket Approval (PMA) with a 180-day timeline (21 CFR 807; 21 CFR 814). FDA considers three classes of devices (class I, II, or III) (FDA, 2009, 2010).

The 510(k) process is used when the new test measures an existing FDA classified analyte (class I or II) where there exists a commercially available predicate test method that has been cleared by the FDA or that was in commercial distribution before May 28, 1976 (21 CFR 860.84). Premarket clearance requires the sponsor to provide information for the new product including its intended use and classification and 'substantially equivalence' to the predicate device. This ensures that a high level of safety and effectiveness is maintained. In addition the sponsor must show characterization of analytical capability of the test (e.g., specificity and accuracy, precision and linearity by correlating patient studies against predicate device) (http://www. fda.gov/ oc/mdufma/coversheet.html).

The PMA process is used when the test is classified as class III; that is, either it is associated with high risk (e.g., when the outcome determines cancer treatment or diagnosis) or the clinical utility of the marker or the technology of the measurement are novel and no predicate device can be identified (21 CFR 814). FDA requires the sponsor to submit the same data required for 510(k) as well as clinical outcomes data, where the level of the marker is related to disease status defined by clinical criteria (http://www.fda.gov/ oc/mdufma/coversheet.html).

In 1997, since some new biomarkers have no obvious predicate devices and do not have safety concerns, FDA created a new hybrid 'de novo' or 'risk-based' classification (21 CFR 814). This process allows a new biomarker to be regulated as in a 510(k), but requires the demonstration of clinical effectiveness.

Therefore, in the absence of a predicate device and depending on the intended use and clinical utility, either a PMA or a 'de novo' process will be required for a new protein of interest before it achieves commercial availability in a kit or device.

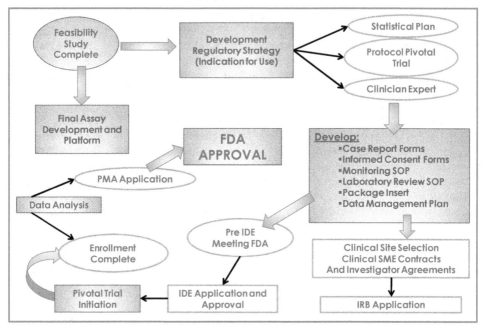

Fig. 4. Regulatory Pathway for PMA Application

6. Conclusion

This chapter provides an introductory review of techniques that have been applied to biomarker identification and clinical validation. Demonstration of clinical utility and compliance with regulatory requirements is critical for the commercialization of novel biochemical markers but also formidable, uncertain and costly.

At present, there are still many unanswered questions in this area of research, however, such as the best statistical methods to analyze the large volume of data generated, the role of potential demographic and clinical confounders, such as age, sex, and on the other hand the broad and complex spectrum of types and severities of brain injuries. In addition, issues such as sample integrity and preservation, normalization, and appropriate control data also must be given careful consideration. A multimarker strategy will probably be needed to provide a greatly expanded approach to the detection of brain injury, elucidating its pathogenesis and making it possible to guide and monitor the therapy in new ways and ultimately to improve outcome.

7. References

Albert, A. (1982). On the use and computation of likelihood ratios in clinical chemistry. *Clin Chem*, Vol.28, pp.1113–1119

Altman, D.G. Practical Statistics for Medical Research (Chapman & Hall, London, UK, 1991)

Anderson, R.E.H.L.; Nilsson, O.; Dijai-Merzoug, R. & Settergen, G. (2001). High serum S100B levels for trauma patients without head injuries. *Neurosurgery,* Vol.49, pp.1272–1273

Anderson, K.J.; Scheff, S.W.; Miller, K.M. et al. (2008). The phosphorylated axonal form of the neurofilament subunit NF-H (pNF-H). as a blood biomarker of traumatic brain injury. *J Neurotrauma,* Vol.25, pp.1079–1085

Beltrao, P.; Kiel, C. & Serrano, L. (2007). Structures in systems biology. *Curr Opin Struct Biol,* Vol.17, pp.378-384

Baydas, G.; Nedzvetskii, V.S.; Tuzcu, M. et al. (2003). Increase of glial fibrillary acidic protein and S-100B in hippocampus and cortex of diabetic rats: effects of vitamin E. *Eur J Pharmacol,* Vol.462, pp.67–71

Berger, R.P.; Dulani, T.; Adelson, P.D. et al. (2006). Identification of brain injury in well appearing infants using serum and cerebrospinal markers: A possible screening tool. *Pediatrics,* Vol.117, pp.325–332

Biberthaler, P.; Linsenmeier, U.; Pfeifer, K.J. et al. (2006). Serum S-100B concentration provides additional information for the indication of computed tomography in patients after minor head injury: a prospective multicenter study. *Shock,* Vol.25, No.5, pp.446–453

Blyth, B.J.; Farahvar, A.; He H.; et al. (2011). Elevated Serum Ubiquitin Carboxy-Terminal Hydrolase L1 Is Associated with Abnormal Blood-Brain Barrier Function after Traumatic Brain Injury. *J Neurotrauma,* [Epub ahead of print]

Bossuyt, P.M.; Reitsma, J.B.; Bruns, D.E. et al. (2003). The STARD statement for reporting studies of diagnostic accuracy: explanation and elaboration. *Clin Chem,* Vol.49, pp.7-18

Boylan, K.; Yang, C.; Crook, J. et al. (2009). Immunoreactivity of the phosphorylated axonal neurofilament H subunit (pNF-H). in blood of ALS model rodents and ALS patients: evaluation of blood pNF-H as a potential ALS biomarker. *J Neurochem,* Vol.111, pp.1182–1191

Brophy, G.M. ; Mondello, S.; Papa, L. et al. (2011). Biokinetic analysis of ubiquitin C-terminal hydrolase-L1 (UCH-L1). in severe traumatic brain injury patient biofluids. *J Neurotrauma,* Vol.28, No.6, pp.861-70

Blennow, K. (2010). Biomarkers in Alzheimer's disease drug development. *Nat Med.* Vol.16, No.11, pp. 1218-22

Burgess, J. A.; Lescuyer, P.; Hainard, A. et al. (2006). Identification of brain cell death associated proteins in human post-mortem cerebrospinal fluid. *J Proteome Res,* Vol.5, pp. 1674-1681

Celis, J. E.; Gromov, P.; Cabezon, T. et al. (2004). Proteomic characterization of the interstitial fluid perfusing the breast tumor microenvironment: a novel resource for biomarker and therapeutic target discovery. *Mol Cell Proteomics,* Vol.3, pp.327-344

Chen, S. S. ; Haskins, W. E. ; Ottens, A. K. et al. (2007). Bioinformatics for traumatic brain injury: Proteimic Data Mining. *Data Mining in Biomedicine.* Ed. Panos Pardalos, Boginski, V.L., Vazacopoulos, A. Springer, pp. 1-26

Code Federal Regulations, vol. 21 CFR807, Available from
http://frwebgate.access.gpo.gov/cgi-bin/getcfr.cgi?YEAR=current&TITLE=
21&PART=807&SECTION=81&SUBPART= &TYPE=TEXT

Code Federal Regulations, vol. 21 CFR814, Available from
        http://frwebgate.access.gpo.gov/cgi-bin/getcfr.cgi?YEAR=current&TITLE=
        21&PART=814&SECTION=1&SUBPART= &TYPE=TEXT)
Davidsson, P. & Sjogren, M. (2005) The use of proteomics in biomarker discovery in
        neurodegenerative diseases. *Dis Markers*, Vol.21, pp.81-92
Denslow, N.; Michel, M.E.; Temple, M.D. et al. (2003) Application of proteomics technology
        to the field of neurotrauma. *J Neurotrauma*, Vol.20, pp.401-407
Ding, Q.; Wu, Z.; Guo, Y. et al. (2006) Proteome analysis of up-regulated proteins in the rat
        spinal cord induced by transection injury. *Proteomics*, Vol.6, pp.505-518
Donato, R. (2001). S100: a multigenic family of calcium-modulated proteins of the EF-hand
        type with intracellular and extracellular functional roles. *Int J Biochem Cell Biol*,
        Vol.33, No.7, pp.637– 668
Douglas-Escobar, M.; Yang, C.; Bennett, J. et al. (2010). A pilot study of novel biomarkers
        in neonates with hypoxic-ischemic encephalopathy. *Pediatr Res*, Vol.68, No. 6,
        pp.531-6
Dumont, D. ; Noben, J. P.; Raus, J. et al. (2004) Proteomic analysis of cerebrospinal fluid from
        multiple sclerosis patients. *Proteomics*, Vol.4, pp.2117-2124
Etzioni, R; Urban, N; Ramsey, S. et al. (2003) The case for early detection. Nat Rev Cancer.
        Vol.3, No.4, pp. 243-52
Fenn, J. B.; Mann, M.; Meng, C. K.; Wong, S. F. and Whitehouse, C. M. (1989) Electrospray
        ionization for mass spectrometry of large biomolecules. *Science*, Vol. 246, pp.
        64-71
Food and Drugs Administration. Electronic code of federal regulations. US Food and Drugs
        Administration [online], Available from
        http://ecfr.gpoaccess.gov/cgi/t/text/textidx?c=ecfr&tpl=/ecfrbrowse/Title21/21
        cfr812_main_ 02.tpl (2006)
Food and Drug Administration. 21 USC 360 c (a)(1). Classifi cation of devices intended for
        human use; device classes, Available from
        http://www.fda.gov/RegulatoryInformation/Legislation/FederalFoodDrugandC
        osmeticActFDCAct/FDCActChapterVDrugsandDevices/ucm110188.htm (accessed
        2010-04-27) (2009).
Food and Drug Administration. Overview of IVD regulation, Available from
        http://www.fda.gov/MedicalDevices/DeviceRegulationandGuidance/IVDRegula
        toryAssistance/ucm123682.htm#4b: (accessed 2010-04-27). Within section "Medical
        devices" (2010)
Ganesalingam, J.; An, J.; Shaw, C.E. et al. (2011). Combination of neurofilament heavy chain
        and complement C3 as CSF biomarkers for ALS. *J Neurochem*, Vol.117, No.3,
        pp.:528-37
Goncalves, C.A.; Leite, M.C. & Nardin, P. (2008). Biological and methodological features of
        the measurement of S100B, a putative marker of brain injury [published online
        ahead of print April 18, 2008]. *Clin Biochem*, Vol.41, No.10/11, pp.755–763
Grant, S. G. (2003). Systems biology in neuroscience: bridging genes to cognition. *Curr Opin
        Neurobiol*, Vol.13, pp.577-582
Grant, S. G. & Blackstock, W. P. (2001). Proteomics in neuroscience: from protein to network.
        J Neurosci, Vol.21, pp.8315-8318

Guingab-Cagmat, J.D.; Kobeissy, F.; Ratliff, M.V. et al. (2009). Neurogenomics and Neuroproteomics Approaches of Studying Neural Injury. In: Essentials of Spinal Cord Injury, (M. Fehlings, et.al ed.).. Thieme, Toronto

Hammack, B. N.; Fung, K. Y.; Hunsucker, S. W. et al. (2004). Proteomic analysis of multiple sclerosis cerebrospinal fluid. *Mult Scler*, Vol.10, pp.245-260

Haskins, W. E.; Kobeissy, F. H.; Wolper, R.A. et al. (2005). Rapid discovery of putative protein biomarkers of traumatic brain injury by SDS-PAGE-capillary liquid chromatography-tandem mass spectrometry. *J Neurotrauma*, Vol.22, pp.629-644.

Herrmann, M.; Vos, P.E.; Wunderlich, M.T. et al. (2000). Release of glial tissue-specific proteins after acute stroke: a comparative analysis of serum concentrations of protein S-100B and glial fibrillary acidic protein. *Stroke,* Vol.31, pp.2670-2677

Herrmann, M.; Jost, S.; Kutz, S. et al. (2000). Temporal profile of release of neurobiochemical markers of brain damage after traumatic brain injury is associated with intracranial pathology as demonstrated in cranial computerized tomography. *J Neurotrauma*, Vol.17, pp.113-122

Herrmann, M. & Ehrenreich, H. (2003). Brain derived proteins as markers of acute stroke: their relation to pathophysiology, outcome prediction and neuroprotective drug monitoring. *Restor Neurol Neurosci,* Vol.21, No.3-4, pp.177-190

Ingebrigtsen, T.; Romner, B.; Kongstad, P. & Langbakk, B. (1995). Increased serum concentrations of S-100 after minor head injury. A biochemical marker with prognostic value? *J Neurol Neurosurg Psychiatry*, Vol.59, pp.103-104

Jonsson, H.; Johnsson, P.; Hoglund, P. et al. (2000). Elimination of S100B and renal function after cardiac surgery. *J Cardiothorac Vasc Anesth,* Vol.14, No.6, pp.698-701

Karas, M. & Hillenkamp, F. (1988). Laser desorption ionization of proteins with molecular masses exceeding 10,000 daltons. *Anal Chem*, Vol.60, pp.2299-2301

Katano, T.; Mabuchi, T.; Okuda-Ashitaka, E. et al. (2006). Proteomic identification of a novel isoform of collapsin response mediator protein-2 in spinal nerves peripheral to dorsal root ganglia. *Proteomics*, Vol.6, pp.6085-6094

Kleindienst, A. & Bullock R.M. (2006). A critical analysis of the role of the neurotrophic protein S100B in acute brain injury. *J Neurotrauma*, Vol.23, No.8, pp.1185-200

Kleindienst, A.; Hesse, F.; Bullock, M.R. & Buchfelder, M. (2007). The neurotrophic protein S100B: value as a marker of brain damage and possible therapeutic implications. *Prog Brain Res.* Vol.161, pp.317-325

Kobeissy, F. H.; Ottens, A. K.; Zhang, Z. et al. (2006). Novel differential neuroproteomics analysis of traumatic brain injury in rats. *Mol Cell Proteomics*, Vol.5, pp.1887-1898

Kobeissy, F. H.; Sadasivan, S.; Oli, M.W. et al. (2008). Neuroproteomics and systems biology-based discovery of protein biomarkers for traumatic brain injury and clinical validation. *Proteomics Clin Appl*, Vol.2, pp.1467-1483

Laser, H.; Mack, T.G.; Wagner, D. & Coleman, M.P. (2003). Proteasome inhibition arrests neurite outgrowth and causes "dying-back" degeneration in primary culture. *J Neurosci Res*, Vol.74, pp.906-916

Lee, J.W.; Devanarayan, V.; Barrett, Y.C. et al. (2006). Fit-for-purpose method development and validation for successful biomarker measurement. *Pharm Res,* Vol.23, No.2, pp.312-28

Lincoln, S.; Vaughan, J.; Wood, N. et al. (1999). Low frequency of pathogenic mutations in the ubiquitin carboxy-terminal hydrolase gene in familial Parkinson's disease. *Neuroreport*, Vol.10, pp.427-429

Mattsson, N.; Andreasson, U. ; Persson, S.; Arai H et al. (2011). The Alzheimer's Association external quality control program for cerebrospinal fluid biomarkers. *Alzheimers Dement*, Vol.7, No.4, pp.386-395

Missler, U.; Wiesmann, M.; Wittmann, G. et al. (1999). Measurement of glial fibrillary acidic protein in human blood: analytical method and preliminary clinical results. *Clin Chem*, Vol.45, pp.138 –141

Mondello, S.; Robicsek, S.; Gabrielli, A. et al. (2010). aII-spectrin breakdown products (SBDPs). diagnosis and outcome in severe traumatic brain injury patients. *J Neurotrauma*, Vol.27, pp.1203–1213

Mondello, S.; Muller, U.; Jeromin, A. et al. (2011). Blood-based diagnostics of traumatic brain injuries. *Expert Rev Mol Diagn*, Vol.11, No.1, pp.65-78

Nylen, K.; Ost, M.; Csajbok, L.Z. et al. (2006). Increased serum-GFAP in patients with severe traumatic brain injury is related to outcome. *J Neurol Sci*, Vol.240, pp.85–91

Nogoy, N. (2007). Neuroproteomics: the hunt for biomarkers of neurotrauma. Andrew Ottens talks to Nicole Nogoy. *Expert Rev Proteomics*, Vol.4, pp.343-345

Oertel, M.; Schumacher, U.; McArthur, D.L et al. (2005). S-100B and NSE: markers of initial impact of subarachnoid haemorrhage and their relation to vasospasm and outcome. *J Clin Neurosci*, Vol.13, pp.834–840

Ottens, A. K.; Kobeissy, F. H.; Fuller, B. F. et al. (2007). Novel neuroproteomic approaches to studying traumatic brain injury. *Prog Brain Res*, Vol.161, pp.401-418

Ottens, A. K.; Kobeissy, F. H.; Golden, E. C. et al. (2006). Neuroproteomics in neurotrauma. *Mass Spectrom Rev*, Vol.25, pp.380-408

Papa, L.; Akinyi, L.; Liu, M.C. et al. (2010). Ubiquitin C terminal hydrolase is a novel biomarker in humans for severe traumatic brain injury. *Crit Care Med*, Vol.38, pp.138-144

Pelinka, L.E.; Kroepfl, A.; Schmidhammer, R. et al. (2004). Glial fibrillary acidic protein in serum after traumatic brain injury and multiple trauma. *J Trauma*, Vol.57, pp.1006 – 1012

Piazza, O.; Cotena, S.; Esposito, G. et al. (2005). S100B is a sensitive but not specific prognostic index in comatose patients after cardiac arrest. *Minerva Chir*, Vol.60, pp.477–480

Piazza, O.; Storti, M.P.; Cotena, S. et al. (2007). S100B is not a reliable prognostic index in paediatric TBI. *Pediatr Neurosurg*, Vol.43, pp.258–264

Pineda, J.A.; Lewis, S.B.; Valadka, A.B. et al. (2007). Clinical significance of aII-spectrin breakdown products in cerebrospinal fluid after severe traumatic brain injury. *J Neurotrauma*, Vol.24, pp.354–366

Price, C.P. & Kricka, L.J. (2007). Improving healthcare accessibility through point-of-care technologies. *Clin Chem*, Vol.53, No.9, pp.1665-75

Raabe, A.; Grolms, C.; Sorge, O.; Zimmermann, M. & Seifert, V. (1999). Serum S-100B protein in severe head injury. *J Neurosurg*, Vol.45, pp.477–483

Redell, J. B.; Liu, Y. & Dash, P. K. (2009). Traumatic brain injury alters expression of hippocampal microRNAs: potential regulators of multiple pathophysiological processes. *J Neurosci Res*, Vol.87, pp.1435-1448

Rifai, N.; Gillette, M. A. & Carr, S. A. (2006). Protein biomarker discovery and validation: the long and uncertain path to clinical utility. *Nat Biotechnol*, Vol.24, pp.971-983

Riederer, B.M.; Zagon, I.S. & Goodman, S.R. (1986). Brain spectrin (240/235). and brain spectrin (240/235E): two distinct spectrin subtypes with different locations within mammalian neural cells. *J Cell Biol*, Vol.102, pp.2088-2097

Ringger, N.C.; O'Steen, B.E.; Brabham, J.G. et al. (2004). A novel marker for traumatic brain injury, CSF aII-spectrin breakdown product levels. *J Neurotrauma*, Vol.21, pp.1443-1456

Romner, B.; Ingebrigtsen, T.; Kongstad, P. & Borgesen, S.E. (2000). Traumatic brain injury: serum S-100 measurements related to neuroradiological findings. *J Neurotrauma*, Vol.17, pp.641- 647

Romner, B. & Ingebrigtsen, T. (2001). High serum S100B levels for traumapatients without head injuries. *J. Neurosurg*, Vol.49, pp.1490

Ross, S.A.; Cunningham, R.T.; Johnston, C.F & Rowlands, B.J. (1996). Neuronspecific enolase as an aid to outcome prediction in head injury. *Br J Neurosurg*, Vol.10, pp.471-476

Sackett, D.L. & Haynes, R.B. (2002). The architecture of diagnostic research. *Br Med J*, Vol.324, pp.539-541

Savola, O.; Pyhtinen, J.; Leino, T.K. et al. (2004). Effects of head and extracranial injuries on serum protein S100B levels in trauma patients. *J Trauma*, Vol.56, pp.1229 -1234

Selakovic, V.; Faicevic, R. & Radenovic, L. (2005). The increase of neuron-specific enolase in cerebrospinal fluid and plasma as a marker of neuronal damage in patients with acute brain infarction. *J Clin Neurosci*, Vol.12, pp.542- 547

Shin, B. K. ; Wang, H. & Hanash, S. (2002). Proteomics approaches to uncover the repertoire of circulating biomarkers for breast cancer. *J Mammary Gland Biol Neoplasia*, Vol.7, pp.407-413

Svetlov, S. I.; Xiang, Y.; Oli, M. W. et al. (2006). Identification and preliminary validation of novel biomarkers of acute hepatic ischaemia/reperfusion injury using dual-platform proteomic/degradomic approaches. *Biomarkers*, Vol.11, pp.355-369

Tanaka, K.; Waki, H.; Ido, Y. et al. (1988). Protein and polymer analysis analyses up to m/z 10000 by laser ionization time-of-flight mass spectrometry. *Rapid Commun Mass Spectrom*, Vol.2, pp.3

Vitzthum, F.; Behrens, F.; Anderson, N.L. & Shaw, J.H. (2006). Proteomics: from basic research to diagnostic application. A review of requirements & needs. *J Proteome Res*, Vol.4, No.4, pp.1086-97

van Geel, W.J.A.; de Reus, H.P.M.; Nijzing, H. et al. (2002). Measurement of glial fibrillary acidic protein in blood: an analytical method. *Clin Chim Acta*, Vol.326, pp.151-154

Vos, P.E.; Lamers, K.J.; Hendriks, J.C. et al. (2004). Glial and neuronal proteins in serum predict outcome after severe traumatic brain injury. *Neurology*, Vol.62, pp.1303-1310

Wang, K. K.; Larner, S. F.; Robinson, G. & Hayes, R. L. Neuroprotection targets after traumatic brain injury. *Curr Opin Neurol*, Vol.19, pp.514-519

Wang, K. K. ; Ottens, A. K.; Liu, M. C. et al. (2005). Proteomic identification of biomarkers of traumatic brain injury. *Expert Rev Proteomics*, Vol.2, pp.603-614

Zweig, M.H. & Campbell, G. (1993). Receiver-operating characteristic (ROC). plots: a fundamental evaluation tool in clinical medicine. *Clin Chem*, Vol.39, pp.561–577

11

The Importance of Restriction from Physical Activity in the Metabolic Recovery of Concussed Brain

Giuseppe Lazzarino et al.[*]
Department of Biology, Geology and Environmental Sciences
Division of Biochemistry and Molecular Biology, University of Catania, Catania
Italy

1. Introduction

Brain concussion is unquestionably the most common form of traumatic brain injury (TBI) worldwide (Bruns & Hauser, 2003; Tagliaferri et al., 2006). In European countries, approximately 235 individual/100,000 people are admitted annually to the hospital following TBI, 80% of which receive a diagnosis of mild TBI (mTBI). (van der Naalt, 2001; Vos et al., 2002). It has been calculated that the ratio in the occurrence of mTBI to severe TBI (sTBI) is approximately 22 to 1, with mTBI accounting for at least 75% of patients who survive after TBI each year (Tagliaferri et al., 2006). These percentages are very similar to those recorded in the United States where it is estimated that approximately 1.5 – 8 million people per year suffer from TBI and, among those requiring hospitalization, a proportion ranging from 75% to 90% are classified as "mildly" injured or "concussed" (Bruns & Hauser, 2003). These wide ranges of annual incidence are probably due to the fact that an unknown proportion of mTBI victims do not seek any medical attention (McCrea et al., 2004) (HEADS UP) but it might also be due to the fact that there is still confusion and inconsistency among researchers and organizations in defining and understanding this type of trauma. (Cantu & Voy, 1995; Cantu, 1998, 2007).

The above reported numbers give the evidence that albeit the incidence of mTBI is tremendously high, the mortality caused by this type of trauma appears to be rather low (6-10 per 100,000/year). To reinforce this concept it has been reported that only 0.2% of all

[*]Roberto Vagnozzi[1], Stefano Signoretti[2], Massimo Manara[3], Roberto Floris[4], Angela M. Amorini[5], Andrea Ludovici[4], Simone Marziali[4], Tracy K. McIntosh[6] and Barbara Tavazzi[5]

[1]*Department of Neurosurgery, Chair of Neurosurgery, University of Rome "Tor Vergata", Rome, Italy*

[2]*Division of Neurosurgery, Department of Neurosciences-Head and Neck Surgery, San Camillo Hospital, Rome, Italy*

[3]*Association of Sports Physicians Parma, F.M.S.I., Parma, Italy*

[4]*Department of Diagnostic Imaging and Interventional Radiology, University of Rome "Tor Vergata", Rome, Italy*

[5]*Institute of Biochemistry and Clinical Biochemistry, Catholic University of Rome "Sacro Cuore", Rome, Italy*

[6]*Media NeuroConsultants Inc., Media, PA 19063, USA*

[7]*Department of Biology, Geology and Environmental Sciences, Division of Biochemistry and Molecular Biology, University of Catania, Catania, Italy*

patients attending the Emergency Departments (EDs) will die as a direct result of this head injury (Vos et al., 2002).

With this in mind, it is evident that this situation represents a really serious public health concern of our time: in fact, the EDs are required to see a massive number of patients, with the most challenging task of identifying the small number of them that will progress to have serious acute intracranial complications. Statistics demonstrate that only 1-3% of all mTBI patients admitted to the hospital with a Glasgow Coma Scale (GCS) score of 14-15 will subsequently develop life-threatening intracranial pathology (the remaining 97-99% of them will be discharged home within 48 hours) (Livingston et al., 2000; Lloyd et al., 1997; Shackford et al., 1992; Swann et al., 1981; Taheri et al., 1993). Furthermore, when a mTBI patient is presenting with a GCS score of 15 and no additional associated risk factors the probability that he may suffer from intracranial hemorrhage, requiring neurosurgical intervention, is below 0.1% (Fabbri et al., 2010).

As a consequence of this very low mortality rate, it is generally and widely accepted that mTBI represents a nosological entity with high frequency but that it does *not* represent a real serious injury. The common feeling that consequences of mTBI are only transient disturbances has slowly grown, mainly supported by the absence of structural lesions on traditional neuroimaging. Therefore, the general idea is that mTBI-affected patients need no intervention other than observation, with no additional clinical examinations nor specific recommendations for the post-injury period. However, a recent report revealed that the diagnosis of an intracranial hematoma in such patients was made with a median delay of 18 hours (Yates et al., 2007), strongly suggesting that the quality of the "observation" that mildly-injured patients receive while in hospital is of utmost concern. If in the USA it has been established that only 50% of mildly head injured patients admitted to the hospital had documentation of neurological observations (Yates et al., 2007) in Europe the situation is even much worse, with mTBI patients who have historically been observed by non-specialist wards by nurses and doctors not experienced in neurological observations. The fundamental issues of whether to image, observe and discharge, each one of these endless patients, focused essentially on identifying those at risk for a hemorrhagic complications has completely obscured the real dilemma of the concussive injury, whose early and late symptoms and sequelae are continuously underreported, underinvestigated, underdiagnosed, and mainly underestimated by the majority of physicians.

1.1 Background: Sports-related concussion
If mTBI were as "mild" as we might think, it would be difficult to explain the actual complex management of these patients that may involve various health care professionals including family practice physicians, behavioral psychologists, clinical psychologists, neuropsychologists, neurologists, psychiatrists, neuro-ophthalmologists, neurosurgeons, physiatrists, nurses, occupational therapists, and physical therapists. Furthermore, long beyond the typical recovery interval of one week to three months, at least 15% of persons with a history of mTBI continue to see their primary care physician because of persistent problems (Alexander, 1995; Bigler, 2003; Gouvier et al., 1992; Kay et al., 1992; Ingebrigtsen et al., 2000). From the aforementioned picture and reminding that the majority of mTBIs are unreported, it is clearly evident how much difficult would be to select a homogeneous population for a study on mTBI, just on the basis of those who refer to the hospital.

Although certainly blended in to the vast world of mTBI, by definition, brain concussion should be considered a discrete and distinct entity, since not all mTBI are truly "concussive"; thus the two terms refer to different constructs and should not be used interchangeably (McCrory et al., 2009). Despite recent efforts, a unanimous definition of concussion has not yet been widely accepted (Cantu, 2007). It is possible to define concussion as a traumatic insult capable of provoking an acceleration-deceleration phenomenon within the skull (Barth et al., 2001). From a clinical point of view, concussion is not necessarily accompanied by loss of consciousness and is associated with various physical (headache, equilibrium, vision disturbances, etc.), cognitive (memory, concentration, etc.), emotional (behaviour) and sleep alterations (Gosselin et al., 2009; Hunt & Asplund, 2010; Randolph et al., 2009). These symptoms are included in the well known post-concussive syndrome and can affect, to various degrees, everyday life, resolving spontaneously within 7-10 days post-injury, in the majority of cases. In concussed subjects, the pathobiology of mTBI can not be defined by classical imaging techniques such as CT scan and MR (Kurca et al., 2006), as it occurs in all mTBI patients. This fact, coupled to the faintness and variability of symptoms, mainly assessed by the patient's self-evaluation, is not certainly of help in diagnosing and monitoring concussed patients.

It is generally accepted that at least 20% of all mTBI are sports-related injuries (concussions), of which 30-45% receives no medical care (McCrea et al., 2004). Athletes, therefore, represent a population at great risk of occurrence of concussive episodes and are, for several reasons, the population of choice with which to undertake trials to study the pathobiology of mTBI (Meehan & Bachur, 2009). It is well established that after the first traumatic episode the probability of recurrence of concussion in athletes increases by 3 times (Cantu, 2003), that currently, there is no agreement as to how many concussions are too many (Guskiewicz et al., 2003; Pellman et al., 2004), nor is there an unanimously approved diagnostic approach to monitor concussed athletes (Delaney et al., 2005; Kissick & Johnstone, 2005; Ponsford, 2005), consequently the criteria to assess a safe return of concussed athletes to play remain unclear (Guskiewicz et al., 2006; McClincy et al., 2006; Lovell et al., 2004).

1.2 Background: Metabolic changes characterizing brain vulnerability following concussion

An increasing number of studies on mTBI have focused attention on concussion-induced changes in brain metabolism (Bergsneider et al., 2000; Praticò et al., 2002) including those related to cerebral energy state (Vagnozzi et al., 1999). Hovda and colleagues first suggested the concept of metabolic vulnerability occurring in brain tissue after any concussive episode (Giza & Hovda, 2001; Hovda et al., 1993). During this transient period of altered brain metabolism and function, a second concussive episode of even modest entity may cause significantly addition and/or dramatic brain damage (Longhi et al., 2005), thereby underlying the so called second impact syndrome (SIS), encountered occasionally in sports medicine (Saunders & Harbaugh, 1984). In fact, the possibility of having a second concussive injury within a not yet defined period of time from the first (i.e., days or weeks) has been reported to be even fatal in some instances (Bowen, 2003; Cantu, 1998; Cobb & Battin, 2004; Logan et al., 2001; Mori et al., 2006; Saunders & Harbaugh, 1984). SIS is clinically characterized by untreatable malignant edema with devastating consequences for the patient up to death. Notwithstanding these reported cases, concerns still exist about the real occurrence of this peculiar pathological condition (McCrory, 2001; McCrory & Berkovic, 2001; Nugent, 2006).

By using a rodent model of closed diffuse mild head injury (Foda & Marmarou, 1994; Marmarou et al., 1994), data from our laboratories confirmed the concept of metabolic vulnerability (Tavazzi et al., 2007; Vagnozzi et al., 2007) and have also produced solid experimental evidence linking the severity of brain injury and recovery with the extent of ATP and N-acetylaspartate (NAA) decrease and recovery (Tavazzi et al., 2007; Vagnozzi et al., 2005, 2007). NAA is the most prominent compound detectable with proton Magnetic Resonance Spectroscopy (^{1}H-MRS) in human brain, making it one of the most reliable molecular markers for brain ^{1}H-MRS studies. Although an exact role of this compound remains to be established, brain NAA was found present in concentrations a hundred fold higher than in non-nervous system tissue and therefore considered a brain-specific metabolite (Miyake et al., 1981; Truckenmiller et al., 1985) and as an in vivo marker of neuronal density. NAA metabolism involves different brain compartments, with neuronal mitochondria taking care of its biosynthesis via the activity of aspartate N-acetyltransferase (ANAT) and oligodendrocytes contributing to its degradation via the activity of N-acetylaspartate acylase (ASPA). NAA homeostasis is finely regulated by three different velocities: 1) rate of neuronal biosynthesis, 2) rate of neuronal outflow in the extracellular space, and 3) rate of oligodendrocyte uptake and degradation (Baslow, 2003a, 2003b). Furthermore, NAA biosynthesis is also strictly dependent on the neuronal energy state and therefore on the correct mitochondrial functioning. In fact, NAA synthesis necessarily requires the availability and the energy of hydrolysis of acetyl-CoA (ΔG = -31.2 kJ/mol), working as the acetyl group and energy donor in the acetylation reaction of aspartate catalyzed by ANAT. It is fundamental to understand that when acetyl-CoA is used for NAA synthesis there is an indirect high energy cost to the cell. In fact, since in this case acetyl-CoA will not enter the citric acid cycle (Krebs' cycle) there will be a decrease in the production of reducing equivalents (3 NADH and 1 $FADH_2$) as the fuel for the electron transport chain. Since the oxidative phosphorylation is stoichiometrically coupled to the amount of electron transferred to molecular oxygen by the electron transport chain, the final result will be a net loss of 11 ATP molecules for each NAA molecule newly synthesized. NAA concentration within neurons is comparable to that of glutamate (~10 mmol/l brain water) but, notwithstanding such a relevant amount and in spite of NAA is known since late '50s, there is no unanimity on the biochemical functions of this still enigmatic molecule. According to different studies, NAA may act as storage form for aspartate, protein synthesis regulator, shuttle of acetate and "amino-nitrogen" from the mitochondria to the cytoplasm, breakdown product or precursor of the neurotransmitter N-acetylaspartylglutamate (NAAG), metabolically inert pool regulating the anion deficit balance, metabolically active pool involved in the production of glutamate. Although NAA might play a marginal role in any of the aforementioned processes, recent studies have suggested that the potentially main roles of NAA might be to participates an acetyl group donor in brain lipid biosynthesis (production of myelin) (Moffett et al., 1991) and to act as a neuronal osmoregulator against cytotoxic swelling (molecular water pump) (Baslow, 2003a). Physiologically, NAA concentration is kept within a strict oscillation range even though NAA is regenerated 1.8 times/24 hours (with a calculated turnover rate of approximately 0.75 mmol/l water/hour). It is therefore evident that a perfect balance of the different velocities involved in NAA homeostasis, should exist. NAA decrease has been observed in association with many neurological diseases causing neuronal and axonal degeneration such as tumors, epilepsy, dementia, stroke, hypoxia, multiple sclerosis, and many leukoencephalopathies. Vice versa, the only known pathologic state characterized by a dramatic increase in cerebral NAA is the autosomic genetic leukodystrophy caused by the synthesis of a defective form of the enzyme responsible for the NAA degradation (N-acetyl-asparto-acylase, ASPA), known as Canavan disease. Due to the enzymatic defect in the NAA degradation, Canavan-affected patients are also characterized by large urinary excretion of intact NAA, up to 2000-fold the normal physiologic excretion (Tavazzi et al., 2005). The morphological alterations in Canavan-affected patients, characterized at MRI by spongi degeneration and structurally defective myelin, can well account for the most accredited roles of NAA: the incapacity to degrade NAA would generate dramatic changes in water extrusion from the brain compartment with consequent spongi degeneration, as well as a drastic decrease in the availability of acetate groups for olygodendrocytes thereby causing deficits in lipid myelin biosynthesis.

1.3 Background: NAA and ^{1}H-MRS as a diagnostic tool to study in vivo brain vulnerability

As already mentioned, the relevance of NAA as a biochemical marker of the metabolic neuronal "wealth" is related to the possibility to measure NAA concentration non-invasively "in vivo" by ^{1}H-MRS. When subtracting the spectral signal of ^{1}H from water (the most abundant molecule containing an atom with an unpaired proton, which is a prerequisite to allow to detect a molecule by MRS), the ^{1}H-NAA resonance returns one the best defined peaks at approximately 2 ppm. Using the clinically safe magnetic fields of the MRS apparatuses (1.5 or 3.0 Tesla) in the range 1.8 to 3.4 ppm to additional, well-resolved, resonance peaks are obtained, one at approximately 3.2 ppm referring to choline (Cho) and the other at approximately 2.9 ppm referring to creatine (Cr). It is worth recalling that the relatively low magnetic fields with no side effects (1.5-3.0 T) do not allow to discriminate in the multitude of compounds that are physiologically present within the brain tissue (acetyl-choline, cytidinediphospho-choline, phospho-choline, glycerophospho-choline, phosphatidyl-choline, free-choline, etc.) having this quaternary ammonium derivative as a characterizing chemical group. The same can be applied either in the case of the creatine-containing compounds (creatine and creatinephosphate) or in the case of the NAA-containing compounds (NAA and NAAG). Actually, in a ^{1}H-MRS the Cho peak represents the choline-containing compounds (with phosphatidyl-choline representing the 90% of the signal intensity), the Cr peak represents creatine-containing compounds (with creatine accounting for the 90% of the intensity signal) and the NAA peak the NAA-containing compounds (with NAA being 12 to 15 fold more concentrated than NAAG). Unless determining the water content within the voxel(s) for a calculation of the absolute concentrations of the different metabolites, it is necessary to quantify at the same time the peak areas of the spectroscopic intensity signals of both Cr and Cho-containing compounds and to then refer to the NAA/Cr and NAA/Cho ratios for the semi-quantitative NAA evaluation in physiopathological conditions (Barker et al., 1993; Brooks et al., 2001; Friedman et al., 1999; Garnett et al., 2000; Mitsumoto et al., 2007). This type of approach assumes Cr and Cho as two unvarying parameters to which relate the NAA changes. The results of a multicenter clinical trial (Vagnozzi et al., 2010) involving 40 concussed athletes and 30 healthy volunteers have been recently published, revealing that, despite different combinations of field strengths (1.5 or 3.0 T) and modes of spectrum acquisition (single- or multi-voxel) among the scanners currently in use in most neuroradiology centers, NAA determination represents a quick (15-minute), easy-to-perform, noninvasive tool to accurately measure changes in cerebral biochemical damage occurring after a concussion.

Patients exhibited the most significant alteration of metabolite ratios at day 3 post-injury, showing a gradual recovering, initially in a slow fashion and, following day 15, more rapidly. At 30 days post-injury, all subjects showed complete recovery, having metabolite ratios similar to values detected in controls. Interestingly, all these 40 patients self-declared symptom clearance between 3 and 15 days after concussion strongly demonstrating differential times of disappearance of clinical gross signs and of normalization of brain energy metabolism. In a previous pilot study carried out in a cohort of singly and doubly-concussed athletes, examined by ^{1}H-MRS for their NAA cerebral content at different time points after concussive events, we demonstrated that the recovery of brain metabolism is not linearly related to time. In this study, two athletes experienced a second concussion between the 10th and the 13th day after the first insult. Although they were not affected by SIS nor showed signs of sTBI, they however had a significant delay in both symptom resolution and NAA normalization (Vagnozzi et al., 2008).

According to the aforementioned data it is clear that concussion causes a reversible change of brain metabolism that can be monitored by ^{1}H-MRS in terms of NAA variations. Furthermore, data recorded in the two doubly concussed athletes suggest that a second concussion might compromise rescue of cerebral metabolism and delaying its normalization. This would in turn cause delaying in return of athletes to play. In the present study, we report data referring to six concussed athletes who received a second concussion at different times during the period of alteration of brain metabolism. The time course changes in their cerebral NAA, evaluated by ^{1}H-MRS up to complete normalization, are presented.

2. Materials and methods

Six non-professional male athletes from different sport disciplines who had suffered from a sport-related concussion, defined as a traumatically induced transient alteration in mental status, not necessarily accompanied with loss of consciousness, were considered in this study. At the clinical examinations they had a GCS greater or equal to 14, normal neurological objective signs and an age ranging between 20 and 33 years (mean age = 26 ± 5 years). According to our previous observations (Vagnozzi et al., 2008, 2010), they were required to restrain from further physical activity during the entire observational period, which lasted until cerebral metabolic normalization. None of the patients had positive MRI for post-traumatic anatomical lesions (the presence of blood, etc.), or suffered from polytrauma, or presented with risk factors for subsequent complications (coagoulopathy, epilepsy, former neurosurgical interventions, alcohol or drug abuse, disabilities). The first clinical evaluation, MRI and MRS were carried out at 3 days post injury; follow-up MRI and MRS analyses, as well as clinical evaluation of concussion-associated symptoms, were performed at different times up to metabolic normalization (15, 22, 30, 45, 60, 90, 120 days post-injury). A group of 10 healthy male subjects matched for age (mean age = 25 ± 6 years) was subjected to MRS and used as the control group.

In controls and athletes, semi-quantitative analysis of NAA relative to creatine (Cr) and choline containing compounds (Cho) was performed in the single voxel (SV) mode, after obtaining proton spectra using a 3.0 T system (Philips, Intera Achieva). For conventional MRI studies, T1 and T2 weighted TSE images were acquired in axial coronal and sagittal planes and, in order to rule out even the smallest amount of intra-cerebral blood, Fast Field Echo (FFE) T2* sequences were used. A multi channel coil (8 ch.) Sense-Head with 4 mm slice thickness, 1 mm gap and a FOV of 230 mm, was used for all MRI sequences. Following localized shimming and water suppression, the spectroscopic examination was carried out using a PRESS (Point Resolved Spectroscopy Sequence) pulse sequence, with the following settings: TE = 144 msec; TR = 2,000 msec; Spectral Bandwidth = 2,000 Hz; acquisition cycles = 128. The optimal positioning of the voxel was determined using the MR images acquired on axial, coronal and sagittal planes to facilitate its three-dimensional placement, adjacent to the cortical-subcortical junction in order to include only the white matter of the frontal lobes, bilaterally and the choice of this location as the region of interest, was made to obtain the most homogeneous data as possible. To this end, a spectrum from a single voxel (SV) customized to sample a volume of interest (VOI) of 3.375 cm^3 (1.5 x 1.5 x 1.5 cm), was obtained (acquisition time about 5 min for each voxel). In follow-up studies, the exact repositioning of the voxel on the same acquisition plane obtained in the previous MRI study was achieved by using dedicated software (SameScan, Philips Medical Systems). Metabolite intensity ratios (NAA-to-Cr and Cho-to-Cr) were automatically calculated at the end of each acquisition using dedicated software (SpectroView; Philips Medical Systems), by which gaussian-fitted peak areas relative to a baseline computed from a moving average of the noise regions of each spectrum were determined. Post-processing of spectral data, using a homemade computed program, allowed us to render uniform calculations of the area under the peaks of NAA, Cho and Cr, using common criteria for peak integration. In the case of a single, well-defined peak (typically the NAA peak), a valley-to-valley integration was performed to obtain the area under the peak. In the case of not fully resolved peaks (frequently the Cho and Cr peaks), a horizontal baseline between the start of the first peak to the end of the second peak was selected; the grouped peaks were then split by a vertical line, drawn from the median point of the common valley between peaks to the horizontal baseline and the area under the peaks calculated. These values were used to determine the metabolite ratios NAA/Cho, NAA/Cr and Cho/Cr.

3. Results

Table 1 summarizes the clinical features of the 6 doubly concussed athletes, including the time interval between concussion and the type and duration of the post-concussive self-reported clinical symptoms after both the first and the second head injury.

Table 1. Demographic data, sport activity and clinical features of 6 non professional athletes suffering from double concussion.

None of these concussions was characterized by loss of consciousness. All athletes declared to suffer from headache following the first concussive episode and each of them suffered from at least one additional post-concussive disturbance. Disappearance of self-reported clinical symptoms after the first concussion ranged between 3 to 8 days (mean duration = 5.8 ± 2.1 days). In two athletes the second concussive event occurred between the first and second ^{1}H-MRS (mean interval between the two concussions = 9.5 ± 0.7 days), whilst in the remaining 4 athletes the second concussion took place between the second and the third second ^{1}H-MRS (mean interval between the two concussions = 18.5 ± 2.1 days). In athletes 1 and 2, the second concussions were characterized by loss of consciousness (< 2 min). Following the second concussive episode, all athletes again declared to suffer from headache and each of them suffered from at least four additional post-concussive disturbances. Self-reported clinical symptoms following the second concussion disappeared with a mean duration = 41.2 ± 13.0 days (p < 0.001 when compared to duration of symptoms observed after the first concussion). Figures 1 and 2 illustrate the time course changes of NAA (reported in the Figures as the NAA/Cr ratio) in the two doubly concussed athletes (Patients 1 and 2) receiving the second head injury between the 1st and the 2nd ^{1}H-MRS, both showing loss of consciousness < 2 min on field.

CASE	AGE	SEX	SPORT PRACTICED	SYMPTOMS AFTER 1st IMPACT	PERSISTENCE OF SYMPTOMS AFTER 1st IMPACT (DAYS)	TIME INTERVAL BETWEEN CONCUSSIONS (DAYS)	SYMPTOMS AFTER 2nd IMPACT	PERSISTENCE OF SYMPTOMS AFTER 2nd IMPACT (DAYS)
1	20	M	Boxe (amateur)	Headache, amnesia	3	10	Loss of consciousness, headache, difficulty in concentrating, irritability, sleep disturbances	52
2	24	M	Rugby	Headache, nausea, retrograde amnesia	4	9	Loss of consciousness, headache, nausea, retrograde amnesia, sleep disturbances, irritability	59
3	32	M	Soccer	Headache, fatigue, nervousness	8	18	Headache, irritability, difficulty in concentrating, "foggy vision", nausea	44
4	27	M	Soccer	Headache, troubling falling asleep	7	16	Headache, nausea, sleep disturbances, irritability, dizziness	35
5	20	M	Kickboxing (light contact)	Headache, sleep disturbances	8	21	Headache, retrograde amnesia, troubling falling asleep, difficulty in concentrating	24
6	33	M	Boxe (amateur)	Headache, anterograde amnesia	5	19	Headache, fatigue, irritability, dizziness, tingling	33

Table 1. Clinical features of doubly concussed athletes. The mean duration of symptom persistence lasted 5.8 ± 2.1 days after the 1st injury and 41.2 ± 13.0 days after the 2nd concussion ($p < 0.001$ when compared to duration of symptoms observed after the first concussion). In both cases, symptoms disappeared much earlier than the time needed for complete NAA restoration.

At the time of the 1st resonance spectrum acquisition (3 days post-injury) both subjects showed a consistent decrease in the NAA/Cr ratio. When effecting the 2nd MRS, notwithstanding athletes were both initially advised to restrain from physical activity, they both declared to have started again their respective sport discipline because of symptom disappearance and to have received a second concussion few days later (mean value between repeat concussions = 9.5 ± 0.7). At this 2nd MRS analysis, the NAA/Cr ratio fell slightly below 1.6 (-23.6% with respect to value in controls), a value very close to that observed in patients suffering from sTBI (Signoretti et al., 2010). In both these athletes, the second concussive episode produced a prolonged loss of consciousness (< 2 min). Both subjects admitted to have experienced, from the beginning up to clinical healing, much more severe and prolonged post concussive symptoms (mean value of symptom persistence = 55.5 days) than those lived following the first impact.

Figures 3, 4, 5 and 6 illustrate the NAA/Cr ratio recorded in four athletes receiving the second concussion between the 2nd and the 3rd MRS.

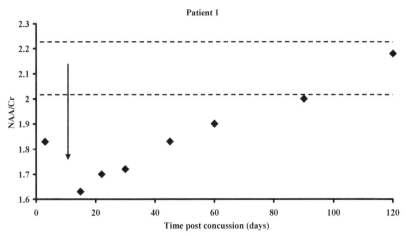

Fig. 1. Change of NAA in doubly concussed athlete. NAA relative to Cr (NAA/Cr ratio) was measured by ¹H-MRS in voxels properly positioned in the frontal lobes. The arrow indicates the approximate time of occurrence of the 2nd concussive episode (see Table 1). Dotted lines represent the range interval of the NAA/Cr ratio recorded in control healthy subjects. Notwithstanding prohibition to sustain physical activity, patient 1 restarted physical training immediately after symptom clearance (3 days after the 1st concussion), when NAA/Cr was about 16% below the value recorded in controls.

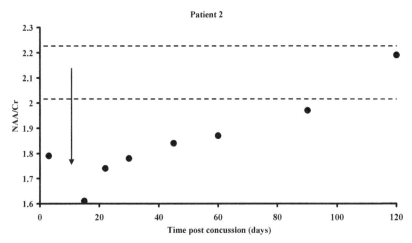

Fig. 2. Change of NAA in doubly concussed athlete. NAA relative to Cr (NAA/Cr ratio) was measured by ¹H-MRS in voxels properly positioned in the frontal lobes. The arrow indicates the approximate time of occurrence of the 2nd concussive episode (see Table 1). Dotted lines represent the range interval of the NAA/Cr ratio recorded in control healthy subjects. Notwithstanding prohibition to sustain physical activity, patient 2 restarted physical training immediately after symptom clearance (4 days after the 1st concussion), when NAA/Cr was about 17% below the value recorded in controls.

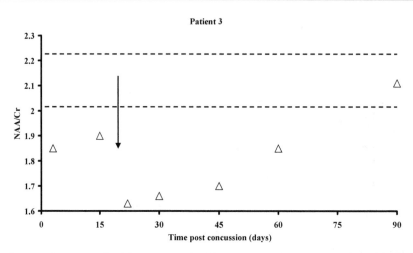

Fig. 3. Change of NAA in doubly concussed athlete. NAA relative to Cr (NAA/Cr ratio) was measured by 1H-MRS in voxels properly positioned in the frontal lobes. The arrow indicates the approximate time of occurrence of the 2nd concussive episode (see Table 1). Dotted lines represent the range interval of the NAA/Cr ratio recorded in control healthy subjects. Notwithstanding prohibition to sustain physical activity, patient 3 restarted physical training immediately after symptom clearance (8 days after the 1st concussion), when NAA/Cr was about 13% below the value recorded in controls.

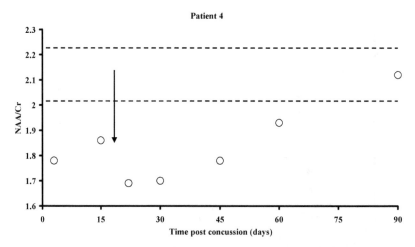

Fig. 4. Change of NAA in doubly concussed athlete. NAA relative to Cr (NAA/Cr ratio) was measured by 1H-MRS in voxels properly positioned in the frontal lobes. The arrow indicates the approximate time of occurrence of the 2nd concussive episode (see Table 1). Dotted lines represent the range interval of the NAA/Cr ratio recorded in control healthy subjects. Notwithstanding prohibition to sustain physical activity, patient 4 restarted physical training immediately after symptom clearance (7 days after the 1st concussion), when NAA/Cr was about 14% below the value recorded in controls.

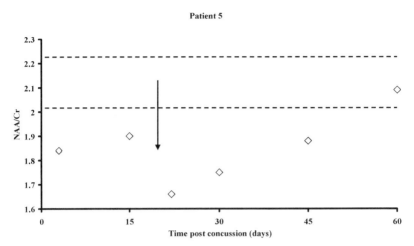

Fig. 5. Change of NAA in doubly concussed athlete. NAA relative to Cr (NAA/Cr ratio) was measured by ^{1}H-MRS in voxels properly positioned in the frontal lobes. The arrow indicates the approximate time of occurrence of the 2nd concussive episode (see Table 1). Dotted lines represent the range interval of the NAA/Cr ratio recorded in control healthy subjects. Notwithstanding prohibition to sustain physical activity, patient 5 restarted physical training immediately after symptom clearance (8 days after the 1st concussion), when NAA/Cr was about 14% below the value recorded in controls.

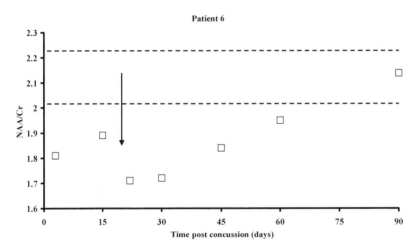

Fig. 6. Change of NAA in doubly concussed athlete. NAA relative to Cr (NAA/Cr ratio) was measured by ^{1}H-MRS in voxels properly positioned in the frontal lobes. The arrow indicates the approximate time of occurrence of the 2nd concussive episode (see Table 1). Dotted lines represent the range interval of the NAA/Cr ratio recorded in control healthy subjects. Notwithstanding prohibition to sustain physical activity, patient 6 restarted physical training immediately after symptom clearance (5 days after the 1st concussion), when NAA/Cr was about 16% below the value recorded in controls.

At the time of the 2nd MRS, the four patients showed a recovery of NAA and affirmed to be symptomless. Both these phenomena allowed athletes to violate the ban on sports so that they started practicing their respective disciplines before completion of brain metabolic recovery. At 22 days post-impact, we found in these subjects a significant further decline in the NAA/Cr ratio, the value of which was even lower than that recorded 3 days post-injury (Figures 3, 4, 5, 6 and 8). During the clinical consult, the four patients declared to have suffered from a second concussion (mean interval between the two concussions = 18.5 ± 2.1 days), interpreted on the field of minor relevance but being of surprisingly remarkable clinical severity and duration (mean value of symptom persistence = 34.0 days). It is worth underlining that in patient 5 completion of brain metabolic recovery was observed at the time of the 6th MRS, i.e. 39 days after the 2nd insult and 15 days after symptom disappearance.

4. Discussion

According to our opinion, data reported in the present study strongly demonstrate that the occurrence of repeat concussion produced a significant increase in the time of recovery of brain metabolism (as evaluated in terms of NAA/Cr variations determined by 1H-MRS), coupled to the appearance of clinical symptoms with increased severity and duration with those reported after a single concussive event (Vagnozzi et al., 2008, 2010). In sports medicine, this finding implies that it should be mandatory for concussed athletes to observe a period of restriction from physical activity until the process of normalization of brain metabolism is completed. Since also in these subjects the clearance of post-concussive clinical symptoms took place much before than the return of NAA to physiological values (Vagnozzi et al., 2008, 2010) it is our advise that monitoring alterations in the biochemistry of post-concussed neurons (NAA changes) by 1H-MRS should be considered a fundamental tool to evaluate recovery of post concussed athletes for their safe return to play.

Supported by abundant literature, it is nowadays worldwide accepted that concussion triggers a cascade of molecular events that transiently alter the biochemistry of the post-concussed neurons, with particular involvement for mitochondrial-dependent energy metabolism. This condition prompted Hovda and coll. to hypothesize the insurgence of a period of brain vulnerability during which a second concussive event may have fatal consequences for the neuronal vitality (Giza & Hovda, 2001; Hovda et al., 1993). Our previous researches in rats undergoing repeat mTBI, using the closed-head weight-drop model of diffuse injury set up by Marmarou and coll. (Foda & Marmarou 1994; Marmarou et al., 1994), clearly demonstrated that, depending on the time interval between injuries, two repeat concussions may cause metabolic cerebral irreversible alterations typical of single sTBI (3 days between concussions) (Tavazzi et al., 2007; Vagnozzi et al., 2007), i.e. cumulative effect of the two concussions. If the two repeat injuries were viceversa spaced by 5 days the changes of brain metabolism are fully reversible and comparable to those recorded in single mTBI, i.e. the two concussions acted as separate events (Tavazzi et al., 2007; Vagnozzi et al., 2007). This strongly indicates the existence of a window of metabolic brain vulnerability during which neurons, when receiving a second insult of even very modest entity, can suffer from dramatic impairment of cell functions. This phenomenon, can be explained by hypothesizing that neurons, after the first mTBI, are deeply involved in the energy-consuming processes to restore cell homeostasis, therefore rendering cells more susceptible to injuries of even very modest entity. The duration for the completion of these "repairing processes" corresponds to the window of brain vulnerability. In a pilot study in a restricted group of concussed athletes, we first monitored the time course of NAA decrease and recovery following concussion, thereby demonstrating the occurrence of the metabolic brain vulnerability status after an mTBI also in human beings (Vagnozzi et al., 2008). In the same study, we also described 2 cases of doubly concussed athletes who received a second impact during the period of energy metabolism recovery and who therefore underwent to a 15 days delay in complete NAA restoration (Vagnozzi et al., 2008). Recently, we provided unquestionable evidences indicating that the determination of NAA by ^{1}H-MRS is a reliable tool with which monitoring post-concussive periods in athletes. In this last study we demonstrated that results of the MRS analyses were independent on the MR apparatus (different MR suppliers), the field strength adopted (1.5 or 3.0 T) and the mode of spectra acquisition (Vagnozzi et al., 2010). Furthermore, the number of athletes enrolled (n = 40) and serially analyzed allowed to demonstrate that it is possible to determine the period of metabolic brain vulnerability for a safe return of athletes to play. Recently, different research groups confirmed our findings and successfully applied NAA evaluation by MRS to monitor the metabolic recovery of mildly-injured patients (Henry, 2010; Gasparovic et al., 2009; Sarmento et al., 2009; Yeo et al., 2011), thereby strongly corroborating the concept that methods capable of investigating at the molecular level are of great clinical relevance in the surveillance of post-concussed patients. On the other hand, the vast data in literature obtained in different models of mTBI (Barkhoudarian et al, 2011; Signoretti et al., 2010) clearly showed that post-concussive brain modifications are caused by a cascade of molecular events involving cerebral metabolism and, more in general, cerebral biochemistry. At present, in addition to the subjective indication of the patient, cognitive neuropsychological tests are widely used to assess the condition of mildly injured athletes. This type of monitoring has been considered one of the cornerstones for return to play after a concussion (Maroon et al, 2000; McClincy et al., 2006; McCrea et al., 2003; Schatz et al., 2006), even though concerns have been raised, including the question of when they should be used in the management and assessment of concussion (Collie et al., 2006; Gosselin et al., 2006; Randolph et al., 2005). Furthermore, none of the currently available diagnostic tests (Broglio et al., 2007; McCrea et al., 2003; Schatz et al., 2006; Register-Mihalik et al., 2008) are capable of measuring the unique, transient and potentially dangerous state of metabolic vulnerability experienced by the post-concussed brain tissue. Therefore, the need to find objective parameters to evaluate the extent of and recovery from concussion-induced cerebral damage has been stressed recently (Cantu, 2000). Our previous studies (Tavazzi et al., 2005; Vagnozzi et al., 2005, 2008, 2010) and the present research demonstrate that ^{1}H-MRS is capable of detecting significant neurochemical changes present in the injured brain despite the normal appearance of neuroimaging, absence of symptoms and normal neurological examination, i.e. we validated the use of a rapid, objective and sensitive diagnostic tool with which evaluating normalization of cerebral metabolism for a safe return of concussed athletes to play outside the window of metabolic brain vulnerability. Therefore, restraint from physical activity following concussion should be mandatory to avoid the risk of insurgence of SIS, with SIS being interpreted as an acute, fatal disease caused by uncontrolled brain swelling (Bowen, 2003; Cantu, 1998; Cobb & Battin, 2004; Logan et al., 2001; Mori et al., 2006; Saunders & Harbaugh, 2006). Results of the present study suggest that the concept of SIS might certainly be revised and could be broaden to any case of repeat concussion in which, after the second injury, a clear disproportion among the entity of the concussive event, the post-concussive clinical symptoms and the cerebral metabolic recovery indeed exists. This restricted cohort of doubly concussed athletes could be included within the aforementioned definition of SIS. In fact, notwithstanding all athletes received two repeat concussions (for each athlete, both events were characterized by the same acute symptoms with no change in GCS and negative MRI), clinical symptoms after the 2nd impact lasted much longer than the 1st one, satisfying our first proposed criterium to diagnose SIS. Moreover, in our previous studies we showed that the time to return the NAA/Cr to normal cerebral levels in singly concussed athletes is within 30 days post-impact. In the present cohort of doubly concussed athletes, the time required to measure values of the NAA/Cr ratio similar to those recorded in controls after the second concussion was of 81.2 ± 24.4 days. This much longer time for NAA recovery satisfy the second criterium we proposed to diagnose SIS. Independently on the inclusion in the SIS category, these athletes definitely showed a prolonged time of clearance of clinical symptoms and brain metabolism normalization. In our opinion, monitoring of brain metabolism in singly concussed athletes should drive the timetable of return to physical activity, especially for those practicing sports at risk of recurrent concussions (American football, boxe, ice hockey, rugby, alpine skiing, martial arts, soccer, etc.), according to this possible steps: 1) if upon first examination, NAA is below the value of healthy controls, i.e. altered energy metabolism, the athlete should rest with no physical activity (approximate post-concussion time interval of 1–15 days); 2) if, at the second examination, MRS suggests an initiation of the process of NAA recovery (i.e. quasi-normal energy metabolism), it is advisable that the athlete begin physical activity of increasing intensity (approximate post-concussion time interval of 16–22 days); 3) if, at the third MRS, progressive NAA replenishment is observed (i.e. normalized energy metabolism), then physical activity might be intensified to a 'return to play' level of conditions (approximate post-concussion time interval of 23–30 days); 4) if, at the fourth MRS, normal NAA, i.e. normal energy metabolism, has been determined, it is suitable that athletes be permitted to return to play (approximate post-concussion time interval 30 days). Such a timetable could be adapted to any post-concussed, non-athlete patient and translated into recommendations differing on personal lifestyle during the recovery of NAA post-concussion: 1) NAA below control values (prolonged altered energy metabolism) would recommend rest, with no physical activity and sedentary lifestyle (approximate post-concussion time interval of 1–15 days); 2) signs of initiation of NAA recovery (i.e. quasi-normal energy metabolism) would suggest normal working activity and moderate physical activity (approximate post-concussion time interval of 16–22 days); 3) normal NAA at MRS (i.e. normal energy metabolism re-established) would implicate return to full normal lifestyle (approximate post-concussion time interval of 23–30 days). Results of this and of previous studies (Vagnozzi et al., 2008, 2010) indicated that the kinetic of NAA recovery, following a single concussion, is non-linear, with a very slow phase of about 15-20 days and a second faster period of 10-15 days. We have recently demonstrated that this non-linear time-course of post-traumatic NAA recovery may be due to the cerebral energy imbalance, assessed by high-energy phosphate quantification (ATP, ADP, AMP, etc.), caused mainly by mitochondrial malfunctioning, as indicated by altered mitochondrial phosphorylating capacity (measured by the ATP/ADP ratio) (Signoretti et al., 2010; Tavazzi et al., 2005). Under these conditions, the remarkable decrease in cerebral NAA, which mirrors the changes in brain ATP, may possibly be attributed to the general energy depression consequent to impaired mitochondrial functions (Lifshitz et al., 2003; Robertson et al., 2006). Incorporating the data obtained in preclinical studies on mTBI, demonstrating decreased ATP concentration for a given period of time post-injury (Tavazzi et al. 2007; Vagnozzi et al., 2005, 2007), it is conceivable that the process of NAA normalization is markedly hindered by an imbalance of neuronal energy metabolism induced by concussion. In fact, NAA synthesis necessarily requires the availability and the energy of hydrolysis of acetyl-CoA (ΔG = -31.2 kJ/mol), working as the acetyl group and energy donor in the acetylation reaction of aspartate catalyzed by ANAT. It is fundamental to understand that when acetyl-CoA is used for NAA synthesis there is an indirect high energy cost to the cell. In fact, since in this case acetyl -CoA will not enter the citric acid cycle (Krebs' cycle) there will be a decrease in the production of reducing equivalents (3 NADH and 1 $FADH_2$) as the fuel for the electron transport chain. Since the oxidative phosphorylation is stoichiometrically coupled to the amount of electron transferred to molecular oxygen by the electron transport chain, the final result will be a net loss of 11 ATP molecules for each NAA molecule newly synthesized. Experimental studies (Signoretti et al., 2010) have shown that spontaneous re-synthesis of NAA occurs only after recovery of mitochondrial dysfunction with consequential return to normal ATP levels; therefore, it appears possible that normalization of NAA concentrations may occur only after the cerebral energy state has fully recovered. The slow normalization of the cell energetic could also be attributed to the drastic decrement of the nicotinic coenzyme pool that was observed in rat models of graded injury. In fact, previous studies (Tavazzi et al., 2005; Vagnozzi et al., 2007) showed the net diminution of the nicotinic coenzyme pool (NAD^+ + NADH and $NADP^+$ + NADPH) that certainly plays a pivotal role in the final result of general depression of cell energy metabolism. This depletion jeopardizes either the reducing equivalent supply to mitochondrial oxidative metabolism, or the catalytic activity of dehydrogenase-mediated oxidoreductive reactions. To date, possible mechanisms for this phenomenon are the hydroxyl radical-induced hydrolysis of the N-glycosidic bond of the reduced forms of the nicotinic coenzymes NADH and NADPH and the activation of the enzyme NAD-glycohydrolase (Lautier et al., 1994). Both mechanisms cause the hydrolysis of these coenzymes and give rise to the same end products, i.e., ADP-ribose(P) and nicotinamide. Independently of the predominant mechanism, the final result is certainly deleterious for the correct functioning of cell metabolism. Finally, the augmentation of poly-ADP ribosylation reactions through the activation of the enzyme poly-ADP ribose polymerase (Du et al., 2003; Nanavaty et al., 2002; Pacher et al., 2002), has been demonstrated to trigger the mechanisms of apoptotic induction (Yu et al., 2002). The overall result should be to significantly contribute to the decrease in the rate of NAA recovery during the time period close to the head insult, when cells are more "metabolically vulnerable" and physical restriction is mandatory to avoid catastrophic consequences.

5. Conclusion

This and previous data (Vagnozzi et al., 2008, 2010) demonstrated that this process can be non-invasively followed in vivo by ^{1}H-MRS giving clinically relevant information concerning the duration of the window of metabolic brain vulnerability. This time interval should be characterized by restriction of physical activity to avoid the occurrence of second concussion with unpredictable consequences, from the delay in cerebral metabolic normalization (such a delay being not yet defined in duration) to the onset of uncontrolled brain edema (i.e., the current definition of SIS). In our opinion, we again provided the experimental evidence in the dramatic discrepancy between the time required for the clearance of post-concussive clinical symptoms and the time needed to restore concussion-perturbed brain metabolism. Since ^{1}H-MRS is the analytical method of choice and NAA the biochemical parameter indirectly representing the brain energy metabolism, it should be strongly suggest ed to determine healing of post-concussed athletes and patients using this potent diagnostic tool. In light of the consequences of a second concussive event during the window of brain vulnerability, potentially catastrophic, it should be strongly recommended that the restriction of physical activity is mandatory and that the removal of this restriction is submitted to the full recovery of the NAA physiological level. Due to the potential catastrophic consequences of repeat concussions and the need to have clear diagnostic tools and protocols to study recovery of the post-concussed brain it is fundamental to undertake further studies to better understand these topics.

6. Acknowledgement

This work has been supported in part by research funds of the three Universities involved (Catania, Rome "Tor Vergata", Rome Catholic "Sacro Cuore").

7. References

Alexander, M.P. (1995). Mild traumatic brain injury: pathophysiology, natural history, and clinical management. *Neurology*, Vol. 45, No.7, (July 1995), pp. 1253–1260, ISSN 0028-3878

Barker P.B.; Soher, B.J.; Blackband, S.J.; Chatham, J.C.; Mathews, V.P. & Bryan, R.N. (1993). Quantitation of proton NMR spectra of the human brain using tissue water as an internal concentration reference. *NMR in Biomedicine*, Vol.6, No.1, (January-February 1993), pp. 89–94, ISSN 0952-3480

Barkhoudarian, G.; Hovda, D.A. & Giza, C.C. (2011). The molecular pathophysiology of concussive brain injury. *Clinics in sports medicine*, Vol.30, No.1, (January 2011), pp. 33-39, ISSN 0278-5919

Barth, J.T.; Freeman, J.R.; Broshek, D.K. & Varney, R.N. (2001). Acceleration-deceleration sport-related concussion: the gravity of it all. *Journal of Athletic Training*, Vol.36, No.3, (September 2001), pp. 253–256, ISSN 1062-6050

Baslow, M.H. (2003a). Brain N-acetylaspartate as a molecular water pump and its role in the etiology of Canavan disease: A mechanistic explanation. *Journal of Molecular Neuroscience*, Vol.21, No. 3, pp. 185–190, ISSN 0895-8696

Baslow, M.H. (2003b). N-acetylaspartate in the vertebrate brain: Metabolism and function. *Neurochemical Research*, Vol.28, No.6, (June 2003), pp. 941–953, ISSN 0364-3190

Bergsneider, M.; Hovda,. D.A.; Lee, S.M.; Kelly, D.F.; McArthur, D.L.; Vespa, P.M.; Lee, J.H.; Huang, S.C.; Martin, N.A.; Phelps, M.E. & Becker, D.P. (2000). Dissociation of cerebral glucose metabolism and level of consciousness during the period of metabolic depression following human traumatic brain injury. *Journal of Neurotrauma*, Vol.17, No.5, (May 2000), pp. 389–401, ISSN 0897-7151

Bigler, E.D. (2003). Neurobiology and neuropathology underlie the neuropsychological deficits associated with traumatic brain injury. *Archives of Clinical Neuropsychology*, Vol.18, No.6, (August 2003), pp. 595–627, ISSN 0887-6177

Bowen, A.P. (2003). Second impact syndrome: A rare; catastrophic; preventable complication of concussion in young athletes. *Journal of Emergency Nursery*, Vol.29, No.3, (June 2003), pp. 287–289, ISSN 0099-1767

Broglio, S.P.; Ferrara, M.S., Macciocchi, S.N.; Baumgartner, T.A. & Elliott, R. (2007). Test-retest reliability of computerized concussion assessment programs. *Journal of athletic training*, Vol.42, No.4, (October-December 2007), pp. 509-514, ISSN 1062-6050

Brooks, W.M.; Friedman, S.D. & Gasparovic, C. (2001). Magnetic resonance spectroscopy in traumatic brain injury. *Journal of Head Trauma Rehabilitation*, Vol.16, No.2, (April 2001), pp. 149–164, ISSN 0885-9701

Bruns, J. Jr. & Hauser, W.A. (2003). The epidemiology of traumatic brain injury: a review. *Epilepsia*, Vol.44, Suppl.10, (September 2003), pp. 2–10, ISSN 0013-9580

Cantu, R.C. (1998). Second-impact syndrome. *Clinics in Sports Medicine*, Vol.17, No.1, (January 1998), pp. 37–44, ISSN 0278-5919

Cantu, R.C. & Voy, R. (1995). Second impact syndrome: a risk in any contact sport. *The Physician and Sport Medicine*, Vol.23, No.6, (June 1995), pp. 27-34, ISSN 0091-3847

Cantu, R.C. (2000). Malignant brain edema and Second Impact Syndrome. In: *Neurologic Athletic Head and Spine Injuries*, R.C. Cantu, (Ed.), 132-137, ISBN 072-1683-39-8, WB Saunders Company, Michigan , USA

Cantu, R.C. (2003). Recurrent athletic head injury: risks and when to retire. *Clinics in Sports Medicine*, Vol.22, No.3, (July 2003), pp. 593–603, ISSN 0278-5919

Cantu, R.C. (2007). Athletic concussion: current understanding as of 2007. *Neurosurgery*, Vol.60, No.6, (July 2007), pp. 963–964, ISSN 1524-4040

Cobb, S. & Battin, B. (2004). Second-impact syndrome. *Journal of School Nursing*, Vol.20, No.5, (October 2004), pp. 262–267, ISSN 1050-8405

Collie, A.; Makdissi, M.; Maruff, P.; Bennell, K. & McCrory, P. (2006). Cognition in the days following concussion: comparison of symptomatic versus asymptomatic athletes *Journal of Neurology, Neurosurgery, and Psychiatry*, Vol.77, No.2, (February 2006), pp. 241-245, ISSN 0022-3050

Delaney, J.S.; Abuzeyad, F.; Correa, J.A. & Foxford, R. (2005). Recognition and characteristics of concussions in the emergency department population. *The Journal of Emergency Medicine*, Vol.29, No.2, (August 2005), pp. 189–197, ISSN 0736-4679

Du, L.; Zhang, X.; Han, Y.Y.; Burke, N.A.; Kochanek, P.M.; Watkins, S.C.; Graham, S.H.; Carcillo, J.A.; Szabó, C. & Clark, R.S. (2003). Intra-mitochondrial poly(ADP-ribosylation) contributes to NAD+ depletion and cell death induced by oxidative stress. *The Journal of Biological Chemistry*, Vol.278, No.20, (May 2003), pp. 18426–18433, ISSN 0021-9258

Fabbri, A.; Servadei, F.; Marchesini, G.; Negro, A. & Vandelli, A. (2010). The changing face of mild head injury: temporal trends and patterns in adolescents and adults from 1997 to 2008. *Injury*, Vol.41, No.9, (September 2010), pp. 913-917, ISSN 1879-0267

Foda, M.A. & Marmarou, A. (1994). A new model of diffuse brain injury in rats: part II. Morphological characterization. *Journal of Neurosurgery*, Vol.80, No.2, (February 1994), pp. 301-313, ISSN 0022-3085

Friedman, S.D.; Brooks, W.M.; Jung, R.E.; Chiulli, S.J.; Sloan, J.H.; Montoya, B.T.; Hart, B.L. & Yeo, R.A. (1999). Quantitative proton MRS predicts outcome after traumatic brain injury. *Neurology*, Vol.52, No.7, (April 1999), pp. 1384–1391, ISSN 0028-3878

Garnett, M.R.; Blamire, A.M.; Corkill, R.G.; Cadoux-Hudson, T.A.; Rajagopalan, B. & Styles, P. (2000). Early proton magnetic resonance spectroscopy in normal-appearing brain correlates with outcome in patients following traumatic brain injury. *Brain*, Vol.123, No.10, (October 2000), pp. 2046–2054, ISSN 0006-8950

Gasparovic, C.; Yeo, R.A.; Mannell, M.; Ling, J.; Elgie, R.; Phillips, J.; Doezema, D. & Mayer, A.R. (2009). Neurometabolite concentrations in gray and white matter in mild traumatic brain injury: an H-1-magnetic resonance spectroscopy study. *Journal of Neurotrauma*, Vol.26, No.10, (October 2009), pp. 1635-1643, ISSN 0897-7151

Giza, C.C. & Hovda, D.A. (2001). The neurometabolic cascade of concussion. *Journal of Athletic Training*, Vol.36, No.3, (September 2001), pp. 228-235, ISSN 1062-6050

Gosselin, N.; Lassonde, M.; Petit, D.; Leclerc, S.; Mongrain, V.; Collie, A. & Montplaisir, J. (2009). Sleep following sport-related concussions. *Sleep Medicine*, Vol.10, No.1, (January 2009), pp. 35–46, ISSN 1389-9457

Gosselin, N.; Theriault, M.; Leclerc, S.; Montplaisir, J. & Lassonde, M. (2006). Neurophysiological anomalies in symptomatic and asymptomatic concussed athletes. *Neurosurgery*, Vol.58, No.6, (June 2006), pp. 1151-1161, ISSN 1524-4040

Gouvier, W.D.; Cubic, B.; Jones, G.; Brantley, P. & Cutlip, Q. (1992). Postconcussion symptoms and daily stress in normal and head-injured college populations. *Archives of Clinical Neuropsychology*, Vol.7, No.3, (March 1992), pp. 193–211, ISSN 0887-6177

Guskiewicz, K.M.; Bruce, S.L.; Cantu, R.C.; Ferrara, M.S.; Kelly, J.P.; McCrea, M. & National Athletic Trainers' Association. (2006). Research based recommendations on management of sport related concussion: summary of the National Athletic Trainers' Association position statement. *British Journal of Sports Medicine*, Vol.40, No.1, (January 2006) , pp. 6–10, ISSN 0306-3674

Guskiewicz, K.M.; McCrea, M.; Marshall, S.W.; Cantu, R.C.; Randolph, C.; Barr, W.; Onate, J.A. & Kelly, J.P. (2003). Cumulative effects associated with recurrent concussion in collegiate football players: the NCAA Concussion Study. *JAMA*, Vol.290, No.19, (November 2003), pp. 2549–2555, ISSN 0098-7484

Henry, L.C.; Tremblay, S.; Boulanger, Y.; Ellemberg, D. & Lassonde, M. (2010). Neurometabolic changes in the acute phase after sports concussions correlate with symptom severity. *Journal of Neurotrauma*, Vol.27, No.1, (January 2010), pp. 65-76, ISSN 0897-7151

Hovda, D.A.; Badie, H.; Karimi, S.; Thomas, S.; Yoshino, A. & Kawamata T. (1993). Concussive brain injury produces a state of vulnerability for intracranial pressure perturbation in the absence of morphological damage. In: *Intracranial pressure VIII*. C.J.J. Avezaat, J.H.M. van Eijndhoven, A.I.R. Maas & J.T. Tans, (Eds.), 469–472, ISBN 038-7559-46-9, Springer-Verlag, Berlin

Hunt, T. & Asplund, C. (2010). Concussion assessment and management. *Clinics in Sports Medicine*, Vol.29, No.1, (January 2010), pp. 5–17, ISSN 0278-5919

Ingebrigtsen, T.; Romner, B. & Kock-Jensen, C. (2000). Scandinavian guidelines for initial management of minimal, mild, and moderate head injuries. *The Journal of Trauma*, Vol.48, No.4, (April 2000), pp. 760–766, ISSN 0022-5282

Kay, T.; Newman, B.; Cavallo, M.; Ezrachi, O. & Resnick, M. (1992). Toward a neuropsychological model of functional disability after mild traumatic brain injury. *Neuropsychology*, Vol.6, No.4, (October 1992), pp. 371–384, ISSN 0894-4105

Kissick, J. & Johnstone, K.M. (2005). Return to play after concussion: principles and practice. *Clinical Journal of Sport Medicine*, Vol.15, No.6, (November 2005), pp. 426–431, ISSN 1536-3724

Kurca, E.; Siva, K.S. & Kucera, P. (2006). Impaired cognitive functions in mild traumatic brain injury patients with normal and pathologic magnetic resonance imaging. *Neuroradiology*, Vol.48, No.9, (September 2006), pp. 661–669, ISSN 0028-3940

Lautier, D.; Hoflack, J.C.; Kirkland, J.B.; Poirier, D. & Poirier, G.G. (1994). The role of poly(ADP-ribose) metabolism in response to active oxygen cytotoxicity. *Biochimica et biophysica acta*, Vol.1221, No.3, (April 1994), pp. 215–220, ISSN 0006-3002

Lifshitz, J.; Sullivan, P.G.; Hovda, D.A.; Wieloch, T. & McIntosh, T.K. (2004). Mitochondrial damage and dysfunction in traumatic brain injury. *Mitochondrion*, Vol.4, No.5-6, (September 2004), pp. 705-713, ISSN 1567-7249

Livingston, D.H.; Lavery, R.F.; Passannante, M.R.; Skurnick, J.H.; Baker, S.; Fabian, T.C.; Fry, D.E. & Malangoni, M.A. (2000). Emergency department discharge of patients with a negative cranial computed tomography scan after minor head injury. *Annals of Surgery*, Vol.232, No.1, (July 2000), pp. 126-132, ISSN 0003-4932

Lloyd, D.A.; Carty, H.; Patterson, M.; Butcher, C.K. & Roe, D. (1997). Predictive value of skull radiography for intracranial injury in children with blunt head injury. *Lancet*, Vol.349, No.9055, (March 1997), pp. 821-824, ISSN 0140-6736

Logan, S.M.; Bell, G.W. & Leonard, J.C. (2001). Acute subdural hematoma in a high school football player after 2 unreported episodes of head trauma: A case report. *Journal of Athletic Training*, Vol.36, No.4, (December 2001), pp. 433–436, ISSN 1062-6050

Longhi, L.; Saatman, K.E.; Fujimoto, S.; Raghupathi, R.; Meaney, D.F.; Davis, J.; McMillan, B.S.A.; Conte, V.; Laurer, H.L. Stein, S.; Stocchetti N. & McIntosh, T.K. (2005). Temporal window of vulnerability to repetitive experimental concussive brain injury. *Neurosurgery*, Vol.56, No.2, (February 2005), pp. : 364–374, ISSN 1524-4040

Lovell, M.; Collins, M. & Bradley, J. (2004). Return to play following sports-related concussion. *Clinics in Sports Medicine*, Vol.23, No.3, (July 2004), pp. 421-441, ISSN 0278-5919

Marmarou, A.; Foda, M.A.; van den Brink, W.; Campbell, J.; Kita, H. & Demetriadou, K. (1994). A new model of diffuse brain injury in rats: part I. Pathophysiology and biomechanics. *Journal of Neurosurgery*, Vol.80, No.2, (February 1994), pp. 291–300, ISSN 0022-3085

Maroon, J.C.; Lovell, M.R.; Norwig, J.; Podelek, K.; Powell, J.W. & Hartl, R. (2000). Cerebral concussion in athletes: evaluation and neuropsychological testing. *Neurosurgery*, Vol.47, No.3, (September 2000), pp. 659-669, ISSN 1524-4040

McClincy, M.P.; Lovell, M.R.; Pardini, J.; Collins, M.W. & Spore, M.K. (2006). Recovery from sports concussion in high school and collegiate athletes. *Brain Injury*, Vol.20, No.1, (January 2006), pp. 33–39, ISSN 0269-9052

McCrea, M.; Guskiewicz, K.M.; Marshall, S.W.; Barr, W.; Randolph, C.; Cantu, R.C.; Onate, J.A.; Yang, J. & Kelly, J.P. (2003). Acute effects and recovery time following concussion in collegiate football players: the NCAA Concussion Study. *JAMA*, Vol.290, No.19, (November 2003), pp. 2556-2563, ISSN 0098-7484

McCrea, M.; Hammeke, T.; Olsen, G.; Leo, P. & Guskiewicz, K. (2004). Unreported concussion in high school football players: implications for prevention. *Clinical Journal of Sport Medicine*, Vol.14, No.1, (January 2004), pp. 13–17, ISSN 1536-3724

McCrory, P.R.; Meeuwisse, W.; Johnston, K.; Dvorak, J.; Aubry, M.; Molloy, M. & Cantu, R.C. (2009). Consensus statement on Concussion in Sport 3rd International Conference on Concussion in Sport held in Zurich, November 2008. *Clinical Journal of Sport Medicine,* Vol.19, No.3, (May 2009), pp. 185-200, ISSN 1536-3724

McCrory, P.R. & Berkovic, S.F. (2001). Concussion: The history of clinical and pathophysiological concepts and misconceptions. *Neurology,* Vol.12, No.12, (December 2001), pp. 2283-2289, ISSN 0028-3878

McCrory, P.R. (2001). Does second impact syndrome exist? *Clinical Journal of Sport Medicine,* Vol.11, No.3, (July 2001), pp. 144-149, ISSN 1536-3724

Meehan, W.P. 3rd & Bachur, R.G. (2009). Sport-related concussion. *Pediatrics,* Vol.123, No.1, (January 2009), pp. 114-123, ISSN 0031-4005

Mitsumoto, H.; Ulug, A.M.; Pullman, S.L.; Gooch, C.L.; Chan, S.; Tang, M.X.; Man, X.; Hays, A.P.; Floyd, A.G.; Battista, V.; Montes, J.; Hayes, S.; Dashnaw, S.; Kaufmann, P.; Gordon, P.H.; Hirsch, J.; Levin, B.; Rowland L.P. & Shungu, D.C. (2007). Quantitative objective markers for upper and lower motor neuron dysfunction in ALS. *Neurology,* Vol.68, No.17, (April 2007), pp. 1402-1410, ISSN 0028-3878

Miyake, M.; Kakimoto, Y. & Sorimachi, M. (1981). A gas chromatographic method for the determination of N-acetyl-L-aspartic acid; N-acetyl-alpha-aspartylglutamic acid and beta-citryl-L-glutamic acid and their distributions in the brain and other organs of various species of animals. *Journal of Neurochemistry,* Vol.36, No.3, (March 1981), pp. 804-810, ISSN 0022-3042

Moffett, J.R.; Namboodiri, M.A.; Cangro, C.B. & Neale, J.H. (1991). Immunohistochemical localization of *N*-acetylaspartate in rat brain. *Neuroreport,* Vol.2, No.3, (March 1991), pp.131-134; ISSN 0959-4965

Mori, T.; Katayama, Y. & Kawamata, T. (2006). Acute hemispheric swelling associated with thin subdural hematomas: Pathophysiology of repetitive head injury in sports. *Acta Neurochirurgica Supplement,* Vol.96, pp. 40-43; ISSN ISSN 0001-6268

Nanavaty, U.B.; Pawliczak, R.; Doniger, J.; Gladwin, M.T.; Cowan, M.J.; Logun, C. & Shelhamer, J.H. (2002). Oxidant-induced cell death in respiratory epithelial cells is due to DNA damage and loss of ATP. *Experimental lung research,* Vol.28, No.8, (December 2002), pp. 591-607, ISSN 0190-2148

Nugent, G.R. (2006). Reflections on 40 years as a sideline physician. *Neurosurgical Focus,* Vol.21, No.4, (October 2006), pp. E2, ISSN 1092-0684

Pacher, P.; Liaudet, L.; Mabley, J.; Komjáti, K. & Szabó, C. (2002). Pharmacologic inhibition of poly(adenosine diphosphate-ribose) polymerase may represent a novel therapeutic approach in chronic heart failure. *Journal of the American College of Cardiology,* Vol.40, No.5, (September 2002), pp. 1006-1016, ISSN 0735-1097

Pellman; E.J.; Viano, D.C.; Casson, I.R.; Tucker, A.M.; Waeckerle, J.F.; Powell, J.W. & Feuer, H. (2004). Concussion in professional football. Repeat injuries — Part 4. *Neurosurgery,* Vol.55, No.4, (October 2004), pp. 860-873, ISSN 1524-4040

Ponsford, J. (2005). Rehabilitation interventions after mild head injury. *Current Opinion in Neurology,* Vol.18, No.6, (December 2005), pp. 692-697, ISSN 1350-7540

Praticò, D.; Reiss, P.; Tang, L.X.; Sung, S.; Rokach, J. & McIntosh, T.K. (2002). Local and systemic increase in lipid peroxidation after moderate experimental traumatic brain injury. *Journal of Neurochemistry,* Vol.80, No.5, (March 2002), pp. 894-898, ISSN 0022-3042

Randolph, C.; McCrea, M. & Barr, W.B. (2005). Is neuropsychological testing useful in the management of sport-related concussion? *Journal of Athletic Training*, Vol.40, No.3, (July-September 2005), pp. 139-152, ISSN 1062-6050

Randolph, C.; Millis, S.; Bar, W.B.; McCrea, M.; Guskiewicz, K.M.; Hammeke, T.A. & Kelly, J.P. (2009). Concussion symptom inventory: an empirically derived scale for monitoring resolution of symptoms following sport-related concussion. *Archives of Clinical Neuropsychology*, Vol.24, No.3, (May 2009), pp. 219–229, ISSN 0887-6177

Register-Mihalik, J.K.; Mihalik, J.P. & Guskiewicz, K.M. (2008). Balance deficits after sports-related concussion in individuals reporting posttraumatic headache. *Neurosurgery*, Vol.63, No.1, (July 2008), pp. 76-80, ISSN 1524-4040

Robertson, C.L.; Soane, L.; Siegel, Z.T. & Fiskum, G. (2006). The potential role of mitochondria in pediatric traumatic brain injury. *Developmental Neuroscience*, Vol.28, No.4-5, pp. 432–446, ISSN 0378-5866

Sarmento, E.; Moreira, P.; Brito, C.; Souza, J.; Jevoux, C. & Bigal, M. (2009). Proton spectroscopy in patients with post-traumatic headache attributed to mild head injury. *Headache*, Vol.49, No.9, (October 2009), pp. 1345-1352, ISSN 0017-8748

Saunders, R.L. & Harbaugh, R.E. (1984). The second impact in catastrophic contact-sports head trauma. *JAMA*, Vol.252, No.4, (July 1984), pp. 538–539, ISSN 0098-7484

Schatz, P.; Pardini, J.E.; Lovell, M.R.; Collins, M.W. & Podell, K. (2006). Sensitivity and specificity of the ImPACT Test Battery for concussion in athletes. *Archives of Clinical Neuropsychology*, Vol.21, No.1, (January 2006), pp. 91-99, ISSN 0887-6177

Shackford, S.R.; Wald, S.L.; Ross, S.E.; Cogbill, T.H.; Hoyt, D.B.; Morris, J.A.; Mucha, P.A.; Pachter, H.L.; Sugerman, H.J.; O'Malley, K. et al. (1992). The clinical utility of computed tomographic scanning and neurologic examination in the management of patients with minor head injuries. *The Journal of Trauma*, Vol.33, No. 3, (September 1992), pp. 385-394, ISSN 0022-5282

Signoretti, S.; Di Pietro, V.; Vagnozzi, R.; Lazzarino, G.; Amorini, A.M.; Belli, A.; D'Urso, S. & Tavazzi, B. (2010). Transient alterations of creatine, creatine phosphate, N-acetylaspartate and high-energy phosphates after mild traumatic brain injury in the rat. *Molecular and Cellular Biochemistry*, Vol. 333, No.1-2, (January 2010), pp. 269-277, ISSN 0300-8177

Swann, I.J.; MacMillan, R. & Strong, I. (1981). Head injuries at an inner city accident and emergency department. *Injury*, Vol.12, No.4, (January 1981), pp. 274-278, ISSN 1879-0267

Tagliaferri, F.; Compagnone, C.; Korsic, M.; Servadei, F. & Kraus, J. (2006). A systematic review of brain injury epidemiology in Europe. *Acta Neurochirurgica (Wien)*, Vol.148, No.3, (November 2005), pp. 255–268, ISSN 0001-6268

Taheri, P.A.; Karamanoukian, H.; Gibbons, K.; Waldman, N.; Doerr, R.J. & Hoover, E.L. (1993). Can patients with minor head injuries be safely discharged home? *Archives of Surgery*, Vol.128, No.3, (March 1993), pp. 289-292, ISSN 0272-5533

Tavazzi, B.; Lazzarino, G.; Leone, P.; Amorini, A.M.; Bellia, F.; Janson, C.G.; Di Pietro, V.; Ceccarelli, L.; Donzelli, S.; Francis, J.S. & Giardina, B. (2005). Simultaneous high performance liquid chromatographic separation of purines; pyrimidines; N-acetylated amino acids; and dicarboxylic acids for the chemical diagnosis of inborn errors of metabolism. *Clinical Biochemistry*, Vol.38, No.11, (November 2005), pp. 997–1008, ISSN 0009-9120

Tavazzi, B.; Vagnozzi, R.; Signoretti, S.; Amorini, A.M.; Belli, A.; Cimatti, M.; Delfini, R., Di Pietro, V.; Finocchiaro, A. & Lazzarino, G. (2007). Temporal window of metabolic brain vulnerability to concussions: oxidative and nitrosative stresses-part II. *Neurosurgery*, Vol.61, No.2, (August 2007), pp. 390–396, ISSN 1524-4040

Truckenmiller, M.E.; Namboodiri, M.A.; Brownstein, M.J. & Neale, J.H. (1985). N-Acetylation of L-aspartate in the nervous system: differential distribution of a specific enzyme. *Journal of Neurochemistry*, Vol.45, No.5, (November 1985), pp. 1658–1662, ISSN 0022-3042

Vagnozzi, R.; Marmarou, A.; Tavazzi, B.; Signoretti, S.; Di Pierro, D.; del Bolgia, F.; Amorini, A.M.; Fazzina, G.; Sherkat, S. & Lazzarino, G. (1999). Changes of cerebral energy metabolism and lipid peroxidation in rats leading to mitochondrial dysfunction after diffuse brain injury. *Journal of Neurotrauma*, Vol.16, No.10, (October 1999), pp. 903–913, ISSN 0897-7151

Vagnozzi, R.; Signoretti, S.; Tavazzi, B.; Cimatti, M.; Amorini, A.M.; Donzelli, S.; Delfini, R. & Lazzarino, G. (2005). Hypothesis of the post-concussive vulnerable brain: experimental evidence of its metabolic occurrence. *Neurosurgery*, Vol.57, No.1, (July 2005), pp. 164–171, ISSN 1524-4040

Vagnozzi, R.; Tavazzi, B.; Signoretti, S.; Amorini, A.M.; Belli, A.; Cimatti, M.; Delfini, R.; Di Pietro, V.; Finocchiaro, A. & Lazzarino, G. (2007). Temporal window of metabolic brain vulnerability to concussions: mitochondrial-related metabolic impairment-part I. *Neurosurgery*, Vol.61, No.2, (August 2007), pp. 379–389, ISSN 1524-4040

Vagnozzi, R.; Signoretti, S.; Tavazzi, B.; Floris, R.; Ludovici, A.; Marziali, S.; Tarascio, G.; Amorini, A.M.; Di Pietro, V.; Delfini, R. & Lazzarino, G. (2008). Temporal window of metabolic brain vulnerability to concussion: a pilot ^{1}H-MRS study in concussed athletes-part III. *Neurosurgery*, Vol.62, No.6, (June 2008), pp. 1286-1295, ISSN 1524-4040

van der Naalt, J. (2001). Prediction of outcome in mild to moderate head injury: a review. *Journal of Clinical and Experimental Neuropsychology*, Vol.23, No.6, (December 2001), pp. 837–851, ISSN 1380-3395

Vos, P.E.; Battistin, L.; Birbamer, G., Gerstenbrand, F.; Potapov, A.; Prevec, T.; Stepan, Ch.A.; Traubner, P.; Twijnstra, A.; Vecsei, L. & von Wild, K. (2002). EFNS guideline on mild traumatic brain injury: report of an EFNS task force. *European Journal of Neurology*, Vol.9, No.3, (May 2002), pp. 207-219, ISSN 1468-1331

Yates, D.; Aktar, R.; Hill, J. & Guideline Development Group. (2007). Assessment, investigation, and early management of head injury: summary of NICE guidance. *British Medical Journal*, Vol.335, No.7622, (October 2007), pp. 719-720, ISSN 0959-8146

Yeo, R.A.; Gasparovic, C.; Merideth, F.; Ruhl, D.; Doezema, D. & Mayer, A.R. (2011). A longitudinal proton magnetic resonance spectroscopy study of mild traumatic brain injury. *Journal of Neurotrauma*, Vol.28, No.1, (January 2011), pp. 1-11, ISSN 0897-7151

Yu, S.W.; Wang, H.; Poitras, M.F.; Coombs, C.; Bowers, W.J.; Federoff, H.J.; Poirier, G.G.; Dawson, T.M. & Dawson, V.L. (2002). Mediation of poly(ADP-ribose) polymerase-1-dependent cell death by apoptosis-inducing factor. *Science*, Vol.297, No.5579, (July 2002), pp. 259-263, ISSN 0036-8075

Permissions

The contributors of this book come from diverse backgrounds, making this book a truly international effort. This book will bring forth new frontiers with its revolutionizing research information and detailed analysis of the nascent developments around the world.

We would like to thank Dr. Amit Agrawal, for lending his expertise to make the book truly unique. He has played a crucial role in the development of this book. Without his invaluable contribution this book wouldn't have been possible. He has made vital efforts to compile up to date information on the varied aspects of this subject to make this book a valuable addition to the collection of many professionals and students.

This book was conceptualized with the vision of imparting up-to-date information and advanced data in this field. To ensure the same, a matchless editorial board was set up. Every individual on the board went through rigorous rounds of assessment to prove their worth. After which they invested a large part of their time researching and compiling the most relevant data for our readers. Conferences and sessions were held from time to time between the editorial board and the contributing authors to present the data in the most comprehensible form. The editorial team has worked tirelessly to provide valuable and valid information to help people across the globe.

Every chapter published in this book has been scrutinized by our experts. Their significance has been extensively debated. The topics covered herein carry significant findings which will fuel the growth of the discipline. They may even be implemented as practical applications or may be referred to as a beginning point for another development. Chapters in this book were first published by InTech; hereby published with permission under the Creative Commons Attribution License or equivalent.

The editorial board has been involved in producing this book since its inception. They have spent rigorous hours researching and exploring the diverse topics which have resulted in the successful publishing of this book. They have passed on their knowledge of decades through this book. To expedite this challenging task, the publisher supported the team at every step. A small team of assistant editors was also appointed to further simplify the editing procedure and attain best results for the readers.

Our editorial team has been hand-picked from every corner of the world. Their multi-ethnicity adds dynamic inputs to the discussions which result in innovative outcomes. These outcomes are then further discussed with the researchers and contributors who give their valuable feedback and opinion regarding the same. The feedback is then collaborated with the researches and they are edited in a comprehensive manner to aid the understanding of the subject.

Apart from the editorial board, the designing team has also invested a significant amount of their time in understanding the subject and creating the most relevant covers. They scrutinized every image to scout for the most suitable representation of the subject and create an appropriate cover for the book.

The publishing team has been involved in this book since its early stages. They were actively engaged in every process, be it collecting the data, connecting with the contributors or procuring relevant information. The team has been an ardent support to the editorial, designing and production team. Their endless efforts to recruit the best for this project, has resulted in the accomplishment of this book. They are a veteran in the field of academics and their pool of knowledge is as vast as their experience in printing. Their expertise and guidance has proved useful at every step. Their uncompromising quality standards have made this book an exceptional effort. Their encouragement from time to time has been an inspiration for everyone.

The publisher and the editorial board hope that this book will prove to be a valuable piece of knowledge for researchers, students, practitioners and scholars across the globe.

List of Contributors

David Dornbos III and Yuchuan Ding
Wayne State University Department of Neurological Surgery, USA

Thomas I Nathaniel
Center for Natural and Health Sciences, Marywood University, USA
Department of Biomedical Sciences, University of South Carolina, School of Medicine-Greenville, Greenville, USA

Francis Umesiri
Department of Chemistry, University of Toledo, Toledo, USA

Grace Reifler, Katelin Haley, Leah Dziopa, Julia Glukhoy and Rahul Dani
Center for Natural and Health Sciences, Marywood University, USA

Effiong Otukonyong
Department of Health Sciences, East Tennessee State University, Johnson City, USA

Sarah Bwint, Katelin Haley, Diane Haleem and Adam Brager
Center for Natural and Health Sciences, Marywood University, USA

Ayotunde Adeagbo
Department of Pharmacology and Physiology, The Commonwealth Medical College, Scranton, USA

Jonathan R. Wisler, Paul R. Beery II, Steven M. Steinberg and Stanislaw P. A. Stawicki
Department of Surgery, Division of Critical Care Trauma and Burn, The Ohio State University, Medical Center,
Columbus, Ohio, USA

Angela N. Hays and Abhay K. Varma
Medical University of South Carolina, USA

Jesús Devesa and Pablo Devesa
Medical Center "Proyecto Foltra", Teo, Spain

Pedro Reimunde
Medical Center "Proyecto Foltra", Teo, Spain

Víctor Arce
Department of Physiology, School of Medicine, Santiago de Compostela, Spain

Dare Adewumi and Austin Colohan
Loma Linda University Medical Center Department of Neurosurgery, Loma Linda, USA

Haralampos Gatos, Konstantinos N. Paterakis and Kostas N. Fountas
Departments of Neurosurgery, University Hospital of Larissa, School of Medicine, University of Thessaly, Larissa, Greece

Eftychia Z. Kapsalaki
Diagnostic Radiology, University Hospital of Larissa, School of Medicine, University of Thessaly, Larissa, Greece

Apostolos Komnos
Department of Intensive Care Unit, General Hospital of Larissa, Larissa, Greece

S. Mondello, F. H. Kobeissy, A. Jeromin, J. D. Guingab-Cagmat, Z. Zhiqun, J. Streeter, R. L. Hayes and K. K. Wang
University of Florida and Banyan Biomarkers, Inc., USA

Giuseppe Lazzarino
Department of Biology, Geology and Environmental Sciences, Division of Biochemistry and Molecular Biology, University of Catania, Catania, Italy

Roberto Vagnozzi
Department of Neurosurgery, Chair of Neurosurgery, University of Rome "Tor Vergata", Rome, Italy

Stefano Signoretti
Division of Neurosurgery, Department of Neurosciences-Head and Neck Surgery, San Camillo Hospital, Rome, Italy

Massimo Manara
Association of Sports Physicians Parma, F.M.S.I., Parma, Italy

Roberto Floris, Andrea Ludovici and Simone Marziali
Department of Diagnostic Imaging and Interventional Radiology, University of Rome "Tor Vergata", Rome, Italy

Angela M. Amorini and Barbara Tavazzi
Institute of Biochemistry and Clinical Biochemistry, Catholic University of Rome "Sacro Cuore", Rome, Italy

Tracy K. McIntosh
Media Neuro Consultants Inc., Media, PA 19063, USA

Printed in the USA
CPSIA information can be obtained
at www.ICGtesting.com
JSHW011423221024
72173JS00004B/656